AT THE BENCH
A Laboratory Navigator

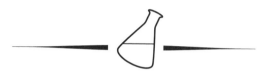

Kathy Barker

The Rockefeller University
New York, New York

COLD SPRING HARBOR LABORATORY PRESS

At the Bench: A Laboratory Navigator

Front cover and interior design by Ed Atkeson
Illustrated by Jim Duffy
Technical Advisor Linda Rodgers
Project Coordinator Mary Cozza

Production Editor Patricia Barker
Desktop Editor Susan Schaefer

Barker, Kathy, 1953–
    At the bench : a laboratory navigator / by Kathy Barker
        p.   cm.
    Includes bibliographical references and index.
    ISBN 0-87969-523-4 (alk. paper)
    1. Medical sciences—Laboratory manuals. I. Title.
    R850.B36 1998
    610'.'24—dc21   98-15662
                                                            CIP

10 9 8 7 6 5

Contents

Preface   ix

Abbreviations   xi

SECTION 1. Getting Oriented

Chapter 1. General Lab Organization and Procedures   3
The Big Picture   4
Laboratory Personnel   5
Lab Routines   7
What to Expect the First Week   10
What to Do the First Week   11
What Not to Do the First Week   13
Survival Through Common Sense and Courtesy   14
Nonnegotiable Safety Rules   17
Resources   19

Chapter 2. Laboratory Setup and Equipment   21
Lay of the Land   22
Using the Equipment   37
How to Buy New Equipment   39
Resources   41

Chapter 3. Getting Started and Staying Organized   43
Setting Up a Functional Lab Bench   44
Setting Up a Command Center   57
Resources   65

SECTION 2. Plotting a Course

Chapter 4. How To Set Up an Experiment   69
Philosophical Considerations   69
Planning an Experiment   71

Interpreting Results   83
Resources   87

Chapter 5. Laboratory Notebooks   89
Type and Format   89
Content   92
Maintenance   93
Ethics   96
Resources   99

Chapter 6. Presenting Yourself and Your Data   101
Communication Tips   101
Oral Presentations   110
Written Presentations   121
Resources   126

SECTION 3. Navigating

Chapter 7. Making Reagents and Buffers   129
Determining What You Need   130
Calculating What You Need   136
Weighing and Mixing   146
Measuring pH   150
Sterilizing Solutions   155
Storing Buffers and Solutions   158
Resources   161

Chapter 8. Storage and Disposal   163
Emergency Storage   163
Storing Reagents   165
Aliquoting   170
Refrigerators and Freezers   172
Discarding Lab Waste   175
Resources   183

Chapter 9. Working without Contamination   185
When to Use Sterile Technique   186
Sterile Technique   187
Protecting the Investigator   197
Sterile Technique in the Class II Biosafety Cabinet   198
Resources   203

Chapter 10. Eukaryotic Cell Culture   205
Types of Cultures and Cell Lines   205

Observing Cells   209
Obtaining Cells   211
Cell Maintenance   215
Freezing and Storage of Cells   228
Contamination   231
CO_2 Incubators and Tanks   236
Resources   243

Chapter 11. Bacteria   **245**
Setting Up   245
Working Rules   247
Obtaining Bacteria   248
Growth and Maintenance   249
Antibiotics   257
Reviving Cultures   255
Obtaining Isolated Colonies   259
Counting Bacteria   263
Storage   273
Freezing Bacteria   274
Contamination   276
Resources   276

Chapter 12. DNA, RNA, and Protein   **279**
Molecular Biology Tips   279
DNA   280
Introducing DNA into Cells and Microorganisms   294
RNA   296
Protein   299
Resources   310

Chapter 13. Radioactivity   **313**
Properties of Radioactive Elements   314
How to Obtain Radioisotopes   315
Doing Radioactive Experiments   320
Experimental Detection of Radiation   329
Storage   338
Disposal   339
Alternatives to Radioactivity   342
Resources   343

Chapter 14. Centrifugation   **345**
Background   345
Working Rules   353
How to Spin   355

Gradients   367
Centrifuge and Rotor Maintenance   368
Resources   371

Chapter 15. Electrophoresis   373

Basic Rules   373
Generalities   374
Specifics   380
Transferring Gel Contents to Membranes   397
Resources   401

Chapter 16. The Light Microscope   403

Background   403
Using the Light Microscope   409
Slides and Stains   417
Fluorescence Microscopy   420
Photography   422
Shared Instrument Facilities   426
Resources   427

Glossary   429
Index   451

Preface

THE FIRST WEEK I SPENT as a graduate student in a laboratory was one of the most confusing weeks of my life. There were no written instructions about anything but specialized experiments. The folklore of the lab was passed down orally, but when to ask, whom to ask, what was reasonable to ask, took enormous amounts of time to figure out. The questions were endless, and I didn't know how to distinguish between the trivial and the critical. Of course, with time, I found my way, as everyone did. And then I became one of the people to whom new people come in and say frantically, "How did you know how fast to spin? How did you know which stain would work? How do you know? How do you know? How do you *know*???" Well, you just know. You yourself asked someone one day: You probably asked three or four times before it sank in. Maybe you wrote parts down on a page of your lab book, or on a napkin that you tossed into a drawer to consult whenever you repeated the procedure, but most of your hard-won expertise was buried deep in the brain, and not always in an accessible part.

But it seemed that the initial unease could have been helped if everyone had access to *something* that explained the social and scientific ramifications of the new and wonderful surroundings. In Friday evening happy hours all over the country people compare notes about lab life, and the same problems and questions keep popping up, and there has still been no way to acquire the knowledge other than by oral absorption over time. Thus, the inspiration for this manual, which is meant to help lab people become familiar with their surroundings and be able, from the first day, to become independent, to know what questions to ask and why, and to function as scientists.

This manual is not a substitute for asking questions: I am not trying to dispense with the oral tradition. One-on-one communication is still the heartbeat of the lab, and it is almost always better to consult a knowing person than a book. But hopefully, the manual can give you a framework within which to work, whether you are the asker or the asked.

The primary audience for this manual is the initiate to the lab bench, one who has had the intellectual but not the practical background to do experiments. This includes physicians, research nurses, technicians, and graduate students. The newcomer has probably had lab experience in college courses or even in rotations, but has not had responsibility for the setup and interpretation of his or her own experiments.

At the Bench: A Laboratory Navigator is divided into three sections, which follow the actual order in which most people will need to understand the laboratory. Section 1 is Getting Oriented, and it describes how to deal with the physical and political setting of the laboratory. Section 2 is Plotting a Course, and it details the rationale and organization involved in setting up an experiment, recording results, and presenting data. Section 3, Navigating, is the most extensive section, containing the details usually hidden behind lab protocols: In these chapters are found topics from the water to use when making buffers, to freezing cells, to washing the rotors of a centrifuge.

To provide the broad base of knowledge, a lot of information has been left out, but there are excellent specialty manuals that cover every topic, many of which are listed at the end of the relevant chapters in the Resources section.

He and she, his and hers are used interchangeably and were chosen randomly: There are no implications in the association of he versus she with a particular job. And of course, there is some fantasy involved… there are some rules that might work in a perfect world, but often fall apart in the real lab. Everyone should go to seminars and never nod off for a minute. Everyone should replace what reagents are missing. Everyone should maintain his or her lab book every week. But life is busy and we all do the best we can.

Thank you to the following people for reading and commenting on one or more chapters of the manual: Alan Aderem, University of Washington, Seattle; John Aitchison, University of Alberta, Edmonton; Jeanne Barker, Merck, Rahway, New Jersey; Linnea Brody, Pathogenesis, Seattle, Washington; Kim Gavin, Cold Spring Harbor Lab, Cold Spring Harbor, New York; Peggy Hampstead, New York University; Sally Kornbluth, Duke University; Danny Lew, Duke University; Bruce J. Mayer, Howard Hughes Medical Institute and Harvard Medical School, Boston, Massachusetts; Esmeralda Party, Rockefeller University, New York.

I also thank Hidesaboro Hanafusa, of Rockefeller University, and Peter Newburger, of the University of Massachusetts Medical Center, in whose labs I learned about research and benchwork; Ralph Steinman, of Rockefeller University , who provided me with the mental and physical space to begin this manual; the many colleagues who patiently shared advice, supplies, and techniques; writers of the wonderful lab books and web sites used for reference; Alan, Zoe, Petai, and Sasha for their tolerance of huge piles of papers; my very supportive family and friends; and finally, Teruko Hanafusa, Ray Barker, and Zan Cohn, for the inspiration they were—and still are—to me.

Working with the people from Cold Spring Harbor Laboratory Press was a complete pleasure. John Inglis supported the idea of the manual and got the whole project going. Linda Rodgers was the most knowledgeable and pleasant scientific foil imaginable. The drawings by Jim Duffy provided inspiration as well as illustration, with a realism and lightness that any lab person will recognize. Mary Cozza, Pat Barker, and Susan Schaefer managed to keep both humor and work flowing efficiently and painlessly. I'm almost sorry the manual is finished.

Kathy Barker

Abbreviations

These abbreviations are not only ones found in this manual, but are some you may commonly hear tossed around casually in the lab.

alkphos	alkaline phosphatase
amp	ampicillin
AMV RT	avian myeloblastosis virus reverse transcriptase
ANOVA	analysis of variance
BAC	bacterial artificial chromosome
BBS	bulletin board system
B-gal	β galactosidase
Bis	N,N′-methylenebisacrylamide
BL 1,2,3, or 4	Biosafety Level 1,2,3, or 4
bp	base pairs
BPB	bromophenol blue
BSA	bovine serum albumin
CAT	chloramphenicol acetyl transferase
CDC	Center for Disease Control
cDNA	complementary DNA
cfu	colony forming unit
CMC	critical micelle concentration
CMV	cytomegalovirus
cpm	counts per minute
CS	calf serum
CsCl	cesium chloride
DEPC	diethylpyrocarbonate

DMSO   dimethylsulfoxide

dNTP   any of the four deoxynucleotide triphosphates: dATP, dCTP, dGTP, dTTP

DOC   deoxycholate

DOS   degenerate oligonuceotide sequences *or* disc operating system

DOT   Department of Transportation

dpm   disintegrations per minute

DTT   dithiothreitol

EHS   Environmental Health and Safety

ELISA   enzyme-linked immunosorbent assay

EPA   Environmental Protection Agency

EtBr   ethidium bromide

EtOH   ethanol

FACS   fluorescence-activated cell sorter

FAQ   frequently asked questions

FCS   fetal calf serum

FISH   fluorescence in situ hybridization

FPLC   forced pressure liquid chromatography

FS   filter sterilize

FTP   file transfer protocol

g generation time

xg relative centrifugal force

G_0, G_m, G_1, G_2 growth phase 1 or 2

GLC   gas liquid chromatography

GMT   good microbiological technique

HEPA   high efficiency particulate air (filter)

HEPES   N-2-hydroxyethylpiperazine-N′-2-ethane-sulfonic acid

HI   heat inactivated

HPLC   high performance liquid chromatography

HRP   horseradish peroxidase

IDLH   immediately dangerous to life and health

IEF   isoelectric focusing

IPTG   isopropyl-β-D-thiogalactoside

kan   kanamycin

kb   kilobase

K_D dissociation constant

LB	Luria-Bertani
LPS	lipopolysaccharide
M phase	mitosis phase
MeOH	methanol
MHC	major histocompatability complex
ml	milliliter
MoMLV or MMLV	Moloney murine leukemia virus
MOPS	3-(N-morpholino)propanesulfonic acid
MSDS	materials safety data sheet
mw	molecular weight
N.A.	numerical aperture
NaCl	sodium chloride
NIH	National Institutes of Health
NFPA	National Fire Protection Association
NK	natural killer
OD	optical density
OHSA	Occupational Safety and Health Administration
ORF	open reading frame
PAGE	polyacrylamide gel electrophoresis
PBL	peripheral blood lymphocytes
PBMC	peripheral blood mononuclear cells
PBS	phosphate-buffered saline
PCR	polymerase chain reaction
PEG	polyethylene glycol
pfu	plaque forming unit
P.I.	principal investigator
pI	isoelectric point
PIPES	piperazine-N,N′ *bis* (2-ethane-sulfonic acid)
pK	equilibrium constant
PKC	protein kinase C
PMA	phorbol myristic acid
PMN	polymorphonuclear leukocyte
psi	pounds per square inch
PVC	polyvinylchloride
q.s.	*quantum sufficiat*

RAM	random access memory
RBC	red blood cell
RCF	relative centrifugal force
RDA	representational difference analysis
RFLP	restriction fragment length polymorphism
RIA	radioimmunoassay
rpm	revolutions per minute
RSO	restriction site oligonucleotide
RT	reverse transcriptase
S phase	synthetic phase
SDS	sodium dodecyl sulfate
S.I.	standard unit
SSC	sodium citrate
TAE	Tris-acetate-EDTA
Taq	*Thermus aquaticus*
TBS	Tris borate EDTA
TCA	trichloroacetic acid
TD	to deliver
TE	Tris EDTA
TEMED	N,N,N′,N′-tetramethylethylenediamine
tet	tetracycline
TLC	thin layer chromatography *or* tender loving care
T_m	melting temperature
Tris	(hydroxymethyl)aminomethane
URL	Uniform Resource Locator
UV	ultraviolet
WBC	white blood cells
w/v	weight per volume
Xgal	5-bromo-4-chloro-3-indoyl-β-D-galactoside
YAC	yeast artificial chromosome

AT THE BENCH
A Laboratory Navigator

Section 1
Getting Oriented

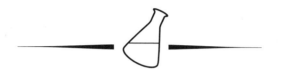

CHAPTER 1

General Lab Organization and Procedures 3

CHAPTER 2

Laboratory Setup and Equipment 21

CHAPTER 3

Getting Started and Staying Organized 43

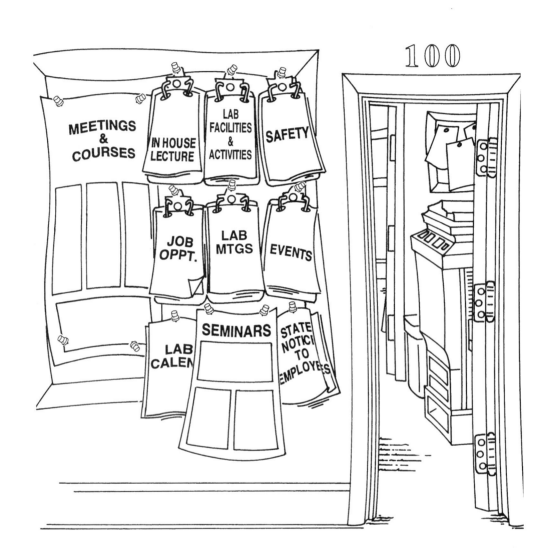

1

General Lab Organization and Procedures

WELCOME TO ONE of the most exciting and enjoyable workplaces ever evolved, the biomedical research laboratory. There is an amazing concept in operation here: You get paid or get credit for doing experiments, surely an almost scandalously delightful way to make a living. The work is worth while. The dress code, if any, is casual. The work hours are often self-determined and based on the needs of the experiment. The lab or department is filled with bright and interesting people, with whom you can discuss the salt concentration needed for a kinase assay or the implications of the latest congressional bill. It can come to have all the psychological comforts of home.

THE BIG PICTURE	4
LABORATORY PERSONNEL	5
LAB ROUTINES	7
Hours	7
Dress code	8
Laboratory tasks, lab jobs, assigned jobs	9
Laboratory meetings	9
WHAT TO EXPECT THE FIRST WEEK	10
WHAT TO DO THE FIRST WEEK	11
WHAT NOT TO DO THE FIRST WEEK	13
SURVIVAL THROUGH COMMON SENSE AND COURTESY	14
Basic survival rules: Attitude	15
Basic survival rules: Courtesy at the bench	15
NONNEGOTIABLE SAFETY RULES	17
RESOURCES	19

Like any complex social organizations, research laboratories have their own customs and rules. The difficulty is that the rules have been unspoken. You are expected to decipher the many obtuse clues and become a law-abiding member of a society in which individualism is highly prized. Although no one is expected to show you how to work the equipment, you will be expected to work it. In a profession in which communication of data is the goal and the reward of the research, not all people can communicate with you clearly and satisfactorily. Don't worry, you will manage! In a short time, the pleasure of working together with colleagues on interesting and similar projects will supplant any initial feelings of unease. But to get your work done well, you must first navigate among sometimes vague and mixed signals and learn how your laboratory beats and hums.

THE BIG PICTURE

A lab is defined by a number of overlapping terms, depending on the audience for whom the lab is being described. A lab may be described in terms of its basic *field*, such as immunology, physiology, or biophysics: This is more of an administrative definition than a functional one. The *experimental model*, the organism used to address the question, is often used to expand the description of the field of research. For example, someone may be a member of a microbial ecology or yeast genetics or a human neuroanatomy laboratory.

The *area of research* is a more practical way to describe a laboratory, since it tells you what the lab actually does: One might say the lab is a cell cycle lab, or a signal transduction lab. The lab probably has a *focus*, a question that binds all the lab members. The entire lab may be working on the proteins involved in secretion from neurons, or trying to understand why and how a particular transcription protein is involved in development. And each lab member has her own *question*, a specific problem that she is trying to solve experimentally.

Another way the laboratory has been defined is by whether it is engaged in *basic or applied science*. Basic science was assumed to be pure science, science done only for the sake of knowledge, whereas applied science has been thought of as the use of a basic science idea for the development of a product such as an antibiotic. Basic science was considered to be the child of academic research, funded by soft money (research support and/or salary funded by competitive grants): Applied science was thought to be performed in companies, funded by hard money (salary and research support are part of the job and are given by the institution or company). These distinctions are not valid. Basic and applied sciences are done in universities and pharmaceutical companies, and research at academic institutions and companies is funded by both hard and soft money. To those who work in labs, the practical similarities are more apparent than the differences.

Some laboratories do *clinical research*, in which human patients or a patient's cells are used to investigate a disease or syndrome, and much of the work is done by medical doctors rather than Ph.Ds. Clinical research labs are usually found only at medical schools or institutions affiliated with a hospital, where there is access to patients.

Each laboratory is usually part of a larger unit, such as a *department* or a *division*, and shares facilities with all department members. Large pieces of equipment such as ultracentrifuges and −70ºC freezers are often departmental, even if they are housed within an individual's laboratory. Cold rooms, warm rooms, dark rooms and film developers, autoclaves and glassware-washers may also be shared, unless they belong to a very large and extremely well funded laboratory. Most departments have a library, where the relevant and current journals of the field are located: This library may often serve as a lunchroom or a small seminar room. And almost every department has a large bulletin board, near the secretary, library, or main office, upon which are posted seminar times and places, job listings, meeting notices, and departmental happenings.

Use the department, and don't hide away in the lab. The department is a resource that can provide you with ideas, equipment, and connections, and your dealings with the members of the department can greatly influence the happiness and productivity of your lab life.

LABORATORY PERSONNEL

Laboratory groups have a dynamic that is fairly unique, in that people work more independently than in other groups, and the organizational structure tends to be rather horizontal. Practically, this means that *everyone is equal,* and it is usually no one's job to show you how to do things. Don't assume that, because a person has a "lower" status than you, you can indiscriminately order that person to make a buffer for you: You might get the buffer, but you might also generate a lot of passive aggression. Antagonizing someone may mean that no one will clear out freezer space for you, take your tubes out of the water bath when you have forgotten them, or help you do a calculation until you change your attitude.

Laboratories have a variety of personnel working in them, with varying levels of commitment and various reasons to be there. The cast of characters commonly includes:

> *Treat all members of the lab with the same respect you give the lab head.*

The principal investigator, or P.I. This person may also be known as the head of the lab, the boss, the advisor. He or she probably spends more time with administrative tasks such as writing grants or research reports than in doing labwork but is the intellectual guide behind most of the projects in the lab. Directly or indirectly, he or she is responsible for funding the laboratory research. The entire atmosphere of the lab—friendliness and camaraderie or vicious competitiveness—will depend on the P.I.'s personality and leadership.

Postdocs. This is short for "postdoctoral" associate, assistant, or fellow (the terms are institution dependent), a person who has received his or her Ph.D. or, more rarely, M.D., and is doing a 2–5-year training period before looking for a position as a P.I. in a university or in industry. A postdoc usually works quite independently on his own project, although he will collaborate with other lab members on particular aspects of the project.

Technician or research assistant. A technician can be a college student who wants to gain more experience in the lab before entering graduate or medical school, or a professional with an M.S. and the appropriate pay and title. In academic establishments the norm is the new college graduate who will stay only for 2 years: In industry or in some medical centers, longer-term arrangements (with more money and prestige) are found. Technicians do a variety of tasks including ordering supplies, preparing media and caring for the lab's

> *A professional technician is often the most skilled and knowledgeable person in the lab.*

cell lines, assisting a particular lab member with his or her experiments, and designing and carrying out their own experiments.

Graduate student. Graduate students are doing lab work required for their M.S. or for a Ph.D. Generally, they work long hours and have a lot of time and emotion invested in their projects. Like postdocs, graduate students have their own project or projects and become increasingly independent during their tenure of 4–7 years in the laboratory.

Rotation student. Many graduate schools require their students to work in several labs before they decide on the lab for their thesis work: These brief weeks of research are known as a rotation. A rotation student is in the lab for 6 weeks to 6 months, usually on a short-term project. He may be required to do rotations, or he may want to pick up techniques in a new field, or he may be testing the waters before making a bigger commitment.

Summer student. Summer students are usually college students, sometimes high school students. A student who has already worked in a lab may be given his own small project, whereas a new student might make buffers for the entire lab or, most typically, be assigned to help a particular person.

Resident. Residents are usually found in a medical center lab researching an aspect of human disease. He or she may spend several weeks to several months in an area associated with his field, usually doing a short-term project. A resident may be known as a fellow in some institutions.

Visiting faculty. During a sabbatical, a faculty member might go to another lab, where she can learn a new technique, try a new field, or collaborate on a series of experiments.

Secretary or administrative assistant. The secretary may be in charge of ordering supplies for the lab, may help lab members with grant applications, and may organize lab seminars and journal clubs, or may work only to serve the P.I. directly. Be especially considerate of the secretary, who is one of the most important and necessary, but undervalued and rudely treated, people in the laboratory.

Laboratory aide. Some jobs in a department or laboratory are done by a laboratory aide, who is hired to perform a set of specific tasks. This person is usually not trained to be a scientist, but helps the lab greatly by doing tedious and time-consuming jobs. Examples of laboratory aids are *medium preparers* and *glassware cleaners*. The medium preparer makes and distributes cell culture media and bacterial broth and plates. A glassware cleaner—the one who washes the dirty glassware and pipets and, perhaps, delivers the cleaned and autoclaved things—is a luxury that small labs may not be able to support. This job is likely to be a departmental one, with several labs being serviced by the same person.

> *Knowing someone's position in the lab can help you understand why he may do certain things that appear inexplicable to you. It can suggest which person might be the best person to consult on a particular scientific or personal problem. But do not define anyone by her title alone, or you may pass by a potential fountain of information. You may also be impressed when you shouldn't be!*

Laboratory supervisor. The day-to-day operation of the lab may be overseen by a laboratory supervisor. The responsibilities of the laboratory supervisor might range from keeping the lab stocked and organizing journal clubs to suggesting experimental approaches. Whatever the situation, don't let the presence of a supervisor prevent you from ever interacting with the P.I.

Laboratory safety officer. A laboratory member, usually one who has been in the lab for a few years, is usually assigned to act as a liaison between the lab and the Environmental Health and Safety (EHS) department. If you have questions about health, safety, or the appropriateness of lab protocols, speak to the lab safety officer before you speak to someone in the EHS department. This is usually a departmental position.

LAB ROUTINES

Although labs have people coming and going through all hours of the day, certain routines and customs stand firmly in the apparent chaos. It will take a number of weeks before the rhythms of the lab are clear and you can make your place in this environment. As much as you can without compromising yourself, initially try to work in with the routines of your particular lab.

Hours

Because experiments don't always fit into a slot of 9 to 5, lab workers often have long, unpredictable, and quite eccentric hours. Most people are allowed to regulate their own hours, with the most trust usually associated with academic departments. But even if the lab is an academic lab, and not a word is said or spoken about hours, *there is probably a standard of time commitment that is expected.* Companies and hospital departments tend to have more traditional hours, whereas academic departments may seem more casual, with more late night action. But in both, working less than the deemed and sometimes unspoken expected hours of work can stigmatize the new worker. Find out what hours of work are expected, and try to conform to this. If most people tend to come in late in the morning, and work evenings, try to do the same: Working hours dissimilar to other workers makes it difficult for you to get to know people and to obtain the help you need.

Position influences hours. Basically, because people are dependent on them, technicians and secretaries are expected to work more regular and predictable hours. But if you are expected to stay to finish experiments or projects, it is only fair that you should have more freedom in choosing hours.

Your personal situation may not allow you to work the lab's hours. Children, classes, commutes, and partners are some of the factors that will also influence the hours you can work. *Try to overlap with other lab members as much as you can.* Be up front about your hours, because you certainly don't want to be in a situation where you sneak around and get into weird behaviors such as leaving on lights or pieces of equipment to show that you were there. Hopefully, your work will speak for itself.

Vacation policy also varies from lab to lab and is usually unspoken. In many places, people are discouraged from taking vacations because it always seems as if it is the wrong time to leave a project: Either the project is going well, and you don't want to walk out on a run of good results, or it isn't going well, and you feel too guilty to leave before you get it back on track. Take the time you deserve, but don't abuse the privilege of independent decisions.

Dress Code

One of the satisfying benefits of working in the lab is the freedom to wear whatever you'd like. People in hospitals and companies often dress more formally than do those in academic institutions, since they must interact with non-lab people and patients. People in academic institutions are more likely to be offended at the thought of having their clothing regulated, even by custom. This is a personal issue, but it is most likely that you can wear whatever you want, and no one will ever question you.

There are few rules on dressing for the lab:

- Don't wear good clothes unless you want to spill phenol or bleach on them. Spills only happen to favorite or expensive clothes.

- If you must wear a tie, keep it out of the Bunsen burner.

Laboratory Tasks, Lab Jobs, Assigned Jobs

In many labs the lab personnel must *share common jobs.* Typical jobs include making liters of a commonly used buffer, picking up the dry ice, changing the CO_2 cylinders on the incubators, or packing up the radioactive waste. These jobs may be permanent or may be rotated at regular intervals. Sometimes the job is a particular piece of equipment which the assigned person is responsible for keeping in good running order.

Take your assignment seriously. Don't let it always come second to your own experiments. Other lab members may be dependent on the buffer you keep forgetting to make, and even if you don't absolutely ruin someone's experiment, you will get a reputation as a bad lab citizen. Try to do this job with cheer.

> *Playing the radio. Most labs have a radio or CD player in the main room, and the debate about the choice of music can quickly escalate into a war. Don't get into it. If you don't like the music, buy yourself earplugs or a Walkman.*

Laboratory Meetings

Meetings are held in laboratories to discuss current research of the labworkers, the current research of the field (since recent journal articles are often discussed, these are known as journal clubs), and organizational problems. These may be combined into one or two meetings: Small labs may not have their own meetings but be participants in departmental meetings. Many labs or departments have a *weekly journal club* and a *weekly research meeting.*

In *research meetings,* one or two people present their data. In some places, all lab members briefly talk. These talks may be casual, over lunch and with only a blackboard or overhead projector, or they may be formal enough to require proper slides and dress.

> *Attend all meetings.* Unless *you have a desperately pressing experiment, arrange your time so you can go to all journal clubs and research presentations. Content aside (and you will probably learn a lot), your attendance shows your support for your coworkers and is important for departmental cohesiveness.*

Journal clubs are almost always quite casual, although local custom will dictate whether photocopies or the blackboard is used to present the paper. Often, the papers to be presented are listed a few days before the meeting so everyone can read the papers and have at least a primitive working knowledge of the topic.

Who participates in lab meetings? The backbone of most lab meetings is the students and postdocs, with participation by technicians, faculty, and short-term personnel being dependent on lab policy. Certainly, if you aren't required to join in but want to participate, you should ask the head of the lab if it is okay.

If you are expected to participate you will usually be given a grace period, especially for research seminars. It is common, if you have previously done research, to give your first research seminar on your past research project. The format of lab meetings varies widely: Chapter 6 contains more details about participation in and preparation of lab meetings.

> *You are probably expected to participate, but you will usually be given a grace period, especially for research seminars. The format of journal clubs and research meetings will vary widely. For your first presentation, at least, follow the lab format. Chapter 6 contains more details about your own presentations.*

WHAT TO EXPECT THE FIRST WEEK

 You will be assigned a lab bench, or a part of a lab bench. You may also be assigned a *desk*, either in the lab or in a common office area. Don't be offended if the place you have been given is very small—space is at a real premium in most labs and, generally, the more successful the P.I., the more crowded the lab, and the less space each person is given. You may well see that many people have more space, but don't complain yet.

 The lab head, or the person responsible for you, will probably sit down with you to discuss the project you will work on. The basics of the project were most likely outlined before you came to the lab, but this is the time you will find out the specifics. *If you are offered the chance to work closely with someone (rather than to work completely independently), grab it!* You will get much more help than if you are patching together instructions on your own, and you can negotiate your autonomy later.

If you can, read literature related to the project you will be working on, or to the theme of the work in the lab, before the talk. Don't worry if everything doesn't make perfect sense, or even if it makes no sense at all—as soon as you do a few experiments, it will all become clearer—it will give you the vocabulary with which to have the conversation.

 You will have an appointment with EHS (also known as Laboratory Safety and/or Radiation Safety), which functions as the overseer of personal safety, radiation use, and biohazard disposal. A film may be shown, or a lecture given, about general laboratory safety precautions and the particular rules of your institution. If necessary, you may be instructed on *radioactivity* usage and provided with a *radiation badge* that is used to monitor your exposure to radiation. If you work with human blood or cells, you will get a *hepatitis B vaccine.* Other vaccines or tests may be needed for working with particular organisms. A *background thyroid scan* should be done if anyone in the laboratory or department will be working with radioactive iodine.

 You will get keys or a keycard for the lab, and an institutional I.D. The keys may not be only for your lab, but also for shared areas for other labs in the department. Don't abuse these keys by wandering around in other labs off-hours.

 You will be assigned storage space in the refrigerator, −20°C freezer, and −70°C freezers. This is in theory: In practice, it may take longer for people to reorganize (for everyone will expand into whatever space is available) to make room for you. Find out where you can keep a few things while waiting for permanent space.

WHAT TO DO THE FIRST WEEK

 Do an experiment! Don't wait until you understand the system to start experiments—you won't be ready to learn effectively until you have done your first experiments. It is magic, but it is the #1 lab truism. It will also help you feel and be considered as a productive member of the lab. The experiment doesn't have to be an earth-shattering one—in fact, *it should be simple* and be used to check your results against others in an assay often done in the lab.

 Set up your lab bench. Order, find, clean, and arrange what you need for your desk and personal lab space. *Think in terms of doing an experiment as soon as possible.*

 Introduce yourself to everyone. Lab workers come and go, people are busy, so don't feel slighted if you don't get the red carpet treatment. *Let everyone know* who you are, and what you are working on. Asking each person about his or her own project is usually a good icebreaker. Go to lunch with lab members at least once during the week.

 Take notes on everything. This is not just a courtesy, but a *necessity*; you will be given so much information this first week that it is impossible to remember all the details. And details can be excruciatingly important when you find yourself alone at night and don't remember where the needed reagent is.

Familiarize yourself with how the lab is run, where things are kept, who does what and when. Watch and ask questions when it isn't too intrusive; don't ask about lunchrooms and telephones when someone is in the middle of an experiment.

 Ask. True, you don't want to bother anyone, especially needlessly. But it is always better to ask a question about a procedure, a reagent, a piece of equipment, than to waste time and money. If you make a mistake, always ask a coworker if the mistake can be rectified. The same mistakes are repeated again and again by new workers, and there is a way out of many apparently botched experiments.

Things to find out about the first week:

Chemicals. Where are the chemicals, how are they arranged, where are they weighed and pH-ed?

Computer usage. Do you have access to a computer? If so, when, and is a password or access number needed? Can you do literature searches on it? Is there a way to get onto the WWW? Can you E-mail? How do you get an E-mail address?

First aid. What is the number to call for an emergency? Where are the chemical spill and first aid kits? Where is the safety shower and how does it work?

Glassware. Where is clean glassware kept? Where does dirty glassware go? Does someone wash all the glassware, or must each person take care of his own?

Institution library. Where is the library, and what do you need to use it? How do you make photocopies in the library? Can you access the library from the lab computer?

Lab coats. Does the institution provide lab coats? If they are cloth, does the institution launder them?

Lab meetings and journal clubs. What is the schedule for lab meetings and journal clubs? Is it posted? What is the format for the meetings?

Lab notebook. Is there a lab rule to follow when writing up experiment results? Are either loose sheets or bound sheets okay? Are the books or sheets provided? Is it necessary to make a copy of each day's data?

Ordering supplies. Does each individual make the phone call, or is someone responsible for ordering for everyone? Is there a strict budget to follow? Can ordering be done by computer? Who picks up the supplies when they arrive?

Photocopy machine. Is a card or number needed, or do you have to keep track of the number of copies?

Telephone calls. What is the phone number in the lab? Is there an answering machine or voice mail, and if so, how do you get messages? Must each person pay for personal calls?

Trash disposal. Who takes away the trash? Where does biohazard material go, and who is responsible for pick-up? Where do you dispose of needles and other sharps? How about recyclable paper?

Work hours. What hours do people tend to work? At what hours are your collaborators in? What is the best time to get first shot at the equipment?

NOT TO DO THE FIRST WEEK

 Don't constantly mention, when being shown something, that "we didn't do it this way in class/my other lab/the hospital." This is an implied insult that won't be appreciated. When you have been in the lab for a while, and have had a chance to really evaluate the lab's way of doing a particular thing, you will be able to introduce an improvement or to make your own decision about a method. But for now, listen.

 Don't read a newspaper or a novel, or play computer games, in the lab. During every day in the lab, especially early on, there is a lot of dead (non-experiment) time, but reading the sports section while others are working hard will create a bad first impression. No, it shouldn't matter, but it does. Use the time to read relevant literature.

 Don't ask or complain about money or salaries. This is a leftover from the science-in-the-sky days, when a serious scientist was supposed to be oblivious to all else but work, and interest in money suggested that person was not content with the beauty of scientific discovery. Scientists have had to become more practical now, but there remains the feeling that money talk is tacky and unprofessional. Negotiate your salary and benefits before you arrive, and keep an ear open for hints of unfairness, but don't cloud the beginning of your job with recitations of what your friends in other labs are receiving as salaries.

 Don't use the telephone or photocopy machine excessively for personal reasons. Try to conduct as much nonprofessional business away from the lab as possible. If you must use the telephone for personal reasons, keep the call as short as possible, especially if you share a phone with other lab members.

In the first week, new lab members tend to photocopy dozens and dozens of articles relevant to their new field of research. Few of these are ever read, even fewer are remembered. Photocopying an article does not imbue you with the power to absorb the information by osmosis! You are more likely to actually learn from papers by reading them immediately and jotting down important points.

Don't suggest that you are working in the lab for any other reason than love of research. If you have another reason, keep it to yourself or you will be perceived as not being serious about your work. By saying things such as "I'm only here to get a better fellowship," you demean most people's reasons for being there.

SURVIVAL THROUGH COMMON SENSE AND COURTESY

Following simple lab courtesy is vital to maintaining a good relationship with your coworkers and getting your work done. This section might also be called "Lab Survival" or "**If you are going to read anything in this book, read this section.**"

Everyone in a lab is generally willing to help but is extremely busy, and respecting that will help you to learn how to ferret out the knowledge you need. These rules sound harsh, but they are common sense in an environment in which group goals are functionally secondary to individual achievement and responsibility.

Even in folklore and fiction, the inconsiderate lab researcher has caused a problem:

"Vergil's dismissal would not have unduly distressed his fellow employees. In his three years at Genetron, he had committed innumerable breaches of lab etiquette. He seldom washed lab glassware and twice had been accused of not wiping spills of ethidium bromide—a strong mutagen—on lab counters. He was also not terribly cautious about radionucleides." (Reprinted, with permission, from Greg Bear 1986, p. 12.)

"Their arrival was viewed as nothing less than an invasion by some workers in Art Riggs's lab. Riggs tended to be meticulous, careful, and considerate; for example, after his technician, Louise Shively, became pregnant, he took over any tasks involving radioactive isotopes. The scientists from San Francisco were different. "It was unbelievable," Shively recalls. "It was clear from the first day that they were random and left a mess piled up behind them wherever they worked. It's like they were whirlwinds." Riggs would occasionally remind them to show some manners at the bench, but as Goeddel admits, "We were so concerned with the project that we weren't really listening too much." To everyone's relief, they did most of their work in a small lab across the hall." (Hall 1987, p. 219)

Courtesy may not always matter—Vergil died in a novel because of his sloppiness, but Goeddel was actually instrumental in the cloning of the insulin gene—but it certainly helps the lab run more efficiently, smoothly, and pleasantly.

Basic Survival Rules: Attitude

1. **Ask, don't command.** The other people in the lab are *co*workers.

2. **Assume nothing.** You should not assume that someone will immediately stop his experiment to help you whenever you need it, that someone else will deal with the alarm on the incubator. Be, at least in the beginning, fairly humble in your expectations. Also, *don't assume that everyone else is always right.*

3. **Write down everything when someone is giving you instructions.** You will be given a lot of information by a variety of people, and you want to avoid asking the same questions over and over. *Record people's names, incubation times and temperatures, locations of reagents, instructions on autoclave use, everything and anything that saves another question.* This has the psychological benefit of not only helping you to remember, but also garnering good will points by making it obvious to people that you are interested in what they are saying.

4. **Make appointments or request time with people.** Time is tight when experiments are running—even 5 minutes of someone's time (and, in a lab, almost nothing takes only 5 minutes) might be impossible to get. Ask someone if, later in the morning, he might show you how to use the balance. Don't wait until your samples are thawing and you have a window of 2 minutes to frantically plead with someone for help.

   > *Don't ask questions of someone who is writing or manipulating tubes. Make your presence known, and wait until she feels able to respond.*

5. **Don't remove journals from the departmental library,** except to photocopy an article. Replace journals exactly where they belong on the shelves. If eating is permitted in the library, remove all crumbs and debris before you leave.

6. **Don't discuss a fellow lab member's results with people not in the lab.** There may be worries about a competing lab, or the data may not have been repeated enough to make it trustworthy.

   > *If a hot result is found in the morning in a lab in New York, everyone in California will know by the afternoon. There are usually far fewer than six degrees of separation between any two lab members, so a sensitive result must be kept completely quiet until the involved researcher is ready to talk.*

Basic Survival Rules: Courtesy at the Bench

1. **Never use reagents or buffers without permission.** The buffers and reagents on people's benches are very precious, and very, very personal. They may be sterile,

they may be RNase free, they may just be private, and you should not even take a milliliter without permission from the owner.

They may also not be exactly what you think they are or what they are labeled, and their use may end up ruining your experiment. There probably are common lab reagents somewhere—but wait until you are explicitly told what they are, and under which conditions you may use them, before you touch them.

2. **If a common reagent is low or runs out, order more.** *Don't put the empty bottle back.* Find out how to place an order to restock the item. It is a good idea to leave a dated note on the shelf to say that the item has been ordered.

3. **Don't ignore a broken piece of equipment or an equipment alarm**. In your early days, you may not be able to deal with problem equipment, but you should *notify other lab members* so the appropriate action can be taken. Don't merely use another centrifuge or gel box, leaving the next prospective user to deal with the problem.

    Immediate action should be taken if you hear a buzzer or alarm in a piece of equipment, as the consequences of ignoring it can be completely disastrous: In particular, loss of power or temperature maintenance in a low-temperature freezer or liquid nitrogen storage tank can mean the loss of the entire department's clones, cell lines, purified proteins, and cDNA libraries. And if it is your fault that this happens, kiss all good will goodbye.

4. **Do not move things around or change the location of any tubes, reagents, or equipment that you encounter in common lab areas.** It isn't the most sensible thing, but people find their reagents as much by location as by label, so put them in a place as close to the original location as possible. If you *must* move something, notify the owner of the material.

5. **Don't leave anything anywhere,** except where it belongs or on your lab bench. This means not a flask in the sink, not a pipet in the garbage, unless it is the correct and designated destination.

6. **If you do something wrong, confess.** Everyone probably knows that you did it, anyway, so tell the truth! It will establish you as an honest member of the community, which is not an insignificant thing in a research profession. Everyone makes mistakes, but sneaking to cover one leaves a nasty taste. Offer to remedy the mistake, if possible.

7. **Clean up immediately after (or better yet, during) each part of an experiment.** Cleanup is *part of the experiment,* not an extra something to do to show you are a nice guy. Be especially careful to keep common areas, such as sinks, cell culture hoods, and electrophoresis areas, free of your paraphernalia and debris. This will help others to expedite their own experiments.

8. **Request the minimum of favors.** It is okay to ask someone to stop or finish an experiment for you, if you really must go, and it will take a minimum of activity on his or her part. Lab workers often depend on each other for this kind of help. But don't present someone with a list of things to finish up because you want to catch a movie.

NONNEGOTIABLE SAFETY RULES

1. Follow the universal lab safety rules:

   - *No eating, drinking, or smoking in the lab.* People often grab a bite to eat at their desks, but it isn't a good idea; not only is it esthetically and healthwise a bad thing, but the lab safety people will get quite peeved if they catch you. There will be a nearby place to eat and drink.

     > *The laboratory may actually be closed down if personnel are found eating in the lab. Usually a warning will be given for the first infraction.*

     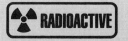 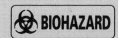

     Be aware of signs that point to potential dangers. Two that are found in many labs are the *yellow radioactive sign,* indicating that radioactive agents are either stored or used there, and the *orange biohazard sign,* which is posted where there may be infectious agents. Don't use anything with these signs, including refrigerators and incubators, until you have checked with the laboratory safety officer.

   - *Avoid open-toed shoes,* because they leave your feet too vulnerable if there is a spill.

   - *Wear a lab coat in the lab.* It isn't considered chic in many labs, but it is too easy to lean on a counter, newly washed down with bleach, and leave a lovely hole in your shirt.

   - *Don't wear the lab coat out of the lab area.* The lab coat protects you from caustic and infectious substances, and it is foolish to then subject other people to the nasty stuff. If it is de rigeur to wear a lab coat to seminars or to lunch, have a clean one set aside for those occasions.

   - *Don't mouth pipet.* Not even sterile water! Ask for a bulb or a mechanical pipetting aid.

2. **Know how to help yourself and other lab members in case of an emergency.**

   - *Memorize the emergency safety telephone numbers.* There may be one emergency number to be used for any sort of crisis. There may be a number for the institutional EHS, as well as a number for the Campus Police or Security: Don't forget the number of the local police and emergency service.

   - *Find out where the first aid kit, the radiation and chemical spill kits, eyewash, and safety showers are.* Be acquainted with the safety rules for your laboratory.

3. **Don't do anything you feel is unsafe.** If you have questions or doubts about any procedure, check with the lab safety officer and the EHS.

RESOURCES

The following books give a flavor for both the professional and personal aspects of biomedical research:

Angier N. 1988. *Natural obsessions. The search for the oncogene.* Houghton Mifflin Company, Boston, Massachusetts.

Bear G. 1986. *Blood music.* Ace Books, New York, New York.

Gornick V. 1990. *Women in science.* Simon and Schuster, New York, New York.

Hall S.S. 1987. *Invisible frontiers. The race to synthesize a human gene.* Tempus Books, Redmond, Washington.

Kornberg A. 1995. *The golden helix. Inside biotech ventures.* University Science Books, Sausalito, California.

Lewis S. 1961. *Arrowsmith.* The New American Library of World Literature, New York, New York.

Teitelman R. 1989. *Gene dreams. Wall Street, academia, and the rise of biotechnology.* Basic Books, New York, New York.

Watson, J.D. 1968. *The double helix.* The New American Library, New York, New York.

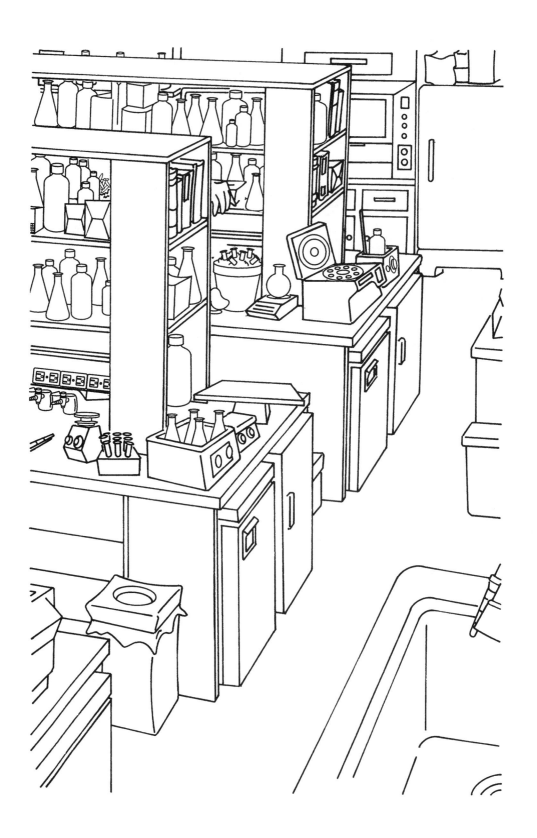

2

Laboratory Setup and Equipment

AT FIRST, THERE WILL SEEM to be a bewildering amount of equipment on the benches, on the floors, sometimes even in the aisles. In most labs, this is very standard equipment, and after a while, all labs will seem to be very familiar places. In certain specialized labs, such as electron microscopy labs or electrophysiology labs, there will be a concentration of certain, atypical kinds of equipment, but a general lab ambiance will still be apparent.

LAY OF THE LAND	22
Main laboratory	22
Other rooms and places	28
Other equipment	31
USING THE EQUIPMENT	37
Basic rules	37
What to do if you hear an alarm	38
HOW TO BUY NEW EQUIPMENT	39
RESOURCES	41

If you don't understand the equipment you are using for an experiment, you don't fully understand the experiment. Start immediately learning what each piece of equipment is, and what it is used for. Not only will this help you feel more at home, but it will also acquaint you with the experimental potential in your back yard. Notice who uses what, so you will know where to find an expert when you need one. When it comes time to use a particular apparatus, be sure to understand the rudiments of its operation: Only then can you properly manipulate conditions or know when an unexpected and apparently Nobel-quality result is merely the result of mechanical failure.

LAY OF THE LAND

Main Laboratory

Laboratory benches predominate, physically and psychologically: These are long or short peninsulas, with drawers underneath, bottles on shelves above, and small equipment and open working spaces on the surface. Often, there is a desk attached to one end. Each person usually has a bench, or part of a bench, and "the bench" is, to its owner, home. The person who shares your bench is your benchmate, observer of all your experimental and emotional ups and downs and thus, the laboratory equivalent of a spouse.

> *Some labs have nothing but "private" lab benches, and lab members are expected to perform all tasks on their own lab benches. Check it out, for the rules are usually very different for private vs public lab areas. On your lab bench, you can probably allow a used paper towel or pipet to remain, but you must be meticulous about removing your supplies and waste from a common area.*

The typical lab bench

A slab of wood, slate, metal, or plastic—this will be the center of your lab life, your primary working area. On the bench are small pieces of equipment, such as a vortex and holders for various pipettors, and supplies such as pipettor tips.

Most lab benches are equipped with a vacuum line, an air line, a gas line, and sometimes, a water line. The *water line* is the most useful in theory but the least in practice: Using it often results in a puddle on the bench. The *air* can be used to blow obstructions from tubes, to dry glassware quickly, and for other brute purposes. But this is dusty air, and it shouldn't be used on glassware that will be used for experiments or buffer preparation. The *gas line* is used to fuel Bunsen burners, needed for aseptic technique at the bench. The *vacuum line* is extremely useful, especially for removing supernatants.

Above the bench are usually shelves. Here are stored personal buffers and reagents. Detergents and Tris buffers often comprise the bulk of the bottles. Pipet tips and containers of microfuge tubes also sit here.

If there are cabinets beneath the lab bench, acids and bases (not in the same cabinet, of course) and large bottles of buffer or solvents will be found. Odd, old, favorite, or infrequently used small equipment might also be here.

There are drawers beneath the lab bench. A casual peek might reveal a terrifying mix of old pH papers, pasteur pipet bulbs, and Sharpies, since these drawers tend to be where harried investigators throw odds and ends, to be organized later. Here might also be found boxes of tips, bags of tubes, and errant pieces of common lab equipment such as gel spacers and combs. These drawers are usually considered to be personal space, so don't just rummage through a neighbor's bench drawers without asking.

Common lab equipment may be found on the bench, usually at the end. Having a piece of common equipment on the bench does not entitle one to preferential use of the equipment! And using a piece of common equipment on someone's bench does not allow you to use the pipets, tubes, or other supplies on the bench.

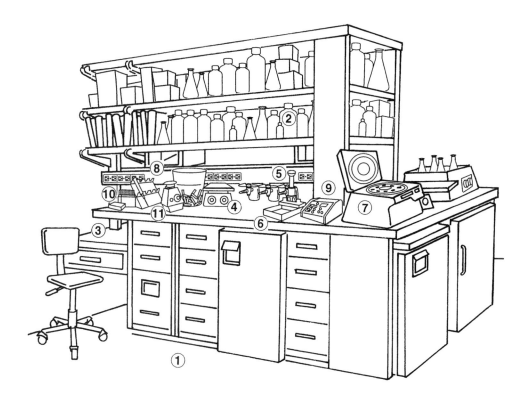

FIGURE 1.

The laboratory bench. **Key:** (1) *Bays.* The area between benches, and more a psychological than a physical entity; sharing a bay with someone is a close and somewhat intimate relationship. Equipment tends to be shared in bays, reagents borrowed and lent, favors asked, stories told. Be kind to your baymate. (2) *Buffers and other reagents.* After being autoclaved, most buffers can be stored at room temperature. These belong to the owner of the lab bench, and should not be touched without permission. (3) *Desk.* Desks, particularly in older labs, may not be part of the lab bench, but may be found wherever there is space. Very few desks are found in some labs, and there are instead rooms filled with desks for all the departmental students and/or postdocs. Sometimes, not everyone gets a desk but must use the department library or conference room to read or to make notebook entries. Usually, however, desks are found at the end of the lab bench and against the wall. (4) *Hot plate.* Used to heat liquids. Samples are usually boiled in a beaker on a hot plate. **Hazards:** Burns, liquids bubbling over. **Alternatives:** Water bath, microwave. (5) *Flame burner* (also known as a Bunsen burner). Vital to aseptic technique, for heating bottles and loops. Hooked up to house gas supply. Turn off after each use. **Alternatives:** Electric loop sterilizers and disposable plastic loops. (6) *Gel box.* Plastic containers used to run protein, DNA, or RNA gels. They range in size from mini-gels to sequencing gels. (7) *Microfuge.* A small, benchtop centrifuge that spins volumes up to 2 ml at approximately 12,000*g*. Used to pellet cells, precipitate DNA ... a workhorse. Some models are refrigerated, most are not. Some units are kept in a refrigerator or cold room. **Alternatives:** Adapters can be used in larger centrifuges and rotors. (8) *Pipettors.* Instruments used to measure and transfer small volumes of liquid. (9) *Power supply.* Used to run electrophoresis, perform transfers of gels to filters. Shocks can result from careless handling. Not all power supplies perform all tasks, so be sure you have the correct one for the job. (10) *Tip boxes.* Pipettors require the right size tips to dispense fluids accurately. These tips are usually autoclaved before use, and are disposable. (11) *Vortex.* Used to mix the contents of tubes. Can have an adapter for multiple tubes. **Alternatives:** Nutator, wheel, shaker.

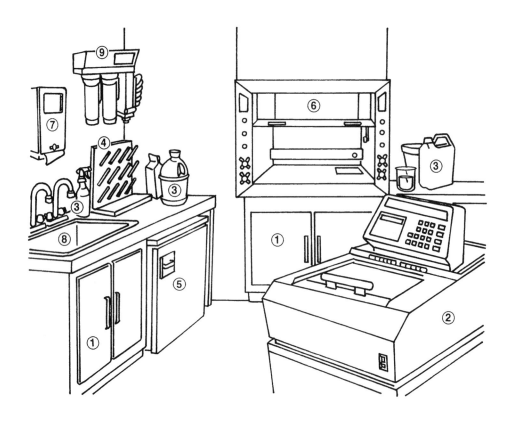

FIGURE 2.

Sink area, centrifuge, fume hood. **Key:** (1) *Cabinets.* Acids or bases or organic solvents are stored in common areas throughout the lab. (2) *Centrifuge.* Spins tubes filled with a liquid/solid mix, separating the mix into (hopefully) distinct phases and concentrating solid phases. There are several kinds of centrifuges, categorized by speed and tube size capabilities. **Alternatives:** No practical alternative. Filtration can remove the media and trap solids for some material. **Hazards:** Generation of aerosols and mechanical failure. Aerosols of biohazard or toxic materials can be produced if good laboratory technique and centrifuge safety and containment equipment aren't used when centrifuging such substances. A mechanical failure can produce fragments moving at great velocity, and if such fragments escape the protective bowl of the centrifuge, they can cause traumatic injury to personnel. (3) *Detergents.* There may be several kinds of detergents and cleaning agents here: for hands, for glassware, and for radioactivity. (4) *Drying rack.* After handwashing, beakers and other labware are placed here. (5) *–20ºC Freezer.* Used to store serum, most enzymes, reagents. There are often several freezers in the lab. (6) *Chemical fume hood.* Air is vented out of a chemical hood, making this the place of choice for working with volatile substances such as chloroform (and phenol-chloroform). Volatile radioactive labeling is done in some hoods, which are certified for this purpose. If this is true of the hood you are using, check for radioactivity with a Geiger counter. (7) *Paper towels.* Used for wiping hands and lab benches, and sometimes, for recording data. Replenish the stock if you use the last one. (8) *Sink.* Keep the sink clear for disposal and work. Be careful what you pour down the sink. Untreated supernatants from cells and bacteria should not be disposed of here, nor should hazardous chemicals. (9) *Water purification unit.* Tap water cannot be used for most laboratory applications. By distillation, or by reverse osmosis and ion exchange, the unit removes particles and other impurities from water. **Alternatives:** Purified water can be purchased in small quantities of 500 or 1000 ml.

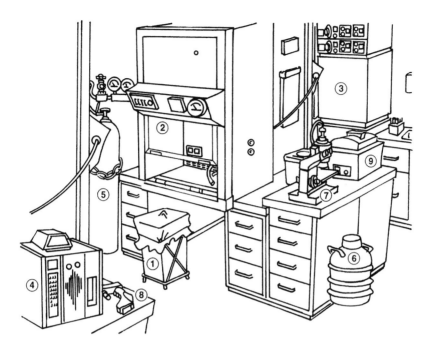

FIGURE 3.

Tissue culture area. **Key:** (1) *Biohazard waste disposal.* Anything living or used to hold anything living must be autoclaved before disposal. (2) *Biosafety cabinet.* Sometimes casually referred to as a hood or a *laminar flow hood*, this has a forced airflow to minimize the entrance of any dust or organisms into the working area. Laminar flow hoods should always be left on. (See Chapter 8.) **Alternatives:** If a biosafety cabinet is not required—if there is not a biohazard associated with the work material—a still-air box or traffic-less and draft-free place can be used for tissue culture. (3) *CO_2 incubator.* Used primarily for tissue culture, CO_2 is piped into an incubator for CO_2-requiring organisms or to maintain pH in the culture medium. **Remarks:** Buzzing may indicate a need to fill the water jacket, or a lack of CO_2. **Alternatives:** CO_2 can be pumped or generated in a container and incubated at the correct temperature. A buffer such as HEPES in a closed system can be used instead of CO_2 to maintain the pH of some cultures. (4) *Coulter counter* (also known as a cell counter). Electronically counts cells or particles. **Alternatives:** A counting chamber can be used with a microscope to manually count cells. (5) *Gas cylinders.* Pressurized gases have many uses in the lab, such as CO_2 for incubators, or nitrogen for disrupting cells. Most gas cylinders in use have a regulator attached to the valve, which is used to close the tank and regulate the outward flow of gas. The tank should always be roped or chained to a wall when standing and should be manipulated carefully when being moved. There is a danger of explosion or fire with oxygen and hydrogen, and you should get instruction from the EHS about the use of these gases. Valves open by turning counterclockwise. (6) *Liquid nitrogen tank.* A metal container filled with liquid nitrogen, it is used for the long-term storage of cells, viruses, and microorganisms. (7) *Microscope.* Used to magnify and observe tissues, cells, and microorganisms; there are two designs found in the lab. A standard compound microscope is used to observe samples that have been removed from culture medium and placed on a slide. An inverted microscope (the objective lens is situated below, not above, the sample) can magnify cells and organisms while they are still in the culture container. Microscopes often have attachments for fluorescence, and a camera. (8) *Pipet aids.* Liquids (volumes over 1 ml) are measured and transferred with pipets. Since no mouth pipetting is allowed, pipet aids such as automatic pipettors or bulbs are used to provide controlled suction. (9) *Water bath.* Used to thaw serum and do enzyme reactions. The contents of test tubes will reach the desired temperature much more quickly in water than in the air of an incubator. **Alternatives:** An insulated ice bucket filled with water at a moderate temperature will maintain a stable temperature for a while.

A water source and sink area are needed in every lab, and some equipment will be placed with access to the sink in mind. Large equipment, such as the fume hood, will be placed wherever there is space, often squeezing into seemingly impossible places.

Many labs are organized into **functional working areas**, and each area may then have its own set of rules. Often there may be a **tissue culture area**, where only cell culture work is done, and where bacterial or yeast work is passionately prohibited. The biosafety cabinet is the center of such a workspace. In such an area, you might

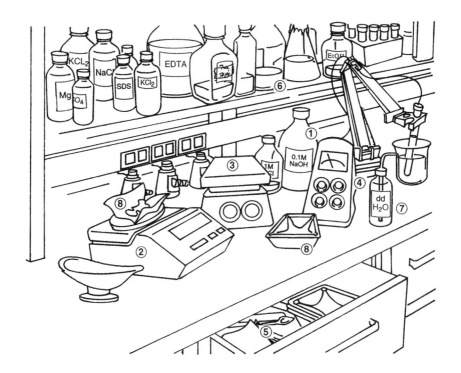

FIGURE 4.

pH and weighing area. **Key:** (1) *Acids and bases.* Concentrated and dilute acids and bases are used to adjust the pH of solutions. (2) *Balance.* A scale used for weighing. There are several kinds, with the top-loading balance being the most useful for weighing lab amounts of solids (and liquids). A two-pan balance is usually used to weigh tubes for centrifugation, and an analytical balance is used for accurately weighing small amounts, usually under a gram. (3) *Hot plate stirrer.* When making solutions, a little bit of heat with mixing is needed to get some materials into solution. **Alternatives:** Hot plate with occasional hand stirring. (4) *pH meter.* Used to measure and adjust the H^+ concentration in a solution. **Alternatives:** pH paper, acid and base addition determined by calculation, but no practical alternative. (5) *Spatulas, scoopulas.* Metal or plastic instruments used to transfer solids from a container to a weighing vessel. These are usually stored in a drawer with weigh boats and stir bars. (6) *Stock reagents.* Supplies of chemicals to be used to make up solutions are kept near the prep area for convenience. (7) *Wash bottle.* A plastic bottle with a spout that delivers distilled water to wash the electrode of the pH unit. (8) *Weigh boats, weigh paper.* Solids must be placed on a support, such as weigh boats and weigh paper, before being placed on the balance to be weighed.

also find an inverted and an upright microscope, CO_2 incubators, a slow-speed centrifuge and microfuge, a refrigerator, and storage for centrifuge tubes, pipets, and tissue culture flasks and plates.

Most laboratories have an **area for preparing reagents.** Here are found the supplies and equipment to weigh chemicals and pH solutions for the buffers needed for experiments.

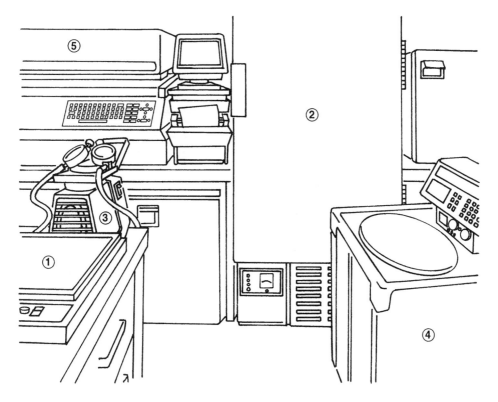

FIGURE 5.

Equipment room. **Key:** (1) *Gel dryer.* After electrophoresis, gels are dried under vacuum to enable autoradiography. **Alternative:** Drying film or vacuum alone. (2) *Low-temperature (usually –70°C) freezer.* The freezer can be upright or horizontal. Used to store bacterial stocks, reagents, samples. **Hazards:** Cold burn. Use at least latex gloves when manipulating samples from a –70°C freezer. *Never walk away from an alarm* on a freezer, as a meltdown could not only destroy years of work, but could also become a biohazard. **Alternatives:** Liquid nitrogen for cell and bacterial cultures. (3) *Pump.* The vacuum pump is the most commonly found pump in the lab, and is used to drive equipment such as lyophilizers and gel dryers. **Remarks:** Oil-requiring pumps must be tended carefully, especially to avoid uptake of fluid into the pump. To prevent volatile substances from a reaction or distillation from getting into the pump and then the lab atmosphere, a cold trap (filled with liquid nitrogen or dry ice) may be installed between the equipment and the pump. Newer pumps don't require oil. (4) *Ultracentrifuge.* A centrifuge that can achieve speeds of over 100,000 rpm; used to separate or pellet small molecules such as viruses and organelles. Since such high speeds are attained, this centrifuge must be used with caution to avoid accidents. (5) *Scintillation counter.* Beta radiation in samples is quantitated. Isotopes commonly counted are ^{3}H, ^{32}P, and ^{14}C.

Other functional working units often found are for **microscopy, electrophoresis, radioactivity, bacterial culture,** or **medium and plate preparation.**

Other Rooms and Places

The lab extends beyond the doors of the main lab or labs. An **equipment room** for centrifuges and other large equipment such as freezers and scintillation counters is usually located quite near the laboratory. The room may be dedicated to one type of

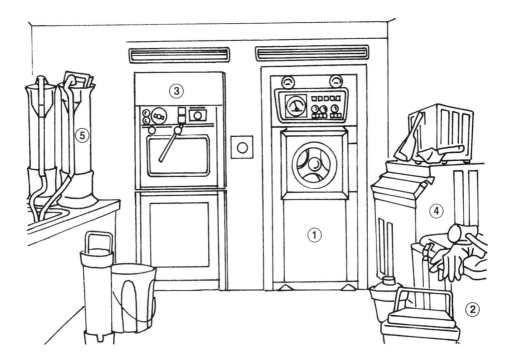

FIGURE 6.

The kitchen. **Key:** (1) *Autoclave.* Sterilizes by subjecting material to saturated steam under pressure. It is used to render glassware, media, and buffers sterile before use, as well as to sterilize biohazard waste before disposal. **Hazards:** *Scalding.* Wait until all steam has been released from the chamber before taking anything out or looking into the autoclave. **Alternatives:** Liquids can be filter-sterilized. Glass and plastic ware can be radiation-treated, but few places have this capability. (2) *Dry ice storage chest.* Dry ice is delivered once or twice a week and is kept in a chest where pieces can be broken off as needed. A mallet and gloves should be beside the chest: Always use the gloves to transfer pieces of dry ice. (3) *Glassware washer.* Washes and dries lab glassware. (4) *Ice maker.* Ice is made constantly as the level of ice goes down. Remove the ice with a scoop, not with your ice bucket. Never eat this ice! People might use ice buckets or other contaminated labware to remove it, and there could easily be hazardous substances in the ice. (5) *Pipet washer.* Water is circulated to wash reusable glass pipets. The pipets may be plugged with cotton and loaded onto canisters at a station in the kitchen.

equipment, such as centrifuges, but most institutions (and particularly, older institutions) have a medley of machines in the equipment room. In some places, safety laws allow big equipment such as freezers to be kept in the hallways. Some of the equipment, such as gel dryers and scintillation counters, handle radioactive samples. Always wear gloves in the equipment room.

The **autoclave** is usually found in a separate room, a room sometimes known as the kitchen. Here may be a glassware washer, a glass-baking machine, storage for glassware, and perhaps an area for medium and plate preparation.

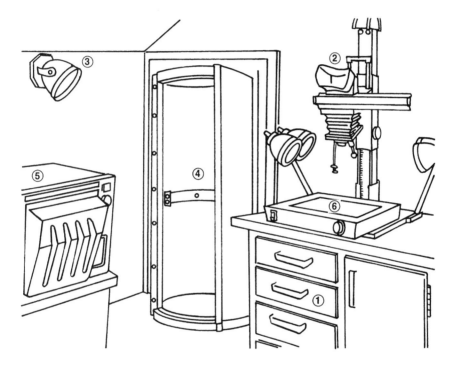

FIGURE 7.

The darkroom. **Key:** (1) *Drawers.* X-ray and Polaroid film are stored in the drawers. Even though the X-ray film is packaged, do not open the drawers unless the room is dark or is lit only by a safelight. (2) *Polaroid camera.* Polaroid film allows one picture at a time to be taken and developed immediately. The most common use is documenting gels whose bands have been stained with ethidium bromide and are seen on a light box. **Alternatives:** Digital imaging systems. (3) *Safelight.* A red light that does not expose film but provides enough light to see by. It is usually operated by a switch as you enter the darkroom. Be sure you know which switch is for the safelight, and which is for the regular light. (4) *Revolving door.* This round door permits entry and exit without allowing light into the room. Step into the opening and slowly push the door around until you come to the entrance or exit. Be sure no one is in the darkroom before you turn on the light. (5) *X-OMAT.* Develops X-ray film used for autoradiograms. **Alternatives:** Manual development of the exposed film. The phosphorimager can be used to document radioactivity without exposure to film. (6) *UV transilluminator or light box.* Ethidium bromide-stained nucleic acid can be visualized; bands on gels can be manipulated. **Hazards:** Eyes and skin can be burned. Always wear glasses or goggles, unless the light box is shielded. Use a shield if you will be manipulating the gel, as your face can easily get burned. When cutting out bands, the wrist area between gloves and lab coat is particularly vulnerable to a burn. **Alternatives:** A handheld UV light.

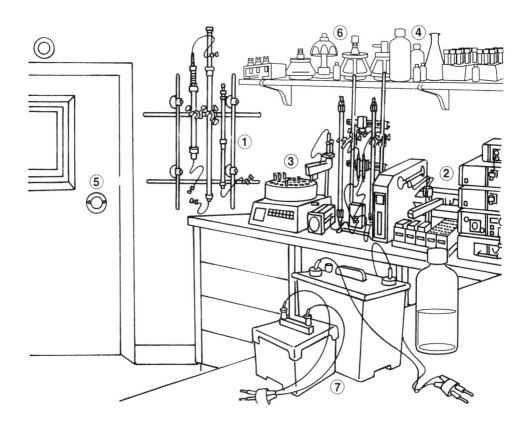

FIGURE 8.

Cold room. **Key:** (1) *Columns.* Contain the solid matrix used for chromatography. They may be smaller than a finger, or almost as tall as the cold room itself. (2) *FPLC.* Automated and pressurized chromatography: High performance liquid chromatography (HPLC) and fast pressure liquid chromatography (FPLC) are used for the separation and analysis of molecules and compounds. Columns, which are the soul of the system and must be carefully tended before, during, and after use, are available for dozens of specific applications. Pump, detector, autosampler, injector, and computer facilitate sample handling and analysis. **Remarks:** The HPLC is kept at room temperature, and the FPLC is usually found in a cold room or a chromatography refrigerator. **Alternatives:** Gravity chromatography with a fraction collector is an alternative for some applications. (3) *Fraction collector.* The fraction collector allows the sequential sampling of the fluid emerging from a column. As the effluent drips from a column, the drops are collected at a preset volume/time into a tube: When that volume has been collected, the old tube is moved and replaced by an empty tube. **Alternatives:** Manual collection. (4) *Prepared media.* Media for cells or bacteria can be purchased ready-made, and must usually be stored cold. Some buffers and reagents are also kept in the cold room. (5) *Release knob for door.* When someone is working inside the cold room, the door should be pulled *almost* closed to maintain the temperature. To open the door, hit the button or switch hard with the palm of your hand or the side of your fisted hand. (6) *Rotors.* Used to hold tubes in a centrifuge. Rotors are often kept in a cold room, to keep the samples cool before the run is begun. (7) *Transfer chambers.* DNA, RNA, or protein can be transferred electrophoretically from a gel to a membrane. During this high amperage transfer, the transfer buffer can heat considerably, and the entire process is often performed in the cold room to reduce the heat. **Alternatives:** Dry or semi-dry transfer apparatuses.

Much of the recording of data is done on film, making access to a **darkroom** indispensable. Darkrooms have a multitude of uses. Of course, they are used to develop and print film, but that may be the least of the uses in a time when most labs send their film out for processing. Instead, the main use of darkrooms is to provide a safe and dark haven for autoradiography and chemiluminescent film loading. A reddish safelight (Make sure you know which light is the safelight, since regular light will ruin the film!) gives enough light that one can take film in and out of boxes and cassettes without risking unwanted film exposure. Some labs keep fluorescent microscopes in the room, even though total darkness is not absolutely required.

Cold rooms are walk-in refrigerators, and are kept at approximately 4°C. Cold rooms are for both working and storage: Many of the shelves will hold plates, film, old bacterial cultures, and bottles of serum, but much of the space will be given over to microfuges, gel boxes, and transfer units, for procedures that sometimes must be performed in the cold. Don't worry if the door closes, there is always a release knob on the inside of the cold room and the warm room.

Warm rooms are kept at 37°C, or at the temperature of the organism that the lab works on. They physically resemble cold rooms, but contain equipment designed to enhance growth and reactions. They are filled with shakers and rollers for aerating growing bacteria, shelves for stacking plates of semi-solid media, and perhaps roller bottle setups for growing hybridomas and other cell lines.

Some departments cluster desks together in a room, called a **desk bay**, instead of scattering them throughout the working lab. Typically, graduate students—and especially, rotation students—and postdocs are given desks here. General use computers might be found and a microwave used for food only. Desk bays are supposed to be working places but tend to be quite social, and deskmates need to be adaptable but considerate of each other.

The **departmental or unit library** has the current and back issues of especially relevant publications, as well as background and how-to books. The library may double as a conference room, and it may also be the only room in the department in which you can make or drink coffee. The photocopy machine is likely to be here.

The coffeepot can be the most controversial piece of equipment in a lab! Find out and follow the rules, which are often extensive and cover perennially touchy topics such as payment, materials replacement, and cleanup. Basically, make a new pot when you have finished the old, clean up after yourself, and don't leave the pot on all night.

Other Equipment

Much of bench work consists of taking a substance or organism, changing it by heating, mixing, and disruption, or adding chemicals, and analyzing the change in the original material. All the changes that are experimentally induced must be quantitated: A signal—often, the signal is light—is measured and transformed into a number.

The machines that quantitate are usually the most complex equipment in the lab. Most of the equipment you see is for specialized variations of measuring and mixing. Equipment will not be grouped as shown in the following figures: It will be scattered throughout the lab and department.

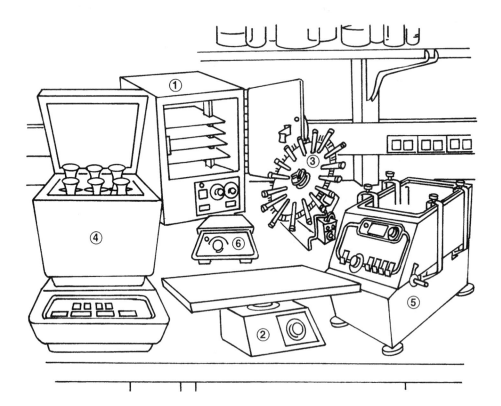

FIGURE 9.

Things that mix and shake. **Key:** (1) *Incubator shaker.* Used for hybridizations of transfer membranes; accommodates trays and has adjustable speed and strokes. (2) *Nutator.* A motorized platform that twists for gentle mixing. Good for microtiter plates. (3) *Roller wheel.* A rotating wheel that is especially good for bacterial cultures. (4) *Shaking incubator.* Used primarily for growing bacteria, shaking incubators agitate the flasks as well as maintain the set temperature. **Alternatives:** A shaker in a warm room. (5) *Shaking water bath.* Usually used for hybridizations, can also be used for microorganisms. Temperature and shaking speed can be controlled. (6) *Stir plate.* These plates can be hot plates only, magnetic stir plates only, or, more often, a plate that can be used as a hot plate and a magnetic stirrer. They are used to boil liquids and mix liquids; the mostly likely place to find one is next to the pH meter.

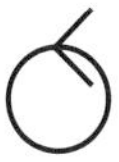

Vibrating. For vigorous mixing of small vessels such as test tubes or microtiter plates.

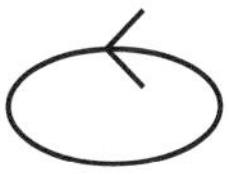

Orbital. Swirling action needed for cultivation of microorganisms and cell and tissue cultures.

Reciprocal. Back and forth motion of vigorous mixing of flasks and separatory funnels in chemical applications.

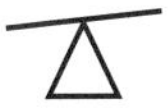

Rocking. Gentle up and down motion for cultivating cell cultures and staining/destaining gels.

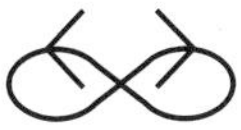

Wave. Three-dimensional motion is ideal for mixing round culture plates, preparing slides and electrophoresis gels.

FIGURE 9B.

Motions of shakers and incubators. Some motions are better than others for particular applications, but most equipment can be adapted to suit your need.

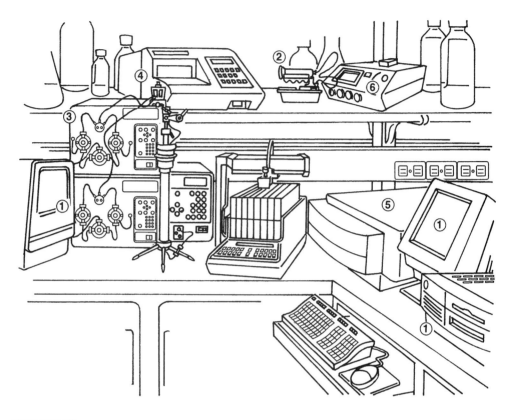

FIGURE 10.

Things that quantitate. **Key:** (1) *Computer.* Computers are part of most kinds of new quantitative equipment and allow fine-tuning of the experiment and thorough analysis of the data. They are indispensable for manuscript generation, data management and storage, and electronic communication. (2) *Geiger counter (ionization chamber).* **Hazards:** Make sure the probe is clean (not radioactive), or the dial may frighten you into thinking you and everything else are contaminated when the counter itself is. **Remarks:** There is a sensitivity dial, which, if turned high, may give such high apparent readings that it appears to be the China Syndrome all over. **Alternatives:** Although a gamma or beta counter can read a wipe test, there is no practical alternative for monitoring a working area on the spot. (3) *HPLC.* Automated and pressurized chromatography: High performance liquid chromatography (HPLC) is used for the separation and analysis of molecules and compounds. Columns, which are the soul of the system and must be carefully tended before, during, and after use, are available for dozens of specific applications. Pump, detector, autosampler, injector, and computer facilitate sample handling and analysis. The HPLC is kept at room temperature, whereas the FPLC is usually found in a cold room or a chromatography refrigerator. **Alternatives:** Gravity chromatography. (4) *Microplate reader, or plate reader.* Basically a spectrophotometer that can test the light emitted through or from samples on plates (usually 96-well plates), and is used for colorimetric assays such as ELISA, cytotoxicity, cell proliferation, and protein determinations. Many have adapters for plates other than 96-well plates. **Alternatives:** Sample-by-sample reading in a spectrophotometer. (5) *Phosphorimager.* Autoradiography is performed by exposure of the radioactive gel, membrane, TLC plates, or tissues to a storage phosphor screen, inducing an image that is collected and digitized. This image is then quantitated and analyzed by computer. Exposure times are much less than for standard film autoradiography. A department may share a phosphorimager, but each lab or investigator usually purchases his own storage phosphor screen. **Alternatives:** X-ray film autoradiography. (6) *Spectrophotometer ("spec").* Measures the transmittance of light through solutions. Used for growth curves, determining the concentration of DNA and RNA, colorimetric assays. Spectrophotometers can vary drastically in size, shape, and complexity. Readings at visible light and UV light require different kinds of cuvets. **Alternatives:** Klett tubes and reader for bacterial cultures.

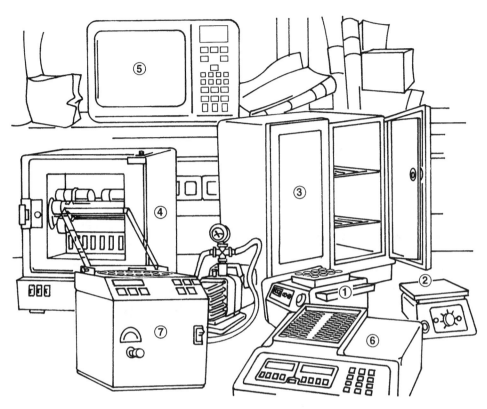

FIGURE 11.

Things that maintain or change temperature. **Key:** (1) *Dry bath.* Samples (tubes) in metal heating blocks, in modules, can be heated to over 100°C. (2) *Hot plate.* Used to heat small volumes of liquids. (3) *Incubator.* Maintains a chosen temperature. Incubators are used for cell and bacterial culture, and may be hooked up to a gas supply. Other incubators are used for sample preparation, such as filter hybridizations. Most incubators are dedicated to a certain temperature. Never change the temperature setting on a laboratory incubator without consulting the other personnel, or leaving a note, if that is the custom. **Alternatives:** Warm room. (4) *Hybridizer incubator.* A set temperature is maintained, and large tubes are rotated to gently agitate samples, usually filters for colony lifts, Northerns, Southerns, and Westerns. **Remarks:** Be sure the tubes have been cleaned before use. **Alternatives:** Filters can be placed in dishes and rocked in a shaking incubator or water bath. (5) *Microwave.* Melting agarose used for pouring electrophoresis gels is the main use of the microwave in the lab. **Hazards:** Agarose gel solutions often contain ethidium bromide, a mutagen. Always use gloves when manipulating objects in the microwave. Never cap bottles tightly, as they can explode. Never use a lab microwave for heating food! **Remarks:** Many eccentric uses, such as lysing cells, drying membranes, and fixing bacteria to membranes. **Alternatives:** Agarose solutions can be melted with a heating plate. (6) *Temperature cycler.* An automated heating block used for the rapid temperature changes of the polymerase chain reaction (PCR). Some models change temperatures, some physically move the sample to a new heating area with a robotic arm. **Hazards:** PCR machines have a high "melting" temperature, which could burn a hand. **Remarks:** Contamination is a major problem, so avoid all pipetting or sample preparation anywhere near the machine. **Alternatives:** None. It is a fancy heating block, but can achieve rapid changes of temperature that an ordinary heating block can't come close to. (7) *Vacuum dryer (speedy vac).* By centrifugation under a vacuum, water or other solvents are removed from a sample. Typical samples are post-ethanol nucleic acid pellets. **Alternatives:** House or simple pump vacuum on a chamber, large unit which may also be used for drying gels and lyophilizing large quantities of material.

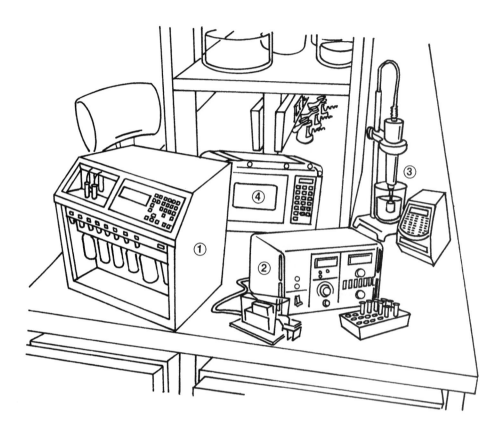

FIGURE 12.

Things that change things. **Key:** (1) *DNA synthesizer.* Oligonucleotides for sequencing and mutagenesis may be made for a lab or department, usually with a dedicated person to run the machine. **Alternatives:** Ready-made nucleotides can be ordered from many companies. **Hazards:** The solvents used are powerful, and empty bottles should be discarded with care. (2) *Electroporator:* The electroporator looks like a power supply and, basically, that is just what it is. Electroporation is a process of applying an electric field to a cell for a brief period of time, temporarily causing small openings to appear in cell membranes, through which molecules can be introduced into cells. Its main use is to transform bacteria and transfect eukaryotic cells with foreign DNA. **Hazards:** This is a high-voltage machine; do not use it without instructions. **Alternatives:** Several chemical and physical methods for transformation and transfections. (3) *Sonicator (also known as an ultrasonic processor).* Sonicators are used to disrupt and fragment biological substances by the emission of high-pitched and powerful sound waves. For example, they can be used to lyse cells or shear DNA. There are two basic types, bath or probe; probe sonicators are generally the most powerful. **Hazards:** Ear damage can result from probe sonicators, so always use with ear protection. **Remarks:** The smaller the tip diameter, the more concentrated the intensity. Keep the tip clean, or it will become damaged. **Alternatives:** Pushing material in and out of a small syringe is not as effective, but can work somewhat. Nitrogen cavitation bombs, detergents, chaotropic agents, and enzymes can be used to lyse cells. (4) *UV crosslinker.* Main use is to covalently bind nucleic acid to a membrane. Also can be used for mutagenesis and to eliminate PCR contamination. **Remarks:** Looks like a microwave. **Alternatives:** Membranes can be baked.

USING THE EQUIPMENT

Basic Rules

- **Get a demonstration of its use** from a lab member, even for a piece of equipment as mundane as the pH meter. At the very least, watch carefully while a lab member uses it, or ask if there are particular rules about that equipment. And *write down* the procedure! You may have been able to pH in your sleep with the pH meter in your old lab (which happens to be the same model as the one in your new lab), but you don't know whether this lab prefers to keep the electrode in buffer or water, whether people take turns making the acids and bases used for pH-ing, where the stir bars go when you are finished... details which, if missed, could drive other lab members quite mad.

- **Wash, return, clean up, turn off** appropriately each piece of equipment you use. Don't change settings. Don't force knobs or levers that don't want to move. Don't ignore alarms or flashing lights.

- **Don't order equipment without consulting with the head of the laboratory.** If your lab doesn't have a piece of equipment you need, he or she can suggest (or you can find) a lab which does have it and will let you use it.

- **Be extraordinarily cooperative when using equipment in another lab.** Check with people there to find the best time for them to demonstrate the use of the equipment and the most convenient time for you to use it.

- **For each piece of equipment in the lab (even the ones you are not using), you should know** (1) what it is, what it *does*; (2) who is in charge of it, whom to approach if there is a problem.

- **For each piece of equipment you use, you should also know** (1) *how* to operate it; (2) *where* the manual, instruction booklet, or protocol is kept. Either there is a central location for all instructions or manuals, or the manual will be in a drawer near the equipment. (3) Is it *turned off after use*, or left on all day? (4) Must it be warmed up before use? Not warming up a machine before use can lead to erratic readings and a decreased work life for equipment components. (5) Is there is a *sign-up sheet?* If there is a sign-up sheet, sign up every time, even if you only use the equipment for 5 minutes.

> *Don't use a piece of equipment without the instructions. If they have been lost, call the manufacturer to obtain another copy.*

- **Respond to all equipment alarms immediately**. Ignoring an alarm can have catastrophic consequences. An alarm on a shaking incubator might merely be a timer: Ignoring this might cause a bacterial culture to overgrow and ruin an experiment. Ignoring an alarm on a CO_2 incubator might allow the complete deple-tion of CO_2, and all the cells in the incubator might die as the pH rises. But the worst-case scenario might be what happens to the whole lab if the alarm on a −70ºC freezer or liquid nitrogen tank is ignored. An alarm on a freezer usually indicates a rising temperature, one on a liquid nitrogen tank a lowering of the liq-uid N_2 level: Eventually, the contents of the freezer or tank would be thawed and the lab's entire stocks of cell lines, viruses, and recombinant bacteria would be ruined. Years of work can be lost.

You must THINK about the equipment you use. The equipment is an important part of your experiments, and its misuse will affect your data in a sometimes unobvious way. Without some thought about the function of the equipment you are using, you won't have a clue why an alarm is suddenly buzzing, or how to know when the bulb has burned out. Some of the most common problems that a moment of thought can help include:

O.D. readings are zero on the spectrophotometer. The bulb may not have been turned on, something that often has to be done in addition to turning on the machine. You may not have chosen the right wavelength. You may have inappropriate cuvettes (not all cuvettes transmit all wavelengths of light). You may have put the cuvette in the wrong sample holder.

The medium covering the cells in the CO_2 incubator has become purplish, indicating that the pH has increased drastically. The CO_2 might have run out. The pan providing humidity may be empty (where did you think the humidity came from?), and with-out humidity, the CO_2 readings may be aberrant.

You cannot see any light on a Gram-stained slide of a sample taken from a patient's wound. The light source may have blown, or the diaphragm controlling the light may be turned down. The potentiometer controlling the light intensity may also be turned down. The objective lens may be turned so that no light is transmitted to the eyepiece. A camera may be attached, and the light set to be transmitted to the camera and not to the eyepiece.

What to Do if You Hear an Alarm

1. **Identify the source of the alarm.** Do this even if you must go into another depart-ment or lab. Don't turn it off until you know that it will be dealt with.

2. **Notify** the person in charge of the piece of equipment. Ask around the lab, or consult a list (if there is one that lists lab responsibilities) to find out. If the responsible person is home, call, even if it is 3 A.M. Once the person has been found, you can relax: Just stand by in case your help is needed.

3. If you can't find the person in charge, **find someone who knows more than you.** Believe it or not, this may not be possible! But try.

4. **If you are left to deal with the alarm:**

    *   First, decide whether there is a *safety* issue. An example of this would be any equipment breakdown that has resulted in a spill of radioactivity. Call the EHS and the Laboratory Safety officer. Another example would be an obviously off-balance ultracentrifuge, for which you should call Laboratory Safety. Do not attempt to deal with a dangerous piece of equipment yourself.

    *   Decide whether there is a *lab emergency.* An example of this would be a rising temperature on a –70ºC freezer, which could destroy the research of an entire department. It is not likely that you can deal with this alone. Call the Laboratory Safety officer, and, if you can't reach him/her, call Laboratory Safety.

        > *Unless you are immediately checking out the situation, leave temperature and atmosphere manipulating devices closed. This will keep the temperature or gas mixture stable for hours, perhaps overnight.*

    *   See whether there is an *experimental emergency.* Will someone's results be ruined? Examine the material involved to find the name of the researcher and call if you can identify the owner. If not, check the experiment to decide where to place any experimental material (see Chapter 8, Storage and Disposal). The equipment can be dealt with later.

    *   If there is no crisis, turn off the alarm, place a note on the equipment so no one counts on it for an experiment, and leave a message for the responsible person.

HOW TO BUY NEW EQUIPMENT

1. **Decide carefully if you need the equipment.** Can you use equipment you already have? Can you borrow it long-term? Will it be used a lot, or will it only be used for one set of experiments? Even if money is not a factor, equipment should never be purchased on a whim.

2. **Check out the options of style and manufacturer.**

    *   Go to a comprehensive directory of suppliers of medical equipment, such as BioSupplyNet, and comparison shop.

    *   Call colleagues to see whether they have used a particular model and can recommend it.

- Browse among the vendors at meetings to see what is available. But unless you have already researched the topic, don't buy yet, even if you are offered (as is the custom at meetings) a sizable discount.

- Post a question about the equipment on an on-line bulletin board.

- Ask the companies for the names and phone numbers of people who have purchased the equipment. Call a few to see if they have been satisfied with their purchase.

3. **Decide which of two or three models you like.** Ask the finalist for a demonstration or trial use of the equipment. Try to use the same conditions you will use for your experiments. Find out how much technical support and advice each company will offer.

4. **Go into final arrangements with your top choices.** Find out what will come with the machine, what you can arrange to have added. Some companies will agree to free software, lessons, supplies, or maintenance contracts to induce you to buy their product. Don't be shy about negotiating the best deal. If price is no object, you probably needn't bother with this.

5. **Purchase the equipment on trial,** if possible. Your purchasing department will handle this.

6. **Try the equipment out, and stay closely in touch with the company.** Ask questions and use their expertise; it should be one reason you chose that particular piece of equipment. Some companies will even provide protocols, and all should troubleshoot with you over the phone.

RESOURCES

Biochemical Resources
    Phone: (517) 381-8269
    http://biores.com (This web site is a database of chemicals, biochemicals, laboratory products, and services that can be searched.)
BioSupplyNet Source Book, BioSupplyNet, Inc., 10 Skyline Drive, Plainview, New York 11803.
    Phone: (516) 349-5595
    Fax: (516) 349-5598
    http://www.biosupplynet.com (The BioSupplyNet Source Book is a comprehensive directory of biomedical research supplies and equipment. The web site allows you to search by key words for product names or categories.)
Chen T. 1997. Glossary of microbiology.
    http://www.hardlink.com/~tsute/glossary/index.html/
Lackie, J.M. and Dow J.A.T., eds. 1995. *The dictionary of cell biology,* 2nd edition. Academic Press, London. Also available in interactive form at:
    http://www.mblab.glac.ac.uk/~Julian/Dict.html/
SciQuest, Research Triangle Park, North Carolina 27709-2156
    Phone: (919) 786-1770
    Fax: (919) 782-3128
    http://www.sciquest.com/catalyst/welcome.cgi (This web site also allows searches by key words, and automatic requests of chosen vendors.)
UW GenChem Pages, University of Wisconsin-Madison, Department of Chemistry:
    http://genchem.chem.wisc.edu/labdocs/labdrwr/labequip.htm/
UW GenChem Pages Dictionary, University of Wisconsin-Madison, Department of Chemistry: http://genchem.chem.wisc.edu/labdocs/mainmenu.htm/

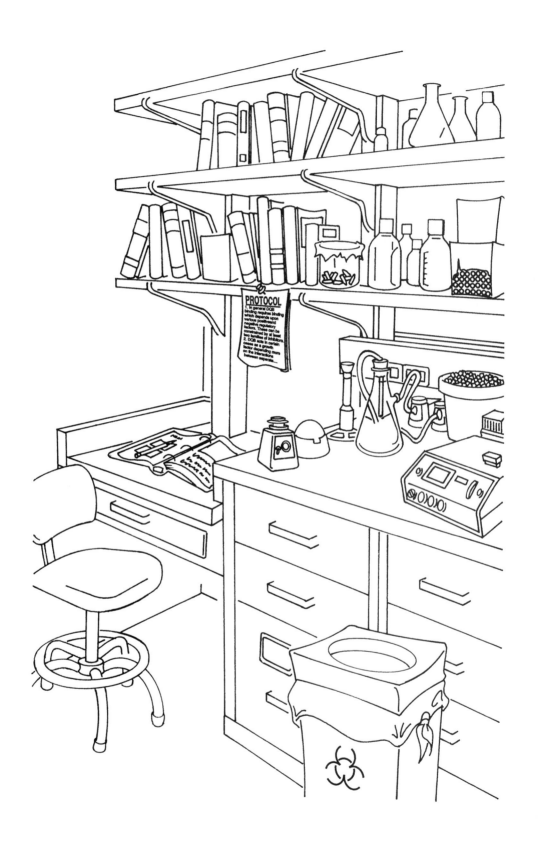

PROTOCOL

1. In general DQB
binding requires binding
which depends upon
various positive and
negative regulatory
factors. These can be
constituted by at least
two families of inhibition
2. DQB acts in certain
cases as a growth
factor depending more
on the interaction
between separate...

3

Getting Started and Staying Organized

YOUR LAB BENCH is your home, your real estate, and its setup and maintenance are integral to the reproducibility of your experiments. Whatever your personal sense of style, try to rein it in and keep your lab bench neat. Ignore the machismo that reigns in many labs, the sense that a Real Scientist doesn't worry about cleaning up junk, and stay organized. At the very least, remove the debris of one experiment before you start another.

SETTING UP A FUNCTIONAL LAB BENCH	44
How to order supplies and reagents	45
Lab bench needs	48
Pipettors, pipets, and pipet aids	51
SETTING UP A COMMAND CENTER	57
The desk	57
Dealing with papers and other stuff	58
Using the computer	61
Basic rules for computer use	64
RESOURCES	65

What will be done on the bench? Will you only prepare samples for gel analysis at your bench, or will you also run the gel —that is, is there a common place in the lab for electrophoresis that you can use? Try to use the common areas as much as possible, and keep your bench space as free as possible: Resist the temptation to do everything on your bench, as it will tend to get fairly messy.

Organization is key. It is no longer possible to incorporate the sheer volume of scientific information available: One can only hope to know how and when to access what you need. Without a system for maintaining references, data, computer files, and journal articles, you will be hopelessly mired in paperwork within weeks. Keeping control of information is as important as IQ in the lab.

SETTING UP A FUNCTIONAL LAB BENCH

To feel as if you have really moved in, set up your lab bench so you can start experiments as soon as possible. It will probably take longer than a week to know exactly what you will be working on and to pinpoint the specific reagents you will need, but there are standard supplies and reagents that everyone needs, and you should set yourself up to do an experiment as soon as possible.

1. **Briefly assess your needs.** Look around the lab, think a bit about the kind of work that goes on, and make a tentative (and perhaps, mental) list of what you think your bench should have.

   > *Don't use opened boxes or bags of supplies. If you find opened pipet tips, pipets, or tubes, use only what can be autoclaved to guarantee cleanliness and sterility.*

2. **Find out what is available at the bench.** Often when you move into a lab bench, you will inherit the equipment that the previous bench user had. Check it out. If it works, use it: Later on, if it is inadequate, you can replace it. Even if it is not exactly what you are used to—for example, people tend to be particular about their pipet aids—give the old one a try.

3. **Get rid of what you don't need.** You need to maximize whatever space you have. After you have gone through the drawers and shelves, get rid of things you won't use. Either ask other lab members if they want it, or put it on a cart for a week with a sign that everyone can take what they want, and then discard what is left after a week.

   > *Immediately dump all buffers you may have found on your shelf. It may be tempting to cut down on your work by using that Tris buffer, but you don't really know if the buffer is okay.*

4. **Clean.** You won't have a chance ever again to have things as clean as possible. Wipe down the shelves and the lab bench with a mild soap mixture. Rinse well.

While you are setting up, and even more so during your experiments, you will create a lot of debris that you will want to get rid of. *Do not throw anything away until the particular laboratory rules for waste disposal have been explained to you.* A lab can be shut down by the Laboratory Safety Department for infractions of the disposal rules.

Chapter 8 gives the particulars of waste disposal, but you should be aware that the following kinds of trash will each have their own method and place of disposal:

Paper, recycled and waste
Biological waste
Radioactive waste
Broken glass
Syringes, needles, pasteur pipets
Chemical waste
Hazardous chemical waste

Use gloves as you are working, since there may be residual radioactivity or hazardous chemicals.

5. **Order what you need for routine lab work.** *Order conservatively.* (Most supplies and equipment needed to do experiments will be in the lab.) You can order as you go along, so order the minimum now. Ask for guidance from the person responsible for ordering (if there is such a person), or from a lab member. Find out what your budget is and, even if it is limitless, order only what you absolutely need. See below to find out how to order.

> *Don't order any major pieces of equipment unless you have discussed it with the P.I. Try to borrow any equipment you need.*

6. **Do an experiment as soon as possible and reassess your needs.** The setup and actual execution of even a small experiment will point out what you need, what you can borrow, what is wrong. Now order what you need to do a specific series of experiments.

> *Although you do want to be as prepared as possible for the first experiment, don't wait until you have everything. Do an experiment the first week, even if you have to borrow supplies.*

How to Order Supplies and Reagents

1. **Find out how to physically place an order.** The ordering procedure will be institute dependent, and your responsibility can range from merely reporting that something is needed, to calling to place the order yourself. Most places have an in-house store for the most commonly ordered items, and the ordering procedure may be different here than for outside orders. Most places have centralized ordering through a Purchasing Department, and that department is responsible for actually making the call and handling the paperwork for all of the lab personnel. It is also the responsibility of the Purchasing Department to find the best deal among the manufacturers on the item you request: If you need the item from a particular manufacturer, you should note this in the order.

> *Most standard supplies that you need for your initial experiments will be in stock in the lab.*

2. **Be sure the item isn't already in the lab or hasn't been already ordered.** Check behind boxes and bottles for a duplicate item. Ask the purchase person if someone else has ordered the item, or ask other lab personnel.

> *More and more institutions are switching to on-line ordering: if this is true for your workplace, you will probably need a password as well as an account number (which you need for all orders). This can take several days, so arrange it before you need an order.*

3. **If the item is standard in the lab, order the exact specifications and amount usually ordered.** For chemicals, the empty bottle itself is the best source of order information. For other items, consult with the person in charge of ordering, or with another lab member.

4. **If the item is new to the lab's repertoire, follow these steps:**

   - *Check with the person who gave you the protocol* or recipe for which the item is needed. The source of a reagent can be critical, especially if you are trying to replicate a result, and an investigator who has used the reagent can give the best advice for type and manufacturer, as well as storage advice.

     > *If there is a senior technician, do consult him or her about ordering and setting up: such a person is usually an exceedingly valuable resource.*

   - If the protocol has no recommendation for the source of a reagent, *ask someone who has done similar experiments to recommend a manufacturer.* You could also ask the purchasing department, or the person who does the ordering, for a suggestion for a manufacturer, and call the manufacturer. There are several *on-line services* that enable you to look up any item, compare prices and specifications, and request information from the manufacturer. Several of these are listed in the Resources, at the end of the chapter. You could also go to one of the many Biomedical Science bulletin boards on line, and pose a question about the item in question to people who might have used it. You could also ask *sales representatives* for help. Most, if you have a good rapport, will tell you fairly honestly about the appropriateness and limitations of a particular item. Just take all such information with a grain of salt.

     > *You must decide how you will deal with sales reps. Most researchers consider it to be a real pain to have to talk with one, and many institutions and companies will not let sales reps onto the floors to harass people. Yet a good sales rep can be infinitely helpful. Most are trained in one of the biological sciences, and they can help make decisions and cut costs. Sales reps have a tough time. Be courteous to all, but be selective when deciding with whom you will speak.*

   - *Buy the minimum amount.* The price per unit of a reagent often drops dramatically with an increase in the size of the order. But a reagent that will not be soon used can go bad, and becomes a very expensive venture. Resist the temptation to buy a whopping big bottle.

   - *Buy the highest quality you need and can afford*—with the emphasis on need. Some reagents come in grades of purity, with a higher price for the more pure reagent. But the most expensive grade isn't necessarily better, and may give different results. If the grade hasn't been specified, call the manufacturer and explain what you need.

- *Keep a record of what you ordered.* This will make it easier to reorder. It is also a good idea to record order numbers and lot numbers under the appropriate experiments in your research notebook.

5. Have the item shipped in the most inexpensive and safe manner. You may, for example, have a choice between a wet ice and dry ice shipment of enzymes. Take the minimum protection needed, according to the manufacturer's advice. Avoid "Rush" orders.

> *For example, bovine serum albumin (BSA) can be used (among other things) to block nonspecific protein binding to a filter, or to stabilize an enzyme reaction. For the latter use, in which any contaminants could inhibit the enzyme activity, the BSA must be much more pure.*

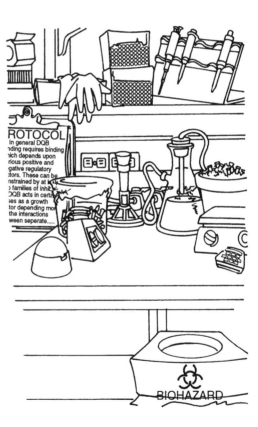

FIGURE 1.

The laboratory bench. The lab bench should have a central area of working space, surrounded by the equipment and supplies you need to set up and perform experiments.

Lab Bench Needs

Space

At least 2 feet should be totally clear lab space for active experiments. Don't store anything here, and clean up the remains of each experiment as it is completed to preserve this area.

> *You could also put down several layers of bench paper at one time, and just strip off the top layer when it is soiled.*

Some people cover the bench with either blue "diapers" or special bench paper which is absorbent on one side, plastic backed on the other side. If you do this, the absorbent side should be up. If you do cover the bench, the paper should be changed frequently, or the entire reason for putting the paper down is nullified.

If you are doing any *radioactive* work on the bench, you must cover the bench with plastic-backed paper. However, this should be done for *each* experiment and the paper should be removed after each experiment (to be disposed of in radioactive waste). Keeping the same paper on after an experiment defeats the whole point of putting it on.

Shelves

> *If the shelves divide a bench in two, be sure that you don't nudge a bottle off the shelf onto your backyard neighbor. Never store acids, bases, or other caustic reagents on the shelves.*

Personal room-temperature reagents are stored above the bench. One of the first things a newcomer to the lab needs to do is to make a supply of buffers needed to start doing experiments.

Reagents typically stored at the bench
10x PBS
Ethidium bromide, 5 mg/ml in water
10x Tris acetate EDTA (TAE) buffer
10x Tris borate EDTA (TBE) buffer
10 % SDS
20x SSC
1 M Tris, pH 7.0, pH 7.5, pH 8.0
0.5 M EDTA, pH 8.0
3.0 M Na acetate, pH 5.2
5 M NaCl
5 or 10 M NaOH
10x Laemmli running buffer

Refrigerated reagents you are likely to need
Chloroform/isoamyl alcohol
Phenol– water saturated
Phenol/chloroform/isoamyl alcohol
Sample buffers for RNA, DNA, and protein gels

See Chapter 7 for methods of buffer and reagent preparation and recipes for commonly needed reagents.

> *Most buffers should be autoclaved before storage at room temperature.*

Bench and drawers: Checklist

Aspirator. A device that uses suction (house vacuum or pump-generated) to remove fluids, usually supernatants.

Biohazard disposal bag. All disposable material in contact with living organisms must be disposed of as biohazard material (Chapter 6). A place next to your bench for a large can or holder for a biohazard disposal bag is essential. A smaller holder for a bag on your bench is not essential, but makes life easier and safer.

Hot plate stirrer. You can boil samples before running them on a gel, stir a hard-to-dissolve reagent to your heart's content, or strip a filter, all at home.

Ice bucket. This is usually a common laboratory item. But since the first thing you will do most mornings is to fill up your ice bucket, be sure you have one always available.

Lab coat. Just about every institution will provide you with one or several lab coats, and most will have them laundered for you. Some labs use only disposable paper coats. Lab coat use is required for certain jobs but you should wear one whenever you are doing lab work, for safety and to prolong the life of your jeans. You need a separate coat for radioactive work.

Latex gloves. Latex gloves come powdered or powder-free. Try several brands of gloves before you order, because many people are sensitive or actually allergic to certain kinds. Make sure you order the right size: Tight gloves hurt, loose gloves get caught in pipettors and make it difficult to manipulate fine items. Used gloves should be disposed of in the biohazard trash.

Microfuge. Okay, this might be more than you should expect. But if you had one, you would use it all the time. You could get a tiny 6-sample personal microfuge, but this doesn't spin fast enough for nucleic acid precipitations.

Microfuge tube racks. Three or four racks will enable you to carry on several manipulations at once. Store them in a drawer so that they don't get "lost."

Parafilm. This stretchy plastic will be used often to seal plates and tubes, so keep it on the bench. Either get a dispenser with a cutting edge, or keep a scissors or covered scalpel always close to the box.

Pasteur pipets, sterile, and bulbs. You can also use disposable transfer pipets. These are used for filling and balancing centrifuge tubes, removing supernatants, and any approximate movement of small volumes.

Pipettors: 0–20, 10–100, and 50–250 or a 10–200, 100–1000 µl. If you inherit a set, have them recalibrated. These can be kept neatly in a shallow drawer, but it is better to either purchase the appropriate rack, or rig up holders by attaching 50-ml plastic centrifuge tubes to the shelf.

Pipets. You need a few glass pipets for measuring solvents and other liquids. Keep the pipets in an autoclavable can or canister. Useful pipet sizes are 2, 10, and 25 ml. Especially if you are doing tissue culture work, most of your pipets will be disposable and sterile plastic ones. Buy individually packaged pipets if you will use them infrequently, the more inexpensive bulk packages if you need pipets often.

Pipet aids. Since there is no mouth pipetting allowed, you need a tool to provide suction. A bulb will work fine, but an automatic pipet aid is more dependable and is easier to use.

Sharpie marker. Keep only one on your bench at a time, with your name on a piece of tape around the barrel; otherwise, you'll never find one when you need it.

Squeeze bottles. One should contain distilled water, for filling balance tubes, etc., and one should contain 70% ethanol for disinfecting tubes, spills, and cleaning the bench. Label every squeeze bottle with its contents.

Sterile microfuge tubes in a covered beaker or another autoclavable container. Have at least two containers filled with the size microfuge tube you will most often be using. The 1.5–1.7-ml and 0.5-ml sizes are the most popular.

Sterile tips in boxes for pipet aid. Although you can purchase prepacked tip boxes, many labs fill them manually. Always have three or four boxes of each size. Not all tips fit all pipettors, so check with the manufacturer of the pipettor (or someone in the lab) for the appropriate tips.

Tape for labeling. If you have plenty of bench space, set up a multiple tape dispenser on your bench so you have easy access to colored or white tape (for labeling reagent bottles), scotch tape (for protecting writing on microfuge tubes), autoclave tape (to put on *everything* you autoclave) and Biohazard and Radioactive label tape. If space is limited, keep a single roll of tape in a dispenser in a drawer.

Timer. Whether you are staining slides for 1 minute, or doing a 2-hour enzyme digestion, you should set a timer. Choose one that has multiple channels, so you can time two or three different procedures at once. Many timers have a magnet on the back, so they can attach to metal shelves, or a clip to allow them to be worn on your lab coat.

Tips/sharps disposal box. Pipet tips and pasteur pipets can pierce plastic bags and should be collected separately in another container. You could use a syringe and needle disposal box for all your sharps, or use a small bag in a holder or beaker to collect them. Check with Laboratory Safety to find out what they recommend (and, perhaps, dispense) for needles and syringes and for other sharps.

Vortex. Usually comes with the bench. An adapter for multiple tubes is available for many models and is very useful.

Pipets, Pipettors, and Pipet Aids

Pipettors

There are dozens of pipettors, so you can find one exactly suited to your particular need. Some have one button for picking up and dispensing samples, and for ejecting tips: Others have separate buttons for each function. Some can be calibrated in the lab, and others must be calibrated professionally. Many can be autoclaved and are ideal for pathogenic organisms.

In addition to the specificity offered through the range of pipettors, flexibility is also given through the wide choice of available tips. Tip extenders allow pipettors to be used in tissue culture, giving the sterile tip access into flasks and jars. Long, flattened tips are made for loading sequencing gels. Other tips have filters that prevent carryover from one sample to another, and are excellent for PCR, infectious, and radioactive samples.

> *For most pipettors, the button must be pushed twice to release the contents of the tips. Push until you meet resistance, and then gently push again. This final push expels the last bit of volume, along with some air, and must be done as gently as possible to avoid creating aerosols.*

Adjustable volume pipettor. Good benchtop pipettors, ideal for a variety of pipetting tasks.

Electronic pipettor. Can be programmed to dispense a set of volumes, and to do dilutions.

Fixed volume pipettor. Fixed pipettors are good as dedicated instruments for particular assays, where the same volume must always be dispensed.

Multichannel pipettor. Constructed to dispense several samples at the same time. They are usually built and used for microplates, with 4, 8, or 12 dispensing outlets. They may be fixed, variable, or repeater dispensers.

Positive displacement pipettor. With a positive displacement mechanism, air space between liquid and plunger is eliminated. These pipettors are extremely accurate, as sample volumes are unaffected by surface tension, viscosity, vapor pressure, or density. Especially coupled with filtered tips, positive displacement pipettors are ideal for PCR, radioactive, and biohazard samples, because there is no aerosol production or sample carryover.

Repeater pipettor. For repetitive dispensing. Dispenses multiple samples without refilling, from an attached reservoir. The reservoir may be an attached syringe or bottle, or may pump from any container through tubing attached to the pipettor. It can be a single-channel or multichannel pipet and may dispense fixed or adjustable volumes.

Pipets

Capillary pipets (also known as micropipets). Small glass tubes that load microliter volumes by capillary action or with bulb suction. Use for samples for thin-layer chromatography, PCR, or electrophoresis.

Measuring pipets. Similar in style and usage to serological pipets, but with a smaller tip opening.

Pasteur pipet. Glass, different kinds and lengths of tips. Good for filling balancing tubes for centrifugation, removing and transferring liquids. Can be plugged with cotton. Often used by being attached to tubing for vacuum aspiration.

Serological pipets. These are your standard, everyday pipets. For most purposes, they are identical to measuring pipets. Glass or plastic, reusable or disposable, plugged or unplugged, single-wrapped, bulk-wrapped, or package-your-own—there are many sizes and options. Glass pipets are needed for organic solvents, and sterile, usually plastic, pipets for tissue culture. Each lab has its own system of choosing and dealing with pipets. Most pipets are made to deliver (marked T.D., to deliver, on the top of the pipet; also marked by double rings) the chosen volume when the fluid is released entirely from the pipet. Other pipets (marked T.C., to contain) are made to release the chosen volume only when the fluid is released to a measured point.

Transfer pipet. Plastic, disposable. With built in pipet bulb. Ideal for filling balancing tubes for centrifugation, or for transferring cells or substances that might stick to glass.

Volumetric pipet. Calibrated to deliver one specified volume. It is not particularly useful in most labs.

Pipet Aids

Pipet aids provide manual suction and are used for ordinary pipets, glass or plastic. They are also used with pasteur pipets, but working with short pipets such as pasteurs may result in fluid uptake into the pipet aid.

Bulb, or pipet filler. Bulbs are chemically resistant, and are a low-tech and useful supply to have around a hood. To pipet, first expel air by squeezing valve "1" (or "A," for aspirate) above the bulb. Then draw liquid up by pressing valve "2" (or "S," for suction) on the stem. To release, press valve "3" ("E," for exhaust) on the side of the stem.

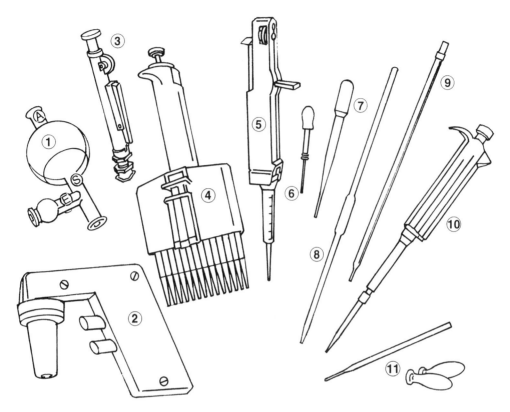

FIGURE 2.

Dozens of pipets, pipettors, and pipet aids are available for benchwork. Only a few examples are shown here. **Key:** (1) *bulb (pipet filler)*, (2) *pipet-aid*, (3) *pipet pump*, (4) *multichannel pipettor*, (5) *repeater pipettor*, (6) *capillary pipet with bulb*, (7) *transfer pipet*, (8) *volumetric pipet*, (9) *measuring pipet*, (10) *fixed volume pipet*, (11) *pasteur pipet, bulb for pasteur pipet.*

Pipet-aid. Attaches to glass or plastic pipets of 1 to 100 ml, handles volumes of 0.1 ml to 100 ml. Filter in tissue culture nose provides protection of electronic components and prevents cross-contamination. Comes with attached power supply or with built-in portable rechargeable power supply.

Pipet pump. Manual, safe, and accurate one-handed pipeting done by rotation of the thumb wheel. For rapid release of the pipet's contents, press the plunger or the quick release bar available for many models.

 Setting up an aspirator. An aspirator is used for removing supernatants, something routinely done in most laboratories. You should have one dedicated for aqueous, nonradioactive material, and you will probably have to assemble it yourself.

You will need:

House vacuum or pump. House vacuum is preferable, since it doesn't require maintenance.

Two 1- or 2-liter filtration/vacuum flasks. To prevent liquids from being pulled up into a pump or house vacuum line, set up two flasks in tandem: The second flask will take any accidental or careless overflow from the first flask.

Vacuum tubing. Tygon vacuum tubing of I.D. (inner diameter) 1/4″ or 5/16″, O.D. (outer diameter) 1/2″ or 9/16″, and wall measurement 1/16″ or 1/8″.

Rubber stopper, with hole. At least 2 cm of stopper should stick out, so the stopper can easily be removed for frequent cleaning. There is a sizing chart in most catalogs. Stoppers can be purchased with or without a hole already present: Unless you really feel like boring a hole, purchase one already bored.

Most of the components for assembling an aspirator will be available either in the lab itself, or in the institutional store. If not, all of the materials can be purchased from one of the large catalog companies.

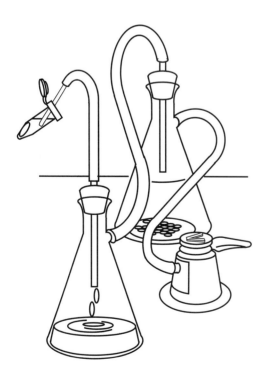

FIGURE 3.

Benchtop aspirator, connected to house vacuum line. (Reprinted, with permission, from Sambrook et al. 1989.)

Glass pipet or hollow glass rod to fit in stopper. Use a thick-walled hollow glass rod. Don't use pipets or pasteur pipets. Pipets are so long that you will not be able to fill the flask as high as you could with a shorter (6–8 inch) glass rod. Pasteur pipets are too short, and are so fragile that they could easily shatter during insertion into the stopper.

0.45-micron filter. In a biosafety cabinet flask setup, this is necessary to prevent aspiration of biohazard material into the vacuum line. If you plan to aspirate bacteria or cells, incorporate one into bench aspiration setup (see Chapter 8).

See "Bench maintenance" for upkeep advice and Chapter 9 for the use of an aspirator to remove supernatants.

 Bench maintenance

Daily
Make sure your "experimental space" is completely clear.
Wipe down the bench at the end of each day with a mild detergent or 70% ethanol, or change the bench paper if it is soiled.
Dump your ice and rinse out your ice bucket.

Weekly
Replenish microfuge tubes, tips.
Dump all biohazard waste.

As needed
Get a new sharps disposal box and deal with the old one as the department requests.

Aspirator
Clean the primary flask regularly, even if you use it infrequently: The fluid may evaporate and leave an impossible-to-clean residue. If you use the suction apparatus often, clean it daily. The method of cleaning will depend on the contents.

• Nonhazardous and nonbiological substances, such as buffers, can be dumped down the drain while the water is running. Rinse the flask several times.
• Biohazard fluid (yes, this includes supernatants from *E. coli*) must be disinfected before disposal. Pour a volume of bleach that is approximately 10% of the volume of the flask fluid into the flask. Swirl gently and let the flask sit for 30 minutes, then pour the contents into the sink while the

water is running. Allow the water to run a minute after you have poured the fluid away, and avoid breathing the fumes. Rinse the flask several times.

> *If you are using and cleaning the suction apparatus often, add the bleach to the clean flask before you replace it on the bench.*

• Solvents and hazardous substances, including phenol, must be disposed of according to the institution's safety rules. Contact EHS or your laboratory safety officer.

Biohazard trash disposal
Biohazard waste must usually be double-bagged, and only certain bags are acceptable at each institution. It must be autoclaved before disposal in regular trash, and this may be an individual, lab, or institutional responsibility.

Tip boxes
Tips can be purchased already sterilized, but it is cheaper to buy tips in bulk and load them into tip boxes. Always wear gloves when you do this, to prevent leaving oil from your skin on the tips. After loading, put a piece of autoclave tape on the box and date it. Autoclave the boxes for 15 minutes.

Some boxes come as towers, with one box on top of the other. Do not stab wildly at the box when getting a tip: If you are a little off center, the entire tower can hit the ground and fall apart.

Microfuge tubes
Like tip boxes, microfuge tubes can be purchased as sterile tubes, or can be autoclaved after being placed in a beaker or receptacle. Don't cap the tubes before autoclaving. Remove tubes by gently shaking the container onto the bench or with a forceps: Never use an ungloved hand to prowl around the container.

Pipet aid
Although some pipet aids are connected to a power source or have batteries, most must be recharged by being plugged in several hours to a power source. When you feel the pipet aid becoming less efficient at pulling liquids, first check to see whether there is a cotton plug from a pipet stuck in the nosepiece. If there is, pull it out with a tweezers. A filter inside the pipet aid prevents aspiration of fluid into the body of the pipet aid. The filter may have gotten wet and need to be replaced. Snap open the nosepiece to check the filter and replace it, if necessary. Order a few filters to keep at your bench. If there is no physical blockage, plug the pipet aid in overnight to recharge.

Pipettors

Pipettors need to be calibrated every few months to a year, depending on the usage. Be aware of the amount in the tip when you are working: You may notice a change in the volume or the feel of the pipettor as it is aspirating. Test the accuracy of the pipettor every few weeks by comparing volumes with a new or newly calibrated pipettor. Some pipettors can be calibrated at the bench, others must be sent away for a check-up. The pipettor must be completely clean and free of radioactivity before it is sent.

Water baths

Change the water if it looks discolored or starts to smell. You could add an antibacterial agent to the water, but it isn't necessary. Use only distilled water in the bath. To prevent evaporation, either use a cover or keep the surface covered with ping pong balls.

SETTING UP A COMMAND CENTER

Most of the research you need to do will be accomplished not at the bench, but at the desk and computer, as you organize information, think, read, and analyze data. Your desk should not merely be the place where you keep your lab notebook and phone numbers. It should be a refuge and a resource, and a powerful place from which you control the direction of your research.

The Desk

It is very convenient to have a desk beside your lab bench. You can monitor experiments while you read, and have a clean place to record experiments in your lab book as you go along. The desk is usually small, and it is good to keep most items in drawers and on the shelves, to keep the desk space clear. Good organization may be all the edge you will have over other scientists, and it starts at your desk.

Bookshelves above the desk are good for library and reference books, journals, and for stacks of papers. Do not keep any chemical or lab equipment here.

One of the drawers should be dedicated to storing papers and articles. If there are no suitable drawers, it is often possible to fit a small file cabinet under or next to the desk.

Another drawer should have a lock. Personal valuables and sensitive data could be kept here, locked. Backpacks, purses, and checkbooks can disappear from the most apparently secure laboratory.

If radioactive work is done on the bench right beside the desk, a plastic shield or plate should be set up between the desk and the bench.

Desk essentials

Calculator. You may have a calculator on the computer, but you need an always reachable one. In some labs you must provide your own calculator.

Calendar/memo book (organizer). This could be the secret to your happiness. Choose whatever format works, but you should have room to record seminars, appointments, ideas, and experiment plans. See pages 59 and 63.

Formatted computer disks. You must always be ready to save files onto a disk, sometimes in a terrific hurry.

Lab notebook. Book or sheets, see Chapter 5.

Paper or notebook to record protocols, freezer contents, etc.

Post-Its. Invaluable for marking sections of books or journals, or leaving notes.

Pencils. Useful for writing on microscope slides, because the marks don't wash off with ethanol or methanol.

Pens. Never be lacking a pen within reach. Use a pen, never pencil, for recording of all data.

Ruler. Clear plastic, for measuring bands on gels, and drawing lines on graphs.

Scotch tape. After writing on tubes with marker, cover with a piece of tape to prevent smudging. Also used for attaching data sheets into your notebook.

Trays. You should have two or three trays to use to organize papers.

Dealing with Papers and Other Stuff

- **All the information at your desk should be accessible within 5 minutes.** Time is too precious to spend finding a method you saw in a paper last week, or trying to figure out if this week's or last week's seminar is the one you shouldn't miss.

  If you aren't vigilant, you could quickly have a desk covered with papers that you will not look at and which will eventually become outdated. Then you can rationalize the afternoon it takes to throw them all away, and feel you accom-

  > Neither neatness nor sloppiness is the key to paper management, nor is quantity the root cause of a paper glut. The real cause of a paperwork crisis is a problem with decision making: picking up the same piece of paper five times and putting it down again because you can't decide what to do with it.
  >
  > *The Organized Executive*, pp 35–36.

  plished something. You haven't.

  The research business is about information, and you need to keep your information...well, informative. And the only way to do this is to:

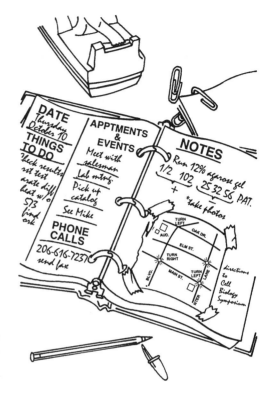

FIGURE 4.

Use the organizer and appointment book to record conversations and planned experiments, as well as seminars and meetings

- **Avoid letting a piece of paper touch your hand more than once.** Deal with each bit of information as soon as you receive it.

- **Establish a filing system.** All the information you have must be either visible or easily found. Some suggested tools are:

    Organizer/appointment book. A large book in which you can record appointments, things-to-do, phone numbers and E-mail addresses, seminar times and meetings. This is vital. You should only have one such book, and put temporary notes in a notebook or a Post-It. You can use a computer program, but only if you have sole use of a computer and only if that is the only organizer you use.

    File cabinet. You will need to have files for journal articles, personal papers (insurance, CV, letters), your reprints, and data (films and sheets that don't fit in your lab book).

> *The only papers you should keep on file are papers with methods you need, important papers relevant to your project, and papers that are difficult to obtain. Most papers are easily available in a library or on-line. A good solution is a literature management program on the computer: You can record the reference and write a summary of the paper.*

Trays for the desktop. Two trays will be fine. One is for incoming papers, yet to be dealt with. The other is for papers that will be handled later. This can be divided by folders into topics—you could have one folder for reprint requests, one for phone calls that must be returned, one for papers you want to read before filing.

- **Set up a regular routine** for dealing with papers and things to do, a routine that is part of a larger routine. (Other tasks that you should set aside time for are reviewing data and keeping up with the scientific literature, both of which are discussed in later chapters.) Consolidate tasks and time as much as possible: Open mail once a day, deal with plasmid requests once a week, look up articles every Wednesday.

- There are only a **few choices** to make for each piece of information. You can: Toss it immediately, file it, act on it, or a combination of the above. Some things cannot be physically dealt with immediately, but should be relegated to a pile to be handled later. For example, you may want to file all the scientific literature you receive daily in a "To read" file. Either set a regular time for your reading, or set a time limit for how long a paper can remain unread. Don't ever let this pile get too big.

> ### Examples of paper triage: Daily mail.
>
> The institution's weekly seminar list. Read the list, decide which seminars you will go to, and write the topic, speaker, and time on your calendar. Don't hang it up, or keep it for reference. Toss it.
>
> An introductory offer for a new journal. Do you want the journal? Will you really read it, can you afford it? Decide now. If you don't want it, toss the paper. (If you change your mind you will always be able to find a phone number for the journal, really.) If you do want it, fill in the form and mail it.
>
> Reprint request. If there are only a few of these trickling in, deal with it immediately. Give it (graciously) to the secretary if it is her job to mail requests, or mail the reprint yourself. If you receive many requests, put the request aside and deal with all requests every 2 weeks.

- **Experiments always take priority,** and there will be times when the most carefully organized system grinds to a halt because there is simply no time to do anything but benchwork. Do the experiments and try to resume control as soon as you can.

Using the Computer

The lab computer is not a luxury, but is indispensable for writing, researching, and communication. You must have access to a computer for (at the very least) word processing and literature searches. Checking out the computer situation should be one of your priorities during your first week in the lab (see Chapter 1).

Word processing

A word processing program is used for text composition and manipulation. Even if you like to write with a number two pencil on a yellow legal pad, the information will ultimately have to find itself on a disk for editing, printing, sending, and sometimes, journal submission.

Word processing programs now come with spelling and grammar checks, table-making and graphing capacity. More importantly, these programs can work with bibliographic, spreadsheet, and database software, and information from other applications can be integrated into manuscripts and presentations.

Find out which word processing program is used by the laboratory and the department, and use that program. Don't hang onto your old program: If you ever need help from the secretary on a grant or manuscript, you'd better be using the program he or she is used to. Most programs are similar enough that it should take less than a day to become quite proficient with a new program.

Bibliographic management

Especially in your early days in the lab, papers and lists of papers you have read or intend to read will accumulate rapidly. A bibliographic management program will help you control this pile by numbering and organizing your references. You can retrieve references by keyword, author, or journal, making it easy to find a particular paper or to make a list of references about a particular topic. This also means that you don't need to keep as many papers, since you can enter a summary or notes into the reference.

If you don't know how to use a computer, or are confused about an application, contact the institution's computer service department. Take any available relevant computer courses offered at your institution. It will require what will seem to be an extravagant investment (a day or two) but it will save you hours and hours of time.

If computer access is a terrible problem, composing may have to be done first on paper, but the more you can compose on the keyboard, the more time you will save.

You must be sure your programs will work together: One way to do this is to use a package of related software from the same manufacturer.

You must be sure that your bibliographic management program can work with your word processing program. Although you can enter all your references manually, it is wonderful to have your reference management program be able to cooperate with reference update programs and all library search programs you use.

The list of references you call up for a manuscript can be formatted in any journal style. And if you redo the paper for another journal, reformatting the references will take a few keystrokes.

References from Medline and other sites, as well as from compatible literature update programs, can be directly downloaded into the bibliographic program.

Internet access

This is not optional. Find out how to get on line from your institution's computer center: There will probably be a form you must fill out, and a password you must apply for. Find out how you can log on at home, using your work account number.

E-mail enables you to keep in contact with colleagues all over the world. You can send manuscripts to collaborators, scan in data and send it to another lab. And yes, you can say hi to your mom. You may need an E-mail password and account, in addition to your on-line account. If you share a computer with other lab members, be sure you have your own password and directory for your own E-mail.

Journals can be found on line. Most free journal web sites only show the Table of Contents and abstracts of the articles, but this is terrific for browsing; the full article is available at some sites.

Literature searches can be done on-line. You can search libraries and databases. Medline, the database of the National Library of Medicine (NLM), is now free, and it is available at any number of sites in addition to the NLM. There are other databases, but Medline will be the most useful

Newsgroups allow you to post questions to technical questions, and to read the answers or participate in a posted "discussion" of the topic on line. If you want ideas on the best electroporator available, or want advice on a particular protocol, ask the question of the appropriate group. You can find a list of groups by searching the Web by key word, or by going to one of the several sites listed at the end of the chapter. Listserv sites also allow you to post questions, but this, and the answers, are sent by E-mail.

Technical literature is available at the Web sites of most companies. This information may not just pertain to the company's products, but also to related basic research.

Literature update programs

Several programs will send you a weekly disk with hundreds of biological journal titles, and sometimes, abstracts, listed. With a saved search strategy, usually by keyword and/or authors, you can search the journals and import the references to your reference management program if the programs are compatible. The alternative to a literature update program is a regular search of the current literature with the same keywords.

Data collection and organization

You can enter your data in a spreadsheet program (for calculations) or in a database (for organization and retrieval). Many instruments, such as beta counters and fraction collectors, are hooked directly to computers with programs that can collect and analyze data. In this case, compatibility with your word processing programs is not likely to be a priority, or even a possibility. However, many programs will be standard and will mesh with your other programs.

Graphics

There are dedicated graphic programs that allow you to enter data and draw a variety of graphs and tables. Data can easily be added or removed, and the graph redrawn. Simple graphics can be done by many word processing, spreadsheet, and data base programs, as well as by drawing and presentation programs.

Presentation programs

Presentation programs are useful for making slides for seminars, but not as useful for illustrations for publications. Text, graphs, and tables are artistically rendered, and can be presented as a slide show on the computer, be printed (and later photographed), or be made directly into slides through a photo or computer department with the appropriate software.

Specialized software

There are software programs that perform a variety of mathematical and theoretical functions, such as designing primers for PCR (see Chapter 12) or modeling protein structure. Unless the lab has a program running, or you are very familiar with a program, don't make a big investment learning a new program now.

Organization and scheduling

Only if you have unlimited access to a computer should you think of using a personal organizer. An organizer and calendar will keep track of and notify you when seminars are and when cells are ready for harvesting: It will keep your phone numbers and dial the phone for you. But you have to use the computer program consistently for it to be worthwhile having it.

You should only have one system of schedule organization. It is almost impossible to use both a computer program and an appointment book to keep track of daily affairs.

Scanner and scanner software

Pictures, text, data, and documents can be scanned into your computer. You can then incorporate the scanned images into your own programs, where you can manipulate them and/or send them by E-mail or over the Internet to other researchers. For example, gels can be scanned in and art or presentation software used to label the lanes and make figures or slides.

Basic Rules for Computer Use

- **Check which computers you can use.** People are very possessive about their computers, and the sight of someone pumping potentially virus-ridden disks into a computer without asking permission can be absolutely infuriating. If there aren't enough computers in the lab, find out if there are departmental computers for you to use. Also check the institutional computing center for available computers.

- **Never use a computer if it is obvious that someone is in the middle of something.** You could lose all of that person's work if they haven't saved it. And the corollary to this, of course, is:

- **Always exit from the program you are working in before you leave the computer.** This makes it clear to other people that the computer is available. It also lessens the chance that someone will (1) read private documents, (2) inadvertently lose your data, or (3) load too many programs and crash the computer.

  > *Turning the computer off while it is reading from or writing to a disk may damage the disk, the hard drive, or both. Be sure the drive indicator lights are off.*

- **Save, save, save.** Save into two places: to a floppy disk, and onto a hard drive. If you save onto a shared hard drive, be sure you have a directory set up to receive your files (for example, ... /yourname/manuscript3). If you have a document that is confidential, save it only to a floppy or your removable hard drive.

- **Check all downloaded software and data, and all floppy disks, for viruses.** The computer should have a virus-check program (if it doesn't, you should get one through computing services) that checks the computer upon start-up and can be used to check every disk put in and every downloaded piece of information. Download only into a temporary directory, check for viruses, and only then, transfer the information to where you want it.

- **Exit all programs before turning off the computer.** The computer should be turned off at night, although relatively harmless custom in some labs dictates that the computer is always left on.

- **Turn on the computer before the monitor: Turn off the monitor before the computer.**

- **No game playing or WWW cruising when someone may need the computer.** Work use always comes first.

- **Don't put floppies into the computer until the computer has been turned on and booted.** In some systems the computer will try to boot from the floppy, usually no big deal, but it is delay.

- **Do not erase or delete anything from the computer, unless it is your files or data.** If the hard drive is getting full, make an announcement to everyone to remove unneeded files or to copy them to another venue. Never remove *anything* without checking with everyone and giving plenty of advance warning!

- **A password is needed for Internet access. Apply for one** (check with the departmental office for the procedure) **and never give it to anyone.** Some programs and computers also require passwords, and these are unlikely to be the same as your Internet access number.

- **Don't eat or drink while working at the computer.** At the least, the keyboard will be sticky. Don't forget that there is no food or drink allowed in the lab.

- **Don't expose your disks or the computer to magnetic fields,** such as the field generated by large stereo speakers. Info on disks is stored magnetically and too close proximity to a magnet can erase the disk.

> *If you spill a drink into the keyboard, turn the computer off immediately and unplug the keyboard. Get as much liquid out as possible and leave the keyboard to dry overnight before you plug it back in.*

Before you panic:
Save your work, if you can.
Check all cables.
Make sure there is power.

RESOURCES

Biochemical Resources
  Tel (517) 381-8269
  http://biores.com   (This web site is a database of chemicals, biochemicals, laboratory products, and services that can be searched.)
BioMedNet, "The World Wide Club for the Biological and Medical Community"
  http://biomed.net.com (Medline is available through this site, as well as discussion groups, a job exchange, and *HMS Beagle*, a science magazine.)

BioSupplyNet source book, BioSupplyNet, Inc., 10 Skyline Drive, Plainview, New York 11803
  Phone: (516) 349-5595
  Fax: (516) 349-5598
  http://www.biosupplynet.com (The BioSupplyNet Source Book is a comprehensive directory of biomedical research supplies and equipment. The web site allows you to search by key words for product names or categories.)
BioTechniques Home Page
  http://www.biotechniques.com (A library of techniques, a buyer's guide, and connections to many biological research sites.)
Glossary of microbiology. 1997. T. Chen.
  http://www.hardlink.com/~tsute/glossary/index/html/
Guide to the Internet. Trends. 1997. Elsevier Science, Cambridge, United Kingdom.
  http://www.elsevier.com/lcate/trendsguidev (A booklet describing how to use the Internet to find scientific information.)
Hancock, L. 1996. *Physician's guide to the Internet.* Lippincott-Raven Publishers, New York.
Horton, R.M. 1996. Using newsgroups: Virtual conferences on specialized topics. *BioTechniques* **20**: 62–64.
Medsite Navigator, Medsight Navigator and Medsite.
  http://www.medsitenavigator.com/ (Tries to integrate and group related medical and science sites together to promote the easy exchange of information. Links to Newsgroups, journals, Internet searches, and Medline.)
National Institutes of Health (NIH)
  http://www.nih.gov/science/journals/ (Pointers to on-line journals are available through many web sites. A comprehensive list can be found through the NIH site.)
Newsgroups, Tips and Techniques.
  http://genome.eerie.fr/bioscience/services/biolnew.html (An extensive list, with links to many biological newsgroups.)
Sambrook J., Fritsch E.F., and Maniatis T. 1989. *Molecular cloning. A laboratory manual.* 2nd edition. Cold Spring Harbor Laboratory Press, Cold Spring Harbor, New York.
SciQuest, Research Triangle Park, North Carolina 27709-2156
  Phone: (919) 786-1770
  Fax: (919) 782-3128
  http://www.sciquest.com/catalyst/welcome.cgi (This web site also allows searches by key words, and automatic requests of chosen vendors.)
United States National Library of Medicine (NLM)
  http://www.nlm.nih.gov
Medline
  http://www.nlm.nih.gov/databases/medline.html (Medline can be accessed in several ways at this site. Once found, papers can be ordered through Loansome Doc, a service which can deliver documents to your library.)
Winston, S. 1983. *The organized executive. New ways to manage time, paper, and people.* Warner Books, New York.

Section 2
Plotting a Course

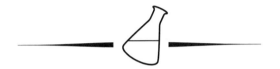

CHAPTER 4

How to Set Up an Experiment 69

CHAPTER 5

Laboratory Notebooks 89

CHAPTER 6

Presenting Yourself and Your Data 101

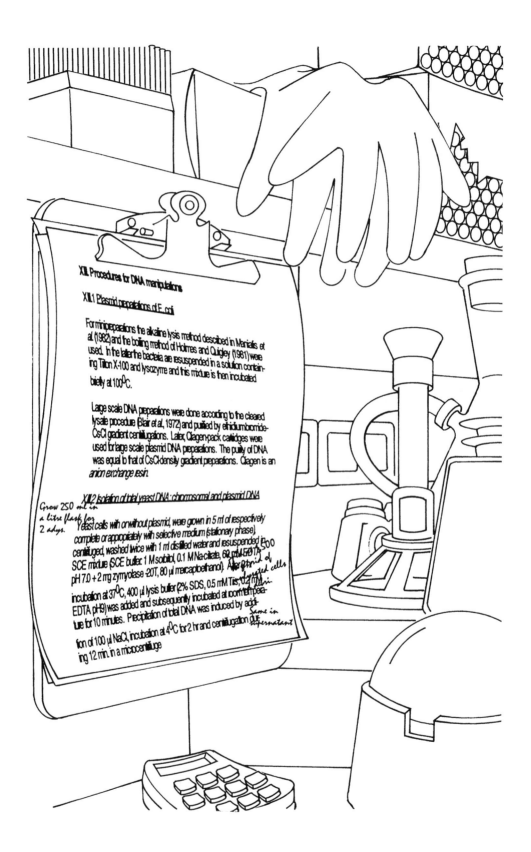

4

How to Set Up an Experiment

A**N EXPERIMENT IS A TEST** made to examine the validity of a hypothesis. Experimentation is the reason you are where you are. If you don't conduct your experiments carefully and thoroughly from the beginning, you'll soon be mired in a bog of half-baked experiments and unclear results that can only be undone by leaving the lab.

There is one extremely important caveat to this advice on organization

PHILOSOPHICAL CONSIDERATIONS	69
PLANNING AN EXPERIMENT	71
Background research	73
Controls	73
Statistics	75
Using a protocol	77
INTERPRETING RESULTS	83
When experiments don't work	84
RESOURCES	87

and clear thinking. DO AN EXPERIMENT DURING THE FIRST WEEK. Don't wait until you think you "know more." Planning experiments is rather like joining a union—you can't join until you have the experience, and you can't get the experience until you are in the union. You may have read every relevant paper, memorized the protocols, talked to everyone in the lab, but still do not really understand the new experiment you are getting ready to do. DO IT ANYWAY. After you have done the first experiment, *everything*—theory, techniques, implications—will become magically clearer. Do read and prepare yourself, but know that a full understanding of your project will not come until you have physically performed the experiments.

Not all experiments will be thrilling. It is terrific to think of doing only very exciting and crucial experiments, but it is more important to first be sure your experiments are reproducible, dependable, and have integrity.

PHILOSOPHICAL CONSIDERATIONS

 Keep the importance of your experiments in mind. Chances are that once you start working, you won't have much chance to think consciously about the universal relevance of your experiments. But as you set up your experiments, it is important to remember why you are doing what you are doing. Think about Science. Sometimes lab work can seem tedious, and remembering why you are repeating the same experiment for the tenth time can keep you going. Keeping the big picture in mind will also help you maintain integrity in your approach.

 Remember that you must publish the results of your experiments. Publications are important—you can't survive without them. If you consider each experiment to be a separate and publishable entity, you are more likely to remember all the needed controls and variables. Thinking about each experiment as potentially publishable can keep you focused on your experiment. It is very easy to drift into other areas, and part of research is following new avenues. But exploration must be done rigorously, and not by default.

> *"...scientists often place at least as much weight on an experimentalist's general reputation for careful, painstaking work as on the technical details of the experiment in assessing whether the data constitute reliable evidence."* (Reprinted by permission of American Scientist, magazine of Sigma Xi, The Scientific Research Society, from Woodward and Goodstein 1996.)

 Set yourself up as a careful and thorough investigator. You will make your reputation not only on your results, but also in the way you set up your experiments. Some people are known as good "bench" scientists, meaning that their experiments are well thought out and well executed. Set up your reputation early, and any unorthodox data you do produce is likely to be believed. If your labmates trust your data, the head of the lab is more likely to, and from this, the rest of the scientific community. Credibility is key.

 Be a critical thinker. As for the rest of science, the theories behind experimentation are not carved in stone, and there are several ways to explain how and why experiments should be done.

Approaches to problem-solving and experimentation

Reductionist. Breaks a problem down into pieces, and solves each piece separately.

Deductive. Proposes a hypothesis and collects data to confirm or disprove the hypothesis.

Inductive. Examines a collection of evidence without prejudice and then proposes a theory to account for all the observed facts.

Falsification. Proposed by Karl Popper. If a prediction that stems from a hypothesis turns out to be false, the hypothesis from which it is deduced is said to be falsified and must be rejected.

Standing alone, every approach is inadequate. Incorporate all the approaches you can. Attack your data from all angles to look for flaws in your thinking or in the experimental approach. Try not to slant your results toward the conclusion you want or expect.

PLANNING AN EXPERIMENT

1. **Define the question.** An experiment should address a hypothesis by answering one or two specific questions. Careful thought and reading, as well as discussion with other scientists, will help define the questions and set up the parameters of the experiment. Be sure not to pick questions that it is not possible to answer.

2. **Design the experiment.**

   • Experimental *variables*. At what do you want to look? Will you look, for example, at an effect over time, or of concentration, or both? What concentrations will you use, and what should the time points be?

   • *Controls.* Every experimental variable needs a control to show that the results obtained are the results of the treatment.

   • *Number of samples.* Should you run samples in duplicate? Triplicate? More? Duplicates are the minimum for any measure of biological activity.

> *"I have often had cause to feel that my hands are cleverer than my head. That is a crude way of characterizing the dialectics of experimentation. When it is going well, it is like a quiet conversation with Nature. One asks a question and gets an answer; then one asks the next question, and gets the next answer. An experiment is a device to make Nature speak intelligibly. After that one has only to listen."* (Reprinted, with permission, from George Wald 1968, © American Association for the Advancement of Science.)

DO SMALL EXPERIMENTS. It is very tempting to get as many data as possible from each experiment, as this will, theoretically, save money and time. Cells have to be grown fewer times, reagents are conserved, and time is maximized. **But the return/effort ratio is actually much higher for small experiments.** Carrying off a large experiment requires a great deal of expertise, as well as luck, and should never be attempted before several small experiments have already been performed.

The determination of what a small or large experiment is is completely subjective. But generally, **if there are so many tubes that you feel hassled or confused, your experiment is too big.** If you feel this happening, divide the experiment into two parts, and only do the first part.

In the end, you won't get rewarded because you managed to pull a huge experiment off, but you can be rewarded by a lovely figure in a published paper, and those are almost impossible to derive from a mind-boggling marathon. Don't get macho.

- *Statistics.* The statistical analysis that is needed will help dictate sample size and other aspects of experimental design. Find out if you will subject your data to statistical analysis—it is too late to do it at the end of the experiment.

3. **Set up the experiment.**

   - Obtain and prepare a *protocol.*

   - *Prepare reagents,* sign up for equipment, grow the cells, and be sure you have all the necessary components.

> *It is a waste of time and reagents to not think carefully before setting up an experiment. Many a beginner (as well as seasoned experimenters) may mistake the busyness and sense of importance one feels when doing many experiments for actually doing something meaningful. Don't be fooled. THERE IS NO SUBSTITUTE FOR CAREFUL PLANNING!*

   - Do a *mental dry run,* to be sure you haven't forgotten anything.

   - If it is a tricky experiment, with precious reagents, do a *physical dry run* first, omitting the reagents. This will ensure that the physical manipulations you have planned are feasible.

   - *Observe* someone else do the experiment. If you will be using a new technique, ask someone who has performed a similar experiment if you could watch her do it next time, or if she could help you.

4. **Do the experiment.** Make sure you have set aside enough time to do it, and add another hour to your estimation. Write down results and observations as they happen.

> *Don't talk while planning or doing a complicated experiment, and don't be afraid to ask people not to talk to you. Some people wear a certain hat, or put on a personal listening device (with or without a tape) to signal coworkers that they need to concentrate.*

5. **Collect and analyze the data.** Inspect all your data as soon as possible—before you do the next experiment! Don't let unread slides or ungraphed time points accumulate. This is a good time to consult with anoth-

---

Common mistakes made when setting up experiments

Not thinking about the necessity for the experiment.

Planning a huge and sloppy experiment intended to wrap up every major question in biology.

Forgetting to evaluate prior experiments.

Not thinking through every control to be sure the experiment will be interpretable.

Not checking to be sure all reagents are ready and available before starting the experiment.

er scientist in the lab or in the field about the results, whether they were "good" or "bad."

6. **Repeat the experiment.** A result must be repeatable or it is completely worthless. And ultimately, it must be repeated by someone else, so you must be sure your result is dependable.

Background Research

Many mistakes in setting up experiments can be avoided by knowing the field. Even if you have a protocol, you still need to understand the details and theories of the experiment. By checking the literature, you can find out what techniques are generally used, what results would be expected, what reagents are most likely to work, and at what concentration they have been used—plus a myriad of details that can help at unexpected times.

Calling or writing one or two of the experts in a field can be a tremendous shortcut for you. Of course, you don't want to waste the other person's time by asking something you could (and should) have looked up yourself (For example, don't call up to ask what the sizes of mammalian ribosomal RNA are). But if you have a question about the specifics of the experiments, E-mail or call.

Start with a few papers, the classics on your topic. Look through the references used in these papers: it is likely that you should read most of them, certainly ones duplicated in other papers. Go to the library and read.

Do a keyword search on Medline or another database. Check not only current papers, but old ones, as an amazing number of good experiments are buried in obscure journals because their value wasn't appreciated. Papers are also found in obscure journals because they are obscure. Use your own judgment about the validity of the data in the papers. Try not to be swayed by reputations or journal names when evaluating data.

Keep up in your field by reading current literature. Most people have a few journals that they read regularly to stay posted on major developments. But experimental ideas and techniques are often found in specialty journals and in other journals not found in your library, so you should systematically search the current literature. Set aside a regular time to search Medline, using a search you define by keywords and authors. Or use one of the literature update programs that send a weekly disk with the latest journals, and search by keywords and authors.

Controls

A control theoretically shows what would happen if you didn't do anything; thus, it shows you what your pretty results really mean. *There must be a control for every different variable in the experiment.* It is not uncommon to have more controls than experimental samples in an experiment. Controls are not extra, they are not a waste of time, they are absolutely integral to the interpretation of every experiment.

Controls are not done once—they must be repeated with every experiment. This includes standard curves for enzymatic assays and molecular weight standards for gel electrophoresis. It is absolutely not valid to go back to an earlier experiment and use the data from those controls, assuming that the controls would have been the same.

Types of controls

Experimental controls. These controls tell you if the basic experimental procedures are working correctly.

Examples of experimental controls are the molecular weight standards used for DNA, RNA, and protein gels (as well as being used to measure molecular weights). From the molecular weight standards, one can tell if the gel was the presumed concentration of agarose or acrylamide, if transfer of the gel to a filter was fairly complete, and if electrophoresis was effective.

Treatment controls. Treatment controls are positive and negative, and show you whether the experimental handling of the cells has elicited an effect. If you have samples that have been treated with multiple factors, the effects of the individual factors must be controlled for independently. Thus, if you are looking at the effect of incubation with factors X and Y, you must have a control incubated with X alone, and one incubated with Y alone.

Positive controls. A positive control is usually an experimental control, which shows you how the data would look if a treatment had an effect.

Examples of positive control are the addition of a cell line expressing receptor X when performing immunofluorescence on cells transfected with receptor X; and inclusion of cells known to respond to factor X by stimulated growth when testing for the effect of factor X on cells never tested.

Negative controls. The negative control shows you what the effect of non-treatment is on your readout.

Examples of negative controls are the addition of a cell line known not to express receptor X when performing immunofluorescence on cells transfected with receptor X; and inclusion of cells known to not respond to factor X by stimulated growth when testing for the effect of factor X on cells never tested.

The negative control is the one most often forgotten, and the one whose omission won't hurt until it counts. It is especially important to distinguish between a positive result and high background when first setting up a system or a set of experiments. Many hopes have been dashed when an initial positive result was found, and the experiment repeated with the same happy results—and then, a negative control showed that absolutely everything, appropriate and inappropriate, tested positively.

Time points. There must be a control for every variation in the time of the experiment. If you are looking at the half-life of mRNA at 0, 5, 15, and 30 minutes after treatment with factor X, you must have a control for incubation of your cells without factor X at 0, 5, 15, and 30 minutes. Don't shortcut by trying to have a control for only time 0 and 30 minutes; every treatment needs a control.

Set up the time points so that the harvesting of one sample is completed before the harvesting of the next sample. If a sample jam does happen, find a "resting place" partially through the harvesting—for example, cells could be held on ice until the end of the experiment. But what you do to one sample must be repeated on the rest: If you hold one set of samples on ice for 5 minutes, you must do the same to all the samples.

Zero time control. You must collect a sample as immediately after treatment as possible. Yes, in many cases zero actually means a lapse of seconds or minutes, but you must get a sample (and the requisite control) as close to Now as possible.

To do a zero time point, it may make the most sense to do it AFTER the other very early time points, only if the "age" of the samples doesn't matter. If you want to collect cells 0, 5, 10, and 30 minutes after the addition of factor X, add factor X to the 5-, 10-, and 30-minute samples and put them aside to incubate. Then add factor X to the 0 time sample and immediately collect the sample or stop the reaction.

What controls should you eliminate if you don't have enough samples?

Despite the best planning, things happen: Some samples may be dropped or become contaminated, there may not be enough treatment factors, you may get called away from the lab and be unable to harvest all the time points, but still, the samples are valuable and you need to get as much data as possible.

The control you leave out will probably turn out to be the most important one, but leave out, in order

1. Procedural controls.
2. Duplicate experimental controls.

If you must leave out more controls than this, it isn't worth doing the experiment. There is no valid experiment without controls!

Statistics

Will your data need to be analyzed statistically in order to be convincing? In biological research, this isn't a straightforward question. Some areas of study apply statistics religiously, but there are entire fields of study which insist that the effects are so big and the results so obviously significant that playing with numbers isn't necessary. Generally, your lab either does or doesn't do statistical analysis on the data it generates.

You will have to decide yourself whether you will analyze your data. It may be an obvious decision, especially if you are trained in statistics. Look at other papers in the lab as well as in the field, and see how the data have been handled. Bring those papers and your experimental plan and talk to a statistician at the institution, perhaps in the computer center. Call one of the many companies that sells statistics software packages, or visit an on-line site and ask. Post a question at a relevant newsgroup.

Be aware that formulas are sometimes different for populations than for samples. This is why you can't simply open a book and pull a formula, unless you understand what you are doing. Better no statistics than bad statistics.

Most of what you will probably be doing is trying to establish whether your data are due to experimental manipulation or chance, and whether the data are consistent with a hypothesis. You may want to predict the characteristics of a sample based on information about the population, or you may want to predict the characteristics of a population based on a sample.

Examples of the uses of statistics in the biomedical laboratory

- To estimate the characteristics of a population on the basis of information about a sample: The Students's *t*-test enables you to establish a confidence interval for the mean for a small, normally distributed population. You can then figure the probability from a table.

The P value, or probability, tests whether the observed deviations from the hypothesis could occur by chance. If the P value is very small, the hypothesis can be said to be true.

- To predict the characteristics of a sample on the basis of information about the population: Find the probability, using a normal distribution curve.

- To see whether the differences between the means of two sets of observations, as for before and after treatment, can be explained by chance: Use difference scores for large sample sizes (over 30), and the *t*-test for smaller sample sizes.

Standard deviation is the measure of the deviation of an individual measurement from the mean of many measurements. The **standard error** (also known as the standard deviation of the mean) measures the mean of all the data observed from the mean of a hypothetical database and is a measure of how close the average is to the "true" mean value (Koch 1994). Standard deviation and the standard error are sometimes (and wrongly) used interchangeably, with the standard error being chosen because it gives a smaller value and apparently minimizes data spread.

Use standard deviation to show how reproducible a particular data point is, based on multiple samples.

- To determine the probability that any given sample was drawn from a population within a given population: Use chi square, a sample distribution. You can also use ANOVA or the Student's *t*-test.

- To predict the effect of one related measure on another: Use linear regression. If the two measures have a linear relationship, you can calculate a correlation coefficient. Calculating doubling times is the most common use of linear regression in the lab.

- To consider data from several samples at the same time and distinguish systematic differences between groups from the chance variations found in each group: Do an analysis of variance (ANOVA). If you want to look at the effect of two experimental treatments on a measure, do a two-way ANOVA.

- To look at the difference between two independent samples, as when Factor X has been added to one group, Factor Y to another: Use the null hypothesis and determine the probability. Use the z-test for large sample numbers, the Student's *t*-test for small sample numbers.

Most computer spreadsheet programs can perform the above statistics (Koosis 1997). Statistics programs can do this as well and will also help you decide what statistics are appropriate.

> *Be sure that the data are linear. There are other models, such as quadratic or exponential, that can be used for calculations. Assuming linearity when there is none is a common mistake that gives inaccurate numbers.*

> *Many statistical tests (for example, ANOVA and the t-test) should not be used if you expect a strong effect to skew the population. Most tests presume a normal distribution of the unknown population.*

> *The null hypothesis is the assumption that experimental results are due to chance. If the probability of obtaining that sample number is less than a predetermined small percentage, the results will be significant, and the null hypothesis is rejected.*

Using a Protocol

1. Obtain a protocol from

   - *Another investigator.* The best place to get a protocol is from another investigator in the lab, especially for your first experiments. The protocol will be tailored to the resources and expertise of the lab, and may contain important

---

Every experiment, no matter how experimental, must have a protocol. *Every* time. Even if you are working a technique out for the first time, or repeating a commonly done procedure, you should do it according to a written protocol. If you have done the experiment 50 times, you should still have a protocol or protocol reference (such as "Protocol for extraction from p 3 followed exactly") for your lab book.

details on the tubes to use in the lab's centrifuge or tricks to get the standards into solution. And you will have an expert on hand.

- *A book of protocols.* There are many laboratory manuals commercially available, with simple and clear protocols given for many fields of biology. Laboratory, course, and departmental lab manuals are also a good source of simple protocols. The disadvantage of using a commercial manual is that you will have to fine-tune the protocol yourself.

- *"Methods" section in published papers.* This is the least reliable place to find a protocol. Methods sections are notorious for the important details that may be left out due to space or other considerations.

2. **Read the protocol to see if it makes sense to you.** Pretend you are doing the experiment, and look for obviously missing steps in logic (yours or the source's) or function. Many assumptions are made in most protocols, but this may not be obvious to you. For example, "phenol extraction" often means one extraction with buffer-saturated and pH-ed phenol, followed by two extractions with phenol:chloroform:isoamyl alcohol.

If you have any questions about a protocol in a paper, do not hesitate to call the author of the paper! The address, phone number, and E-mail address of the person to whom correspondence should be addressed are on the first or last page of the article. E-mail with a followup phone call if there is no electronic response is the preferred sequence of communication.

3. **Change the protocol as you require and rewrite it.** This only refers to making steps more understandable to you, or changing specific equipment as needed. If a protocol said a sample was centrifuged for 13,000*g*, you must find the appropriate centrifuge to use and record that on the protocol.

4. **Prepare all reagents listed on the protocol and be sure you have everything you need.** Everything! Nothing is too obvious. It could be a drag to race to the centrifuge with your tubes, only to find that someone else had just started an hour run. Have a backup lined up, or sign up for a centrifuge. Sign-ups are risky on first experiments, as it is hard to define the time you will need, so it is probably safer to have a backup plan. Be particularly sure you have the radioisotope you require. This may need to be ordered several weeks before the experiment.

*Should you use a kit? The reagents are assembled, the directions are clear, and in most cases, yes, you should, if the price isn't prohibitive. But there is an important caveat: **Don't let a kit substitute for thinking.** Know every component of the kit, and be sure you understand just what the kit is doing.*

5. **Follow the protocol exactly the first time you do the experiment.** Why? If someone gives you a protocol and you do not follow it exactly, that person cannot

(and might not want to) help you interpret the data. You must be able to reproduce the usual result before you can start to vary conditions. You must know that you are measuring the effect of a variable, not of your technique. You must try not to be a variable in your own experiment!

6. **Modify the protocol based on your experience with it.** As you proceed through the experiment, note down any improvements to the protocol that would make sense. When you are evaluating your data, rethink the alterations and check with someone in the lab to see if they make sense. Rewrite the protocol for the next go. Usually, you have a printed protocol on which you make changes over several experiments. It is worth modifying, scanning, or even typing new protocols into your own computer files, and the sooner you computerize your protocols, the better. Then as the protocol continues to evolve, you can add changes and still have a legible protocol.

> *Don't worry if you don't have immediate success. Everyone who has been around a lab knows this: A new experiment doesn't work the first time. You repeat it, carefully. It still doesn't work. You repeat it again, and maybe, again. It still doesn't work. But on the next try, although you are sure you are doing exactly as you had been doing, the experiment works. And it always works, from then on.*

Examples of Protocols

6-12-92

ELECTROPORATION OF M. SMEGMATIS
B.Jacobs,Meth.Enzymol:204,527,1991

Make sure 10% glycerol is cold

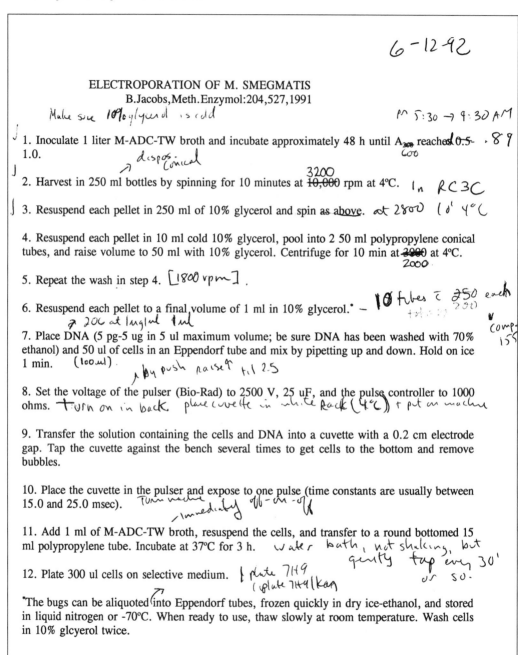

M 5:30 → 9:30 AM

1. Inoculate 1 liter M-ADC-TW broth and incubate approximately 48 h until A~~600~~ reached 0.5- .8 ?
1.0.   *600*   *dispos. Conical*

2. Harvest in 250 ml bottles by spinning for 10 minutes at ~~10,000~~ *3200* rpm at 4°C. *In RC3C*

3. Resuspend each pellet in 250 ml of 10% glycerol and spin ~~as above~~. *at 2800 10' 4°C*

4. Resuspend each pellet in 10 ml cold 10% glycerol, pool into 2 50 ml polypropylene conical tubes, and raise volume to 50 ml with 10% glycerol. Centrifuge for 10 min at ~~3000~~ *2000* at 4°C.

5. Repeat the wash in step 4. [1800 vpm].

6. Resuspend each pellet to a final volume of 1 ml in 10% glycerol.* — *10 tubes ⊂ 250 each* *tot: 2000*   *comp. 155*
→ 200 at 1mg/ml 1ml

7. Place DNA (5 pg-5 ug in 5 ul maximum volume; be sure DNA has been washed with 70% ethanol) and 50 ul of cells in an Eppendorf tube and mix by pipetting up and down. Hold on ice 1 min. *(100 ul).* *by push raiseth til 2.5*

8. Set the voltage of the pulser (Bio-Rad) to 2500 V, 25 uF, and the pulse controller to 1000 ohms. *Turn on in back place cuvette in white Rack (4°C) + put on machine*

9. Transfer the solution containing the cells and DNA into a cuvette with a 0.2 cm electrode gap. Tap the cuvette against the bench several times to get cells to the bottom and remove bubbles.

10. Place the cuvette in the pulser and expose to one pulse (time constants are usually between 15.0 and 25.0 msec). *Turn machine* *on - on -off* *immediately*

11. Add 1 ml of M-ADC-TW broth, resuspend the cells, and transfer to a round bottomed 15 ml polypropylene tube. Incubate at 37°C for 3 h. *water bath, not shaking, but gently tap every 30' or so.*

12. Plate 300 ul cells on selective medium. *plate 7H9 (plate 7H9 (kan*

*The bugs can be aliquoted into Eppendorf tubes, frozen quickly in dry ice-ethanol, and stored in liquid nitrogen or -70°C. When ready to use, thaw slowly at room temperature. Wash cells in 10% glcyerol twice.

PROTOCOL 1.

A copy of the protocol can be used as a template upon which to record the particulars of the experiment and any changes you make to the procedure.

Immunoprecipitation of the 68K Protein—^{32}P-Labeled 68K protein was immunoprecipitated from cell lysates containing equivalent amounts of protein using an antiserum directed against the bovine brain 87K protein as previously described (4). In some cases, an antiserum directed against purified mouse brain 68K protein was used. The two antisera gave identical results. Immunoprecipitated 68K protein was separated by electrophoresis on 8% SDS-PAGE gels according to Laemmli (9), and ^{32}P-labeled 68K protein was visualized by autoradiography using Kodak X-Omat x-ray film and intensifier screens. Where indicated, autoradiograms were scanned on an LKB Ultroscan densitometer.

IMMUNOPRECIPITATION PROTOCOL

Start with cell lysates in approximately 100 μl lysis buffer on ice (protein concentration 1.5 μg/μl). Keep samples at 4 degrees for all subsequent steps.

Preclear with 50 μl Protein A Sepharose beads (Sigma #P-3391) (50% slurry in PD). Add beads and nutate 15 minutes at 4C.

Spin tubes at 7000 rpm, 2 minutes, 4C, in TOMY with swing out Rotor.

Carefully transfer supernatants to new eppendorf tubes.

To supe, add 5μl antibody/150 μg protein. Nutate 1 hour at 4C.

Add 50 μl Protein A Sepharose beads and nutate 15minutes 4C.

Spin as before. Save the supernatant for gel to confirm depletion by antibody.

Wash beads two times with Wash Solution A

    Once with Wash Solution B

    Once with Wash Solution C

ie, add 1 ml buffer, vortex, spin as before, discard supernatant.

Resuspend beads in SDS sample buffer, boil 5 minutes and run on SDS Page gel.

Preparation of Protein A Sepharose Beads

To 1.5g Protein A Sepharose Beads add 30ml PD

Nutate 15min. at 4C

Centrifugre in Kneewell 1500 rpm, 10min, 4C

Aspirate Supe

Repeat this Wash procedure 2 times

Add 6ml fresh PD to washed beads so that final volume is 12ml.

Add 2.4mg Sodium Azide (final concentration is .2mg/ml)

PROTOCOL 2.

These immunoprecipitation protocols are from the same lab. The first is from a published manuscript (Rosen et al., *J. Biol. Chem. 264: 9118–9121*), the other from the actual protocol used in the laboratory. (Protocol courtesy of Alan Aderem, University of Washington, Seattle.)

TO TAKE BEAUTIFUL FLUORESCENCE PICTURES WITH THE ZEISS

Turn on microscope (knob on right, back)

Load camera (on right):
    Align red line and red dot and pull out cannister
    Slide out of holder
    Use crank to be sure there is no film in cannister (! button on front, right should have a steady
        light is there is a film in, and a flashing light if there is no film)
    Take off cannister
    Push silver button to open film holder
    Slide film in place, pull across, and thread
    Close film holder
    Slide film holder into holder and cannister
    Slide cannister into microscope with red dot and red line aligned
    Rotate cannister up
    Push B (front button) 3 times to advance film
    Set ASA (front of microscope)

Turn on fluorescent bulb (box on right)

Cut off visible light source (black knob on left)

Set fluorescence filters (black knob on right, 2nd from top)
    1st stop, 4 lines = green for rhodamine
    2nd stop, 3 lines = blue for fluorescein
    DO NOT PULL FILTER ALL THE WAY OUT WHEN FLUORESCENCE BULB IS ON
    - YOU CAN HURT YOUR EYES

Focus

Cut off light to ocular (black knob, on right, top). You will see crosshairs, and use it to be sure focus
is okay, but light will be very dim.

Press A (button on front, right) to take picture. Exposure meter on right tells you what proportion
of the exposure is completed, exposure is complete at 1. 3200 ASA will take approximately 15-30
seconds, and 160 ASA will take more than 3 minutes.

Slide filter (behind objective) to block fluorescence. Use this, with visible light button (left, back) to
take visible light picture.

Unload camera:
    Slide out cannister
    Use crank to wind film completely
    Remove film from cannister and holder and replace cannister

To turn off:
    Fluorescence bulb off
    Power off
    Wipe objectives gently and completely with lens paper only

PROTOCOL 3.

A protocol can be made for a procedure as well as for an experiment, and may be posted near the
particular piece of equipment whose use it describes.

INTERPRETING RESULTS

You must examine your data with the same attention to detail that you give to analyzing the experiments of a competitor. Lay out the data and ask yourself:

1. **Did the experiment work?** Check your *controls*. Look at your procedural controls first to ensure that your equipment worked. Did the cells eat? Did the molecular weight markers run as you expected? Examine your positive control. If this worked, your experiment was probably properly executed. Now look at the negative control. If there is an effect where you didn't expect one, you must decide whether this is a real effect or background. If your negative control appears to be negative, all is probably well. If it is positive, either the experiment was not planned correctly or another variable asserted itself during the experiment.

2. **What are the results?** Compared with the controls, and minus the background, *did you get an effect?* How much of an effect? Two fold? Fifty fold? Do all the computation and graphing, so you are comparing data rather than subjective effects. Are two effects synergistic or additive? Did the effect vary over time?

3. **What does the experiment mean?** Does the result make sense? Is the result what you expected? Do you have any explanations for spurious results? Would additional controls help toward an understanding?

4. **Do other investigators understand the experiment?** Talk to other lab members. Discuss the results with the person from whom you obtained the protocol, or from someone versed in the technique. Go back and read background papers again. Don't get too excited yet, until the results have been repeated.

5. **Is the result repeatable?** Do the experiment again. Include controls that would strengthen the result and solve any questions you have about the result.

> The only way to learn to interpret experiments is to do a lot of them. You will develop a feel for what an experiment means, or for what it needs. Experience with different kinds of experiments will enable you to "know" instantly when an experiment has or hasn't worked. DO a lot of experiments.

When Experiments Don't Work

You did the experiment, and got a completely unexpected result.

1. If it is a procedural problem, *check your equipment.* Make sure plugs were attached, that you used the right buffer. Go carefully through your notes to see if you omitted anything.

2. *Redo the experiment.* This often takes care of the problem, because many mistakes with positive and negative controls are manipulation mistakes.

3. *If the problem recurs, redo only that part of the experiment* that is in question. An experiment with only positive and negative controls is usually what is needed.

> For example, if a negative control gave a strong signal in your assay, check only the negative control and a negative control obtained from another source in a very small repeat experiment, against a positive control. If only the original negative control "behaved" incorrectly, there is a problem only with the negative control, and not the rest of the experiment. If both negative controls give a positive result, you must begin to check buffers and other components.

4. When you have identified a probable source of the problem, *do a small experiment* to see whether the problem is fixed. Do not be tempted to jump in and repeat the original experiment yet—wait until the result has been explained.

5. When you cannot find the source of the trouble, when you have asked advice and done everything you can, *repeat the experiment.* And repeat. And repeat.

> The difficulty is in distinguishing between an experiment that has yet to work, and one that never will. It takes practice and experience, and it will get easier—but it will always be a part of life at the bench.

Switching projects

Most projects start out with hope and excitement. As they are nurtured and explored, as so many hours are poured into experiments, the investigator can lose perspective. Emotion and ego are involved in the success of a project. It sometimes seems impossible to give a project up.

It is imperative that, as a scientist, you learn when to stop a project. And since, with such emotional investment, you won't always be able to make such a decision, you should solicit and accept advice.

Knowing when to halt a project is not always clear. In fact, it is very seldom clear. Some indications are:

> *An idea often precedes the available technology. No matter how spectacular and important the idea is, if you can't reliably prove it, you should not work on it.*

- *The data are not reproducible.* If you cannot replicate your results, even if you heartily believe in them, you cannot further the project. It may be that there are problems with a particular assay or piece of equipment, and this should be investigated before the project is dropped. It may also be that such variations are inherent in the system, or that the effect is not important, or that the effect you are studying is too small to be explored with the technology available.

- *The project has no support from the P.I.* Laboratories vary greatly in the amount of independence each lab worker has. In some places, you will choose your own project and how to go about it, and will receive very little actual instruction from the P.I. But you will probably get advice or opinions, and you should listen. Even if you have been given complete free rein, it makes no sense to continue with a project that the P.I. does not believe in: It is very difficult to work well on a project the lab head does not like. Of course, try to convince him or her with your data. If that doesn't work, consider a change of project.

> *There are P.I.s who care little for personnel and assign projects with little chance of success. This is usually done because he or she has an idea that he is interested in, but has no real chance of working. If you feel you are being sacrificed, do something immediately. Talk to the P.I., and talk to others in the department: It is a character assessment as well as scientific acumen you must judge. If he or she refuses to remove you from a project that is obviously doomed, you should consider leaving the lab.*

- *The direction of the project has changed.* Unexpected results may send the project down a path that neither the lab nor the investigator wants to follow. An example would be a student who started working in a fly lab on a protein thought to be critical in *Drosophila* physiology. After cloning and sequencing the gene, he discovers that the protein is involved in mammalian neurogenesis, and that the role in *Drosophila* is of minor importance. The project has changed, and the student must decide whether to study neurogenesis in a lab equipped for fly genetics, join or collaborate with another lab, or drop the project.

- *The project is too difficult.* The difficulty of a project has to be judged against the time you have to work on it. If your visa will expire in 2 years, you don't want to work on a project that will take 4 more years to continue. One option is to have someone ready to take over the project, and share in the kudos. It is not a failure to switch projects! Most failure-to-thrive problems come from inexperienced researchers clinging to a nonviable project.

"Waiting for the bus in the rain" or "I've invested too much time in this project to quit now."

You arrive at the bus stop. You wait for the bus. It is late. You look at your watch, you look at the rainy streets, you look at your watch. This bus is never late—usually. But it is today. There is another bus you could take, if you hurry around the corner. But yet...you have invested so much time in this bus, what if it comes just after you have left?

Well, what if it does? What have you really lost if you get on the other bus? Research is like waiting for the bus in the rain. There will be no neon sign telling you when to change projects, but you must make an informed decision. You can't worry about time you think you have wasted if you switch projects. Think about the time you will waste if you don't switch when you should.

RESOURCES

Bausell R. Barker. 1994. *Conducting meaningful experiments: 40 steps to becoming a scientist.* Sage Publications, Thousand Oaks, California. (Covers the philosophy of experiments, deciding whether an experiment is worthwhile, and analyzing and reporting the results.)

Brown S., McDowell L., and Race P. 1995. *500 tips for research students.* Kogan Page, London. (Intended for students but useful for all researchers, especially ones in an academic environment. Contains not only tips on setting up experiments, but practical advice on such topics as coping with uncertainty, attending conferences, and developing your institutional know-how.)

Carey S.S. 1993. *A beginner's guide to scientific method.* Wordsworth Publishing, Belmont, California.

Carr J.J. 1992. *The art of science: A practical guide to experiments, observations, and handling data.* Hightext Publications, San Diego.

Jacobs, Jr. W.R., Kalpana G.V., Cirillo J.D., Pascopella L., Snapper S.B., Udani R.A., Jones W., Barletta R.G., and Bloom B.R. 1991. Genetic systems for mycobacteria. *Methods Enzymol.* **204:** 537–555.

Koch A.L. 1994. Growth measurement. In *Methods for general and molecular bacteriology* (ed. Gerhardt P. et al.), pp. 249–276. American Society for Microbiology, Washington, D.C.

Koosis D.J. 1997. *Statistics. A self-teaching guide.* John Wiley & Sons, New York.

Rosen A., Nairn A.C., Greengard P., Cohn Z.A, and Aderem A. 1989. Bacterial lipopolysaccharide regulates the phosphorylation of the 68K protein kinase C substrate in macrophages. *J. Biol. Chem.* **264:** 9118–9121.

Stent G. 1982. Prematurity and uniqueness in scientific discovery. In *Readings from Scientific American. Scientific genius and creativity,* pp. 95–104.

Wald G. 1968. Molecular basis of visual excitation. *Science* **162:** 230–239.

Woodward J. and Goodstein D. 1996. Conduct, misconduct and the structure of science. *Am. Sci.* **84:** 479–490.

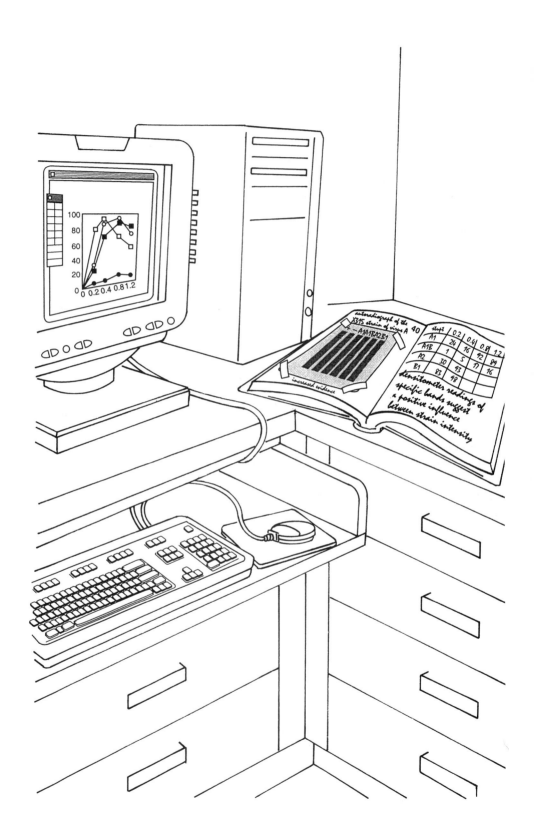

5

Laboratory Notebooks

THE LABORATORY NOTEBOOK is the record you keep of the methods and results of your experiments. *If there is a fire in the lab, grab your lab notebook.* Leave the computer, the plasmids in the freezer, the special apparatus the glass shop rigged up for you—*nothing*

TYPE AND FORMAT	89
CONTENT	92
MAINTENANCE	93
ETHICS	96
RESOURCES	99

is as valuable as your raw data. With it, you can write papers, plan experiments, and build on your results: Without it, you might as well have not been in the lab.

Your lab notebook should be clear and thorough. If something goes wrong, you must be able to go back and figure out what happened: Did you use older cells in the previous experiment? Was the incubation buffer made correctly? Did the enzyme suddenly stop working from one day to the next? Your lab book should be packed with clues that will help you solve the problem. Furthermore, *another scientist* should also be able to interpret your notes. A scribbled record, interpretable only by the writer, is not only obscure but is actually suspicious. Your lab book should be a defense against, not a proof of, fraud. It is proof of who you are, as a scientist.

TYPE AND FORMAT

Sheets versus book? There are many ways to record data. Before you invest your time in a particular method, be sure to *find out if the organization or P.I. requires a certain format.* Some companies and organizations have extremely stringent rules: This is not only because of issues of fraud, but also for protection, in the case of drug development and/or lawsuits.

For example, in one international pharmaceutical company, numbered notebooks must be signed out of the office. The lab book, with numbered pages, must be kept every day, and countersigned every day by someone not connected with the project. The lab books are locked every night. They are kept indefinitely, and are microfiched once a year: They are never considered to be personal property. When a compound is being considered for human trials, the data and calculations in the notebooks are checked for errors by a group of people.

Needless to say, not all of these rules are followed in every laboratory. But if you are required to stay on top of your data this way, just do it. You'll never regret having organized data, and you will just have to cope with the sometimes tedious attention to detail.

Academic laboratories tend to be much more liberal in their lab book requirements, and many have no rules or guidelines whatsoever. Here you may find everything from data kept on paper towels to bound notebooks with carbon paper. Check with the P.I., and follow his recommendations. Most will recommend a book.

There are advantages and disadvantages to all styles of lab notebooks.

Type	Advantages	Drawbacks
Bound book	No lost sheets Proof against fraud	Experiments entered as done, no logical order

Loose leaf sheets/
folders
	Can group by experiment,
	  maintain order
	Easy to record data
	  during experiments
		Can lose sheets, harder to prove
		  authenticity

Computer/ spread sheet	Easy to read Easy to do calculations	Can lose data, harder to prove authenticity

Looseleaf sheets are good for organizing multiple projects. They are also good for manipulations during experiments, since you can use a clipboard and not worry about the bulk of a notebook. Entering data directly into a computer makes further manipulations, such as graphing and statistics, quite simple. But accountability is an issue that only a bound notebook can address. If you have a choice of notebook type, *go with the bound book.*

What to look for in a bound lab notebook

- Large, 8 1/2 by 11 inches. You can attach photographs and some printouts, and have room for notes.

- Bound pages. It should be impossible to rip pages out without destroying the integrity of the book.

- Numbered pages.

- White, gridded pages. Lined pages are too confining, blank pages become messy quickly.

- Duplicate pages. The second page is usually yellow, with perforations that allow it to be torn out easily.

Effective use of a bound lab notebook

Use pen only, never pencil. Write on the white page, with carbon paper to record a copy on the yellow page. The white page remains in your notebook.

The yellow pages will be your second copy. Set up a file system for these pages, in folders. Put all data that don't fit into the notebook into the corresponding folder with the yellow pages.

Write the date and the experiment on *all* pieces of data, including printouts and photographs.

Keep your notebook and folders in different places.

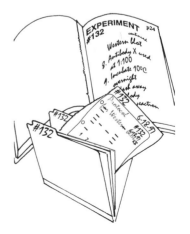

FIGURE 1.

Set up a file system for printouts, photographs, X-rays, duplicate (yellow) lab notebook pages, and for all data that cannot be neatly taped onto a notebook page. Each experiment should have its own folder.

CONTENT

The record of every experiment should contain:

- **Date of the start of the experiment.** Put a complete date (including the year) on every page, even on continuation pages.

- **Title of the experiment.** *Brief* is best. Examples are "Mini-preps of library clones" or "PMA effect on chemokine release from fibroblasts."

- **Brief statement of purpose.** This is an extension of the title, with a bit more detail. For the titles above, one might add "To check the insert sizes of the chicken cDNA library" and "Compare sparse vs dense cultures for IL-8 release." The title and purpose may be combined.

- **Description of the experiment.** *The protocol for the experiment* could be written out in the book before you begin, and amended as you do the experiment. A copy of a protocol could be pasted in, and also amended as you go. Always give a reference for the protocol you are using. This may be a journal article or a protocol from a book, or a reference to a protocol you developed ("as done on 9/5/97; see page 13").

Record *calculations* on an empty, adjoining page. Include calculations for concentrations, dilutions, molecular weights, and molarities.

Everything that happens—and doesn't happen—is *data*. Include all controls as data, including standard curves and 0 time point numbers.

As you go, tape what *print-outs and pictures* will fit into the notebook. Keep everything else together, well-labeled, so that the origin can be determined if they are separated from the rest of the write-up. File in folders with the yellow copies.

If it makes it easier for you to keep track of the data points, draw a scheme of the layout of the samples. For example, if you often use a 96-well plate, photocopy a plate or a template, tape it into your book, and record the sample descriptions onto it.

At the end of the accumulation of all data, write a *one-sentence summation of the results* of the experiment. Note any oddity or aberration, and add any comments about why the experiment may or may not have worked.

> **Table of contents.** At the beginning of the lab notebook, or on a separate blank sheet, keep a table of contents, with experiments listed by title, date, and page number. It seems like a pain, but it will always save you time when you are searching for a particular set of data.

YOU WILL NOT BE ABLE TO REMEMBER EVERYTHING. YOU MIGHT NOT BE ABLE TO REMEMBER ANYTHING.

Record everything. There is nothing too minor to record. Write so anyone (including yourself) can pick up your notebook and duplicate the experiment (and the results) perfectly.

Information commonly omitted that you might need later:

Serum lot number
Antibody titer
Other people involved
Centrifuge model, speed, and temperature
Incubation time
Number of washes
Tube type and sizes
Unanticipated delays in incubations, washes, and treatments
Growth medium used
Buffer pH
Calculations
Initial number of cells
Age and passage number of culture
Agarose or acrylamide percentage of gel
Growth stage of bacteria
Condition of the cells used: sparse vs overgrown culture, granular cells, floating cells in an adherent culture

MAINTENANCE

It is not enough to record data as you go along. Unless you update and review the notebook, you will not have a good grasp of the contents.

Record everything as soon as you can. Try to record the experiment as you proceed through the experiment. If this is not possible (for example, when you are working with radioactivity), do it at the end of the experiment. And if you can't do this, do it the next day, at the latest. DO NOT save one day a week to record your data. The 20+ experiments that you might do in a week can become a mental muddle by the end of the week.

Do weekly check-ups. Set a regular block of an hour to go through your notebook. Even if you are working all weekend, Friday is often a convenient time. Use this time to do the following (see p. 96):

Lab notebook styles can be very individualized, but must still contain the essential elements. (See sample notebook pages on pages 94 and 95; courtesy of Jian Guo, University of Washington, Hongxia Fan, Rockefeller University, and Clare Carroll, Rockefeller University.)

March 15, 1993. [155 RNA]

Using LEEs DNA, inoculate the rest of DNA #3 ☀ (overnight)
into 500 ml LB/AMP. → SHAKE 37°C. Maxi-Prep tomorrow.

RNA ISOLATION

Kb grew up G 500-600 mls 155. Isolated RNA in
Guth, low acetate etc.

Reprecipitated 2x in GuHCl. Pellet look big but Kb added
glycogen. (we'll see after OD reading.)

Wash 2x in 70% ETOH. Spin 10', 13K. 4°C.
Pellets are a nice size (could be DNA?)
Reprecipitated in 1/10 vol KAcet 3M, 100% ETOH 2 vol.

3-16-93.
Spin down 12M 30', 15K, 4°C.
Small pellets

PHOTOMETRIC   SET SAMPLE, PRESS START KEY
λ 260.0   5ul → 600ul ddH₂O
No. A1
 1   0.130 →→ LEE DNA   500ul TE.
 2   0.068 →→ RNA 1st 155. 50ul DEPC
 3   0.029 →→ RNA 2nd

DNA = 121 × .130 × 50 = 786.5 ug/ml in 600ul → 393.25 ug

RNA   121 × .068 × 40 = 329.12 in 50 ul → 16.5 ug.

RNA   121 × .029 × 40 = 140.36 ng/ml in 50ul → 7.8 ug.
RNA at 20 in salt/alcohol.

15:31 3/17 '93   260.0NM   0.029A

June 3, 1992 COUNTS of ³H-uracil uptake. Merlos 5-26 D1, D2, D5

	TCA D.1	TCA D.2	TCA D5	D.1	D.2	D.5
-	3101.5	1529.4	187.7	4688.1	1496.8	322.6
	1408.5	1633.6	309.9	4288.6	1496.0	2692.3
1:1 155	274.9	489.9	99447.0	3921.5	4672.1	40883.3
1:1 155	275.7	3828.4	55954.2	274.5	3616.Y	35166.9
5:1 155	17460.4	10168.0	96931.7	15998.3	11483.8	92499.5
5:1 155	16787.9	10901.8	101587.1	7843.9	11055.0	81683.5
10:1 155	965.8	14157.4	100727.0	6587.9	28667.0	98439.9
10:1 155	621.5	22503.8	101739.4	601.7	34246.9	76547.8
20:1 155	873.6	67394.5	146437.4	11641.8	64448.2	140389.3
20:1 155	778.4	78718.4	146041.4	800.2	64456.4	121926.8
5:1 coli	1988.0	1470.3	36800.3	20536.4	4480.8	5644.4
5:1 coli	903.3	27148.3	45760.6	23151.1	6158.7	3717.0
10:1 coli	15204.2	20207.2	46085.1	12424.0	6603.3	4740.7
10:1 coli	14104.7	26543.3	46387.4	16603.1	15867.3	4540.5
5:1 BCC 10s	1346.5	25314.0	2434.5	681.8	31837.3	1083.9
5:1 BCC 10s	1318.6	34581.4	1434.2	4192.8	31948.9	1113.4
10:1 BCC 10s	5222.3	2499.8	87481.0	4027.9	30749	7026.4
10:1 BCC 10s	3397.3	21707	81634.3	21299.8	26757	8199.4
5:1 BCC 20s	9905.0	1677.1	5110.7	11151.3	2059.8	1575.8
5:1 BCC 20s	8990.8	1520.2	1801.7	7213.7	1779.5	1170.2
10:1 BCC 20s	472.8	4390.7	5738.9	581.3	6743.0	1943.2
10:1 BCC 20s	428.1	25548	3714.7	419.7	6456.2	1932.5

Added 1250 ul TCA

TCA samples washed w/ETOH only. (Kept at 4°C)
Plain samples washed w/ H₂O & ETOH. (kept frozen at -20°C)

Immunoscreen — 16 day mouse embryo cDNA library in λEXlox® vector

1. titer library ~ 1.3 x 10⁴ pfu

2. make BL21
   ① grow BL21 O/N
   ② spin 20' at 2000 rpm 4°C
   ③ resuspend the cells to OD_{600} = 0.5 in 10mM MgSO4

3. plate (15cm 2xYT/liter)
   ① { 2.5ul original / ∅
       747.5 ul 5M
       750 ul BL21   (OD_{600} = 0.5)
   ② mix well, at 37°C for 15'-20'
   ③ add ~8ml 2xYT top agar
   ④ plate. and incubate at 37°C for 7 hrs
      just until small plaques become visible (0.5 – 1mm size)
   ⑤ apply the numbered IPTG-treated membrane to the plates
   ⑥ freeze at 4°C O/N

4. treat the membrane with 10mM IPTG before apply the membrane to plate
   ① dilute IPTG in sterile ddH2O to 10mM
   ② 30' prior to use, wet the membrane in IPTG sol
      place the membranes on Whatman 3mm paper to air dry

→ count colonies
→ grow up 10 colonies in 2ml of LB/0.2% Maltose/kan, 37°C, O/N
→ miniprep DNA

Dilution	cfu (5ul)
10⁻³	20 50
	600 3000

5.0 λ	DNA
1.5	#3 NEB
0.5	BamHI (20 u/λ)
5.0	RNase A
3.0	ddH2O
15.0	37°C, 1 hr

∴ Vector is not pT4ø 78.

- Transformation of .155
  200-400 µl   .155 competent cells
  0.5 µl   each of 10 colonies
  10'   4°C
  → electroporate at

	②	③	⑤	④	⑥	⑦
	10 µl	pNVα06 (0.14 µg/λ)	for ①,③,③	①	⑤	④
T=	2.5 KV	2.5 KV	2.5 KV	2.5	2.5	2.5
R=	129 Ω	480 Ω	480 Ω	189	129	720
S=	1.45 KV	2.45 KV	1.45 KV	1.25	1.25	1.25
Gap=	0.2 cm	0.2 cm	0.2 cm	0.2	0.2	0.2
FS=	5.18 KV/cm	2.78 KV/cm	1.38	1.36	1.34	1.38
t=	1.33 msec	16.8 msec	3.44	8.05	4.08	2.95	10.09

→ inc on ice, 10'
→ add 400 µl of comp 7H9, 37°C, shake

- *Attach all data, printouts, and X-rays to the appropriate experiments.* If the paper or picture is small, tape it into the book. If it is large, place it in the experiment file. Most films need to be held up to the light to be seen properly, so file even small films instead of putting them in the book.

- *Make tables and graphs.* Try to do this during the week, but certainly do it before the week is over. A graph or a table makes all data easier to interpret; it looks "real," and will validate your position in a discussion far better than a wordy explanation. You also want to avoid making dozens of graphs and tables only when you are writing the paper or giving a lab seminar. If the table or graph is small, tape it into the notebook; otherwise, file it in the folder.

> *If you don't know your data, the experiments are useless. Only by knowing your results can you plan your course, discuss your conclusions, and be in control.*

- *Write summaries for all the week's experiments.* Go through every experiment, and be sure there is a sentence or two summarizing the results at the end of every one. Feel free to write more—interpretations, recommendations for other experiments—but always write your summary where you can flip through the notebook and find it.

- *Record the experiment in the table of contents.* By simply recording the titles and dates of the experiments you will greatly boost your organization, since you can much more quickly find any experiment you want. If appropriate, record the page number.

- *Make a plan for the following week.* While the data are fresh in your mind, think a bit about what they mean and what you need to do next. A written summary is probably unrealistic, but would be amazingly helpful.

Solicit feedback on your data and your plans. Once you know your data, discuss them with coworkers or your P.I. You don't need to completely understand what all the results mean to initiate a discussion, but you certainly must know what the data are.

ETHICS

Ownership. *The lab notebook belongs to the laboratory, not to the labworker.* If you are terribly attached to your book and want to keep it when you leave, discuss it with the

P.I. He or she may be happy with a copy, but that would be unusual. Ask whether you may take the yellow copies.

> *It is considered to be an invasion of privacy for one lab worker to read another person's lab notebook without asking.*

Don't be afraid to make your lab notebook personal, with remarks, lamentations, and peeves noted, as long as the data are reported clearly and thoroughly. But too much deviation from the data is unprofessional and could be embarrassing, so minimize the emotional information.

Public versus private. The lab notebook is a curious document, a mixture of a public and private record. In most places, it is left on desks or lab benches, but is never looked at by anyone but the "owner." Don't sneak a peek at another lab member's book, even (or especially) if you want to check on suspected fraudulent data. If you suspect fraud, speak to the P.I. And if you suspect someone is examining your book, lock it up or give it to the P.I. to lock up at night.

P.I. access. Generally, the P.I. will read technicians' and summer students' notebooks freely, but will not read graduate students' or post-docs', as this is viewed as intellectual infringement by many. But don't be offended if your book is examined, especially if the P.I. is helping you troubleshoot an experiment. It is technically a public document and should be able to stand up to scrutiny.

Archives. How long should a lab notebook and raw data be kept? Because of space limitations, most labs cannot keep all lab notebooks indefinitely. They should be kept for *5 years,* and disposed of only at the discretion of the head of the laboratory.

Don't dispose of

- Old notebooks you find when you start in a lab
- Your own notebooks, even after 5 years
- Any notebooks for an ongoing project
- Data found in drawers and on the computer

> *Omitting a result is falsifying data.*

Recording data. A "mistake" made in your notebook will be amplified by the time it makes it into the literature, so be absolutely rigorous about recording everything as accurately and honestly as you can.

Never omit a data point from your notebook! There are statistical criteria for eliminating data points, and these should be followed. Some kinds of data do not lend themselves to this kind of analysis, and the decision to jettison a data point is harder to justify.

> You may be pushed to obtain certain results. In many cases of fraud, the perpetrator has blamed the P.I., saying that the P.I. expected a particular result, and the researcher felt compelled to produce it. It is true that a P.I. may want a result. **But your data are your responsibility,** and it is up to you to be sure the data are recorded honestly and accurately.

If you drop a data point, note in your lab book the reason you have eliminated it from calculations and graphing. Write "since I think I had jiggled that plate," or "because such a result was not seen in 6 other experiments," or "the cells didn't look healthy." No matter how weak your reasoning seems to you (and if it does seem weak, perhaps you shouldn't be doing it), you must make clear what data you discounted and why.

RESOURCES

Broad W. and Wade N. 1992. *Betrayers of the truth. Fraud and deceit in the halls of science.* Simon and Schuster, New York.

Carr J.J. 1992. *The art of science. A practical guide to experiments, observations, and handling data.* HighText Publications, San Diego.

Schrader-Frechette K. 1994. *Ethics of scientific research. Issues in academic ethics.* Rowman & Littlefield, Lanham, Maryland.

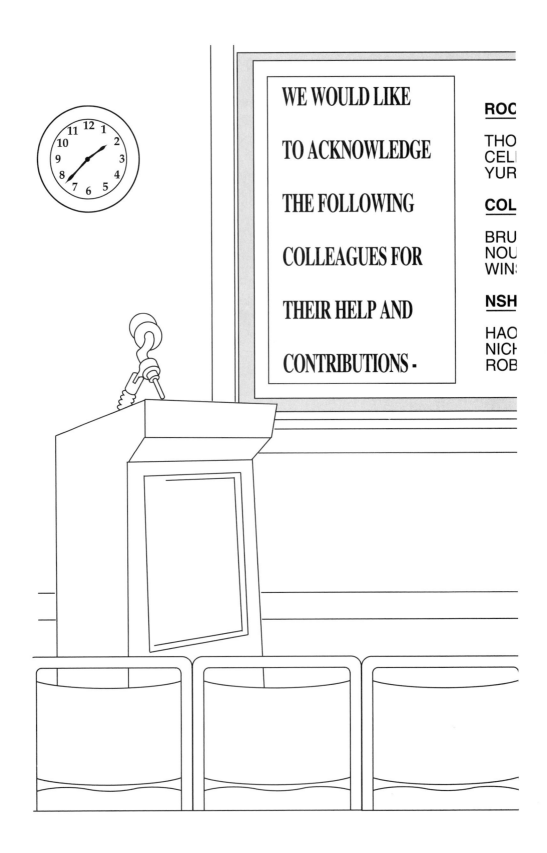

6

Presenting Yourself and Your Data

IF YOU CAN'T COMMUNICATE your data, they don't exist. You must be able to explain your results and the implications of those results to people with more and less knowledge than you have. This is done orally, through discussions and seminars, and on paper, through journal articles and grant submissions. You should become comfortable—or appear comfortable—with both. If your first language is not the language of the lab, presenting yourself well can be an even more difficult task, but it still must be done.

COMMUNICATION TIPS	101
Getting along in the lab	102
Networking	106
Attending seminars	108
ORAL PRESENTATIONS	110
Research seminars	111
Journal clubs	116
Presentation tools	118
WRITTEN PRESENTATIONS	121
Manuscripts	121
Grants	123
RESOURCES	126

Presenting your data well is not something merely for the ambitious. It is necessary for your survival.

COMMUNICATION TIPS

Forget the still-cherished image of the scientist struggling alone in the lab at midnight, shunning the world. For sure, there will be plenty of late hours with you alone with your tubes, but it is not possible to practice modern science in a vacuum. As many discoveries and connections are made in conversations as in biochemical assays, and you must be open to contact with other scientists to make the most of their—and your own—research.

Getting Along in the Lab

The first and most important situation in which you will present yourself is to the people in your own laboratory. Most of what you make of yourself in science has its basis in how your fellow researchers perceive you and your data, and it is well worth expending energy to deal with the other lab members.

Chapter 1 describes some of the usually unspoken rules to follow when you first start work in a new lab. But the nature of your communication with other lab members will evolve as weeks turn into months, and new issues will take on importance.

- **Absentee P.I.** People in labs complain that either the P.I. is oppressively present and wants to know every detail of what is going on, or is never around. If the P.I. of your lab isn't around a lot, take it upon yourself to stay in touch. Leave a note about a good result, pop into her office for 5 minutes, try to have lunch together. It's your career, and you are the one to be hurt if the P.I. can't remember you when it is time to write a recommendation.

- **Bay- and benchmates.** These are your physically (and often, emotionally) closest colleagues in the laboratory. Your bench- and baymates will be the first to see great raw data, the first to know that the Big Experiment didn't work, the first to hear your ruminations and give advice on your experiments. And you will offer the same services to your benchmates. Enjoy the scientific expertise and companionship so close at hand. But in this intimate situation, you must sometimes allow for privacy: There are times when you must just back off and leave your bay- or benchmate alone.

- **Collaborations and credit.** Although most collaborations are worked out before the experiments really begin, they can move in unplanned directions. The usual problem is that the importance of the individual experiments has changed, and the assumed first author will be relegated to another position on the credit list. Ask the P.I. to mediate all disputes.

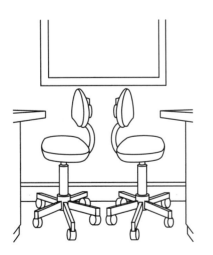

- **Confrontations.** Most lab confrontations involve a lab member angry because another lab member broke a piece of equipment and didn't deal with it, didn't do the assigned lab job, used up a reagent without ordering more, or used a "private" reagent or equipment without permission. If you are the offended party, deal only with the immediate issue, and don't make personal

remarks or ascribe an evil agenda to the perpetrator. If
you are the guilty party, confess and deal with the
problem as soon as possible, without excuses or resentment.

> *It is helpful to have an occa-sional lab meeting dedicated to airing complaints about lab equipment.*

    Another class of confrontation deals with intellec-
tual (and emotional) property. Someone may be angry because she believes another lab member infringed on her project, or discussed sensitive data with an outside person. It is worth the two parties trying alone to fix this, but it is usually
necessary to ask the P.I. to mediate. Don't bring personal disagreements to the P.I.

- **Deadlines.** Follow deadlines, your own and others, religiously. It keeps you organized, and it helps everyone to whom you have made a commitment. Try to set a
deadline when someone asks you to do something (or when you ask someone for
a favor): For example, if you ask someone to read a manuscript, you could say
"Can you read this manuscript this week? If not, let me know and I'll ask someone else."

- **Difficult P.I.s.** The P.I. has a lot of control over the path of a researcher's career,
and there will always be some people who deal badly with this kind of power.
Although you should have checked out the personal dynamics of the lab before
joining (by asking others in the lab and department how well they enjoy working
there), you may find yourself in a nasty situation. The difficulty can take many
forms, and you must be able to sort out the trivial from the important. If you
think there is a serious problem, document all complaints, include witnesses for
confrontations, and seek collaboration of the problem from other lab members
before deciding what to do.

- **Favorites.** In a lab, there always seems to be someone who has the P.I.'s attention
and admiration. Look carefully. Is it deserved? Maybe you can learn something.
And if it isn't deserved, mind your own business and learn to not let it bother you.
It is only a problem if you feel it results in detrimental treatment to yourself.
Concentrate on your experiments.
    The favorite could be you! If so, don't abuse the situation, and don't let it get
to your head. You might be out of favor tomorrow.

- **Gossip and bad-mouthing.** It is true that the line between gossip and information isn't clear. People do talk about people. But be careful. You have to live with
your labmates, so don't sabotage the relationships by passing on information that
isn't anyone's business. The intimate atmosphere of the lab demands a high level
of respect and consideration, even for people you may not like.
    Most large labs find a scapegoat, someone to blame for the missing gel
combs, radioactive ice buckets, and dearth of good results. Don't jump on the
bandwagon. The talk may be true, but it is also possible that a long-ago personal

problem with one person became unfairly expanded. Make your own unbiased judgments as time goes on.

It is also common for labs to dislike the work of certain other labs, usually competitors. Do not assume this idea is right, and continue to assess competitors' work honestly and fairly. Don't disparage other people's results without good cause. It is not true that making someone look bad makes you look good. Nothing is to be gained by bad-mouthing anyone.

- **Harassment.** The atmosphere can cause one to assume too much and get quite sloppy. Never be casual about racist or sexist remarks. If you feel you are the target of harassment, speak your mind firmly and in front of other lab members before you think about official action.

For the nonnative English speaker

- Resist the urge to speak your native language in the lab, even if the majority of the lab members speak the same language. Speak only English at work.

- Keep your lab notebook in English.

- Take a speaking or writing class in English. Many universities have conversation groups, where you can practice English once a week with other nonnative English speakers. You could also start your own conversation group.

- Practice speaking with people who are willing to correct you. Let other lab members know that you want mistakes to be pointed out to you.

- Always ask a native English speaker to read through and correct everything you write.

- Ask lab members to clarify what you don't understand. For experimental protocols, this is particularly important. If a repeated explanation still isn't satisfactory, ask the person to write down what they are saying.

- Before any oral presentation—even for an informal lab seminar—go through your talk with a native English speaker. Incorporate that person's comments, and practice the talk again in front of the same person.

- Ask a person who speaks your native language, but speaks and writes English well, to comment on your speech and on your written work. People speaking the same language tend to make many of the same mistakes, and this person could point out patterns of mistakes.

- For your first seminar, write out exactly what you are going to say. Have someone correct it. If you feel you are too nervous to memorize or ad lib a good talk, read your lecture.

- Socialize with other lab members. Go to lunch or to happy hour once in a while, and try to join in the conversation. Don't forget to ask people to correct you.

- **In or out.** Your data are good, the P.I. thinks you are good. The data are nonexistent, the P.I. thinks you are nothing. Have a thick skin, and don't rely on results as the sole basis for your feeling of self-worth.

- **Language.** If English is not your native language, it is imperative that you learn to speak and write English as well as you can. Most people in the lab will respect your scientific skills and admire you tremendously for assuming the task of doing science in another language. But some, in the lab and outside, might still avoid working with you if they can't understand you. Without good language skills, it will be difficult to advance in your job or obtain a new job that you are otherwise qualified for.

- **Letters of recommendation.** Letters of recommendation will be an issue for many years, because they are required for many grant and job applications, even at the full professor level. This is not to say that you should curry favor with people because of the letters you may need. But keep in mind that you should be enough a member of the scientific community that you could easily give several names of scientists who know you and know your work. If you can't think of three people from whom you could expect a good letter, you are probably not interacting enough with other scientists.

- **Personal and political differences.** Almost everything gets discussed in labs, sometimes quite heatedly. Try not to let disagreements get in the way of lab interactions.

- **Socializing.** Very important! This is especially important if you have children or commute, and don't get to hang out in the lab at night. Many collaborations are forged over lunch or a beer. Make it a point to join, at least occasionally, in lab parties or outings.

- **Time.** There is no unit of time smaller than half an hour in the lab. If you are arranging a time to get together with someone, always add 30 minutes to your most generous estimation of when you will be ready.

- **Vacations.** There is probably an unofficial vacation policy, as well as an official one. Find out what the lab policy is, and try to conform to it. If it is the custom to take no vacations (a strange and macho custom in some academic institutions), you should take one anyway, but be prepared to deal with sullen resentment and snide remarks.

  Try not to arrange any vacation at a particularly bad time for the laboratory. Give the P.I. plenty of notice about the date and extent of your vacation! Tell her, in person. Then write down the dates of your departure and return, and give it to the secretary. It is also useful to post a notice on your desk or bench, so others in the lab know when to expect you back. Even if you decide to take just one day off, always let someone in the lab know.

Networking

Networking is a fancy term for staying in touch with people in your field. It is necessary. It takes energy. But don't worry if you aren't terrifically extroverted. It certainly helps, but there are many ways in which you can interact with other scientists.

- **Chatrooms and newsgroups on the WWW.** Scientific chatrooms and newsgroups allow you to exchange information, scientific or otherwise, on the Internet. You can do anything from getting a recipe for a buffer to asking advice about a job offer at another institution.

- **Collaborations.** A good collaboration is exhilarating. Two or more people, with different and complementary expertise, can achieve much more than the sum of the parts. And it is fun, it is everything one expects from science, but a bad collaboration is a drain without compensation.

  Don't make any collaboration, even a casual one, without discussing it first with the P.I.!

  All collaborations take more time than you think. The agreement starts out with the promise of "just one experiment," but this almost always expands and expands into multiple controls and experiments. If you can't afford the time, if participation has become one-sided or unfair, or if results are not forthcoming, end the collaboration as soon as you can.

- **Confidence.** Don't be intimidated by titles and long C.V.s: Don't let fear of not knowing as much as someone else stop you from discussing data with that person.

- **Conflict of interest.** Multiple collaborations can lead you here, so be on the alert that your collaborators are not in competition with each other. Be up front with everyone you are working with.

  Reviewing a competitor's grant or manuscript is another conflict of interest. If you will be influenced by the data you will read about, you should not review the grant or manuscript. It is perfectly permissible to return something you have been asked to review with a note saying that you are unable to do so, and why.

- **Good data.** Great results are a passport to the scientific community. When you are a winner, everyone wants to know you. If sudden success happens to you, take advantage of the opportunity to meet as many people as you can: Promote your data and yourself enough to last through the inevitable dry times. But don't rest on your laurels, and don't assess your self-worth based on your good data any more than on your "bad" data.

- **E-mail.** E-mail is an easy way to request a plasmid or ask for a protocol. Sending a quick note to someone you met at a meeting, or complimenting someone on a

How to "give" a poster session

- If someone appears interested in your poster, ask him or her "Would you like me to walk you through this?" Don't just stand quietly beside the poster.
- If the person says no, just remind him that you are available for questions, and fade back.
- Most will say yes, and you should then give a very brief, figure-by-figure summation of the poster.
- Stop when you have finished, let the person move on if he or she pleases: People like to maneuver quickly at poster sessions. Don't be offended at quick comings and goings.
- If you become very engaged with someone, and other people come to see the poster, let everyone know that you are aware of them, and will get to them as soon as possible. Exchange addresses and phone numbers, or arrange another meeting with the (pleasantly) monopolizing person if it is clear that 5 minutes won't be enough time.

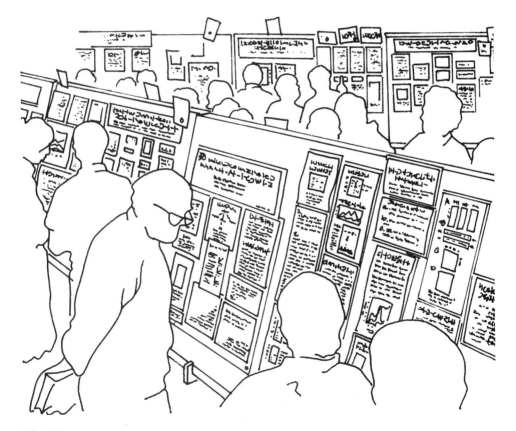

FIGURE 1.

Data set up for a poster session. The actual session, during which the investigators are available to explain the data, is 1 or 2 hours. The boards may be left up for a morning or afternoon.

talk, is relatively painless for sender and recipient and maintains contact with the outside world.

- **Interdepartmental seminars and journal clubs.** Theme meetings with scientists outside of your own group are an easy way to network in your geographical area. If there isn't a cross-institutional meeting in your field, think of starting one.

- **Meetings.** Attend at least one meeting a year. Don't pass up an opportunity to give a talk, but go even if you are not presenting. Once you are at the meeting, be as active as you can about learning the field and meeting people. Poster sessions are the best places at meetings to meet and interact with other scientists. Go to as many posters as you can. Ask questions. Take addresses. Give a poster, if you have a chance.

Attending Seminars

Rule # 1—Stay awake! It is sometimes hard to avoid the Thursday afternoon, 4 P.M. slump. You sit in a crowded seminar room, "listening" to a lecture. The lights are out, the room is warm, the topic is tepid… but be active and pull yourself together! It is rude and grotesque to fall asleep and to lean, slack-jawed and snoring, on the shoulder of the guy next to you. It is insulting to the speaker, and it is an image the rest of the department won't be able to get out of their heads, maybe forever.

Choose carefully the seminars you attend. Don't go to seminars you know you won't listen to.

Furthermore, it really is a complete waste of time to go to a seminar and not then listen actively. Unless there is a political reason that your body had to be at the seminar, bring your mind also: You don't learn anything by merely showing up.

Even if it is a terrible seminar (it happens), don't give into the temptation to call yourself out with your beeper—this is too obvious a ploy. If you really must go, get up and leave.

Stay involved with the seminar by

- **Listening** actively, trying to understand what the speaker is saying.
- **Anticipating** where the speaker is going with the data.
- **Weighing** what the speaker says versus what you know. Relate his experiments to what is known in the field.
- **Reviewing** and **summarizing** what is being said.
- **Looking** at the speaker. It is tempting to just look at the slides, board, or overheads, but you should look as long as you need to take in the data and return your gaze to the speaker.

- **Taking notes.** But listen while you take notes: It is all too possible to take beautiful notes without hearing a word.
- **Sorting** out evidence and facts from statements unsupported by evidence. Make judgments, but remain open-minded. Be ready to ask a question about something you don't understand.
- **Asking questions.** In an informal seminar, you can ask the questions as they occur to you, but you should wait until the end of a formal meeting to ask most questions.
- **Sitting up.** Don't get too comfortable, and keep your gaze focused on the speaker.

Asking questions

Questions and answers are the very heart of scientific research, so you must let go of

At most seminars, the same few people ask questions. Why? Does no one else have a question? Of course they do—if they were listening, that is. The reason more people don't ask questions is insecurity. Oh, it is masked behind reasonable explanations, such as

- My question won't interest anyone else, so I'll ask the speaker after the seminar.
- I won't be able to express my question, it is too complicated.
- I'm probably supposed to know the answer, it is my field.
- It is too obvious a question. Everyone else knows the answer.
- I don't want to look stupid or unread.
- I don't want to have a confrontation in public.
- I must have missed the slide that would explain. I can't let on that I wasn't paying attention.

any baggage that prevents you from asking questions freely.

Formulate questions as the seminar progresses. Try to ask at least one question a seminar. Listen to the answer. You may have a follow-up question.

Acknowledge the answer. Nod, smile, or say something to thank the speaker for the answer. Question, don't attack. If you must ask a hostile question, do it very politely and professionally.

Ask only questions you want the answer to! Don't ask a question because you want everyone to know that you

You may be nervous, but learn to live with it. It is important that you be an active rather than a passive participant in all laboratory meetings and discussions.

know your stuff, and that your own experiments are exciting and brilliant ("That was a very interesting talk. Now, in *my* lab......") This is a very transparent maneuver.

ORAL PRESENTATIONS

Consider that you are giving an oral presentation every time you discuss your data with someone. Not to say you should be stiff or formal, but you must be organized and thoughtful. The same rules apply to conversations as to international meetings.

 Preparation

- **Prepare what you are going to say** before you say it whether you are having a one-on-one conversation with the P.I., or are giving a seminar at an international meeting. Learn as much as you can about the topic to be discussed.
- **Know your audience.** It is your responsibility to get an idea across. If you are speaking in a place you don't know, ask several weeks beforehand about the composition of the listeners. Are they students, physicians, chemists? It will (it should!) make a difference in the preparation of the talk.

- **Practice** your talk. Practice it alone. Practice it in front of critics, at least 3 days before the seminar so you will have time to calmly make changes. Practice with your visual aids. Shorten the seminar if it runs over time

 Execution

- **Don't worry about nervousness**—think of it as excitement and channel it into enthusiasm. Most people get nervous.

- **Speak clearly and distinctly.** Avoid mumbling, speaking too fast, speaking too slowly, and mispronouncing words.

- **Be alert for conversational tics** and eliminate them. Don't say "Uhhhh," "Uhmmm," or "Okay" at the end of every sentence.

- **Watch the timing** of the seminar. If it is supposed to be a 45-minute seminar, make sure the seminar is 45 minutes or less, even if you have to jettison some of your slides to make it. Less is more.

- **Inject your personality** into the talk. It keeps you and the audience more attentive, and it reminds everyone that a seminar is really a large conversation.

Research Seminars

The laboratory seminar is the forum in which you will present your own data to your lab or department members. Although you should be constantly talking to the head of the lab and other coworkers about your data, the laboratory seminar is where you will really put the whole picture together for everyone in the department. Too often, the preparation for a lab seminar is the first time a researcher actually sits down with the data and tries to make a story. Try to avoid this by routinely analyzing your data, but be sure to give yourself enough time for preparation of your seminar to organize yourself.

This seminar will either be *formal* or *informal,* and each type is organized quite differently. Each laboratory has its individualized format, which you should follow for your presentation.

> *Data from lab seminars are confidential.*

A formal laboratory seminar

- Is usually for the entire department and is handled as a seminar at an international meeting would be.

- Is held in a lecture room or hall.

- Is usually 45 minutes to an hour long.

- Has data presented as slides.

- Should be a slick presentation.

- Focuses on an understanding of the problem and the approach, as well as the data.

- Has few technical problems.

- Is devoid of jargon.

- Has a question and answer period at the end of the seminar.

An informal laboratory seminar

- Is only for the members of the laboratory.

- May be held in the lab or lab library, as well as in a meeting room.

- Is 30 minutes to an hour in length.

- Has actual gels and films shown on an overhead projector or passed around and often uses blackboards.

- Is a forum for problem solving.

- Focuses on the data. Technical difficulties are brought up for discussion.

- Permits jargon.

- Allows questions to be asked throughout the seminar.

Informal laboratory seminars

- **Objectives.** Informal laboratory seminars are really working meetings, and you should approach yours as an opportunity not just to impress, but to learn. You should be as prepared for an informal seminar as you would be for a formal one. Orchestrate the meeting, stay in control! Your major concern should be in explaining your experiments—what they are, what the results are, what went well or wrong, and why.

> *Avoid the making-more-data-before-the-seminar-syndrome. Instead of wildly running sequencing gels the day before the seminar, use the time to organize and prepare the data you have. No one will care about the extra 500 bases you sequenced, but they will mind a messy seminar. Everyone knows that experiments done just before meetings seldom work, anyway.*

- **Introduction.** Give a brief description of the theory and background to your experiments. It is assumed that the audience knows the field, but you should mention where the experiments fit into the field. You should not give more than 5 minutes of background. Recap your experiments that led up to the research you will discuss. Describe any esoteric methodology.

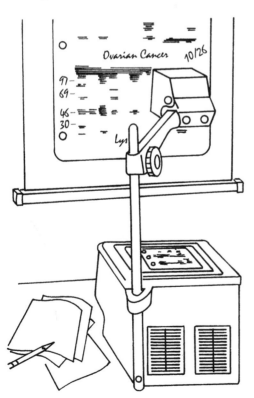

- **Data presentation.** Have your data—slides, gels, graphs, and photographs—ready and stacked in order. Show films on an overhead projector. Hold up photographs. Draw graphs on the blackboard.

  Show data basically in the order it was generated, but keep to a logical progression of thought. Each time, explain why you did the experiment.

  Unless you want to prove a point about technological difficulties, show only good data. State whether that exquisite gel is typical or unusual, and be honest about the reproducibility of the data.

Have statistics and other analysis ready. You don't have to show it all, but you should have solid numbers available.

Know your data. If you are showing a complicated gel, be sure you know what every lane is, even if only lanes 1–3 are relevant to the experiments you are discussing.

Know your methodology. This is not the place to say, "I don't know" too many times. In this little world of your work, you should know everything.

Acknowledge any help you received with experiments as you discuss the experiment. Don't forget to acknowledge intellectual contributions.

Make a conclusion for every piece of data you show.

Summarize your mini-conclusions of each experiment. Have your experiments been successful? Discuss whether you have met your objectives and if not, why. Remind the audience of your goal, and the experiments you need to do to achieve it.

- **Answering questions.** Answer questions about the experiments as you go along. If someone asks a lot of background questions, appears to be the only one missing the point, and your time is short, ask that person to hold questions until after the seminar. Use the question time to answer your own questions. You can ask the audience for suggestions about a particular experiment, or advice about a protocol.

Formal laboratory seminars and meetings

- **Objectives.** A formal seminar is a story and should be a tidy package in itself, without loose ends. The background, the rationale, the methods, data, and conclusions should be internally logical, sensible, and attractive to a varied audience. You are not so much trying to educate as to convince and entertain.

> *Start with the whole story; let people know where they are going. The seminar as a gradually unfolding puzzle is only good in theory.*

- **Introduction.** The introduction should be at least 10 minutes long. In a very few sentences, give the overall problem you are working on. Say why this problem is important. Let the audience know why this topic is worth researching (and why it is worth listening to).

Give the relevant background to this problem. The audience will probably be varied, and you must explain the theory and experimentation that led to your research in a way that everyone can understand. State what you will be talking about for the rest of your seminar. Basically, give the outline of your talk.

> *Memorize the first few sentences of your talk. The initial moments of a seminar can feel awkward, and knowing exactly what you will say in your opening will ease the initial tension.*

- **Data presentation.** Present data in a logical sequence, building on the data of each previous slide. Even if your experiments were not done logically, present them that way. Interpret each slide carefully, lane by lane, point by point. Clearly state the point shown by every data slide.

    At formal seminars, a projectionist or a friend will usually operate your slides. Just say "Next slide, please" when it is time to change. Thank the projectionist at the end of the seminar.

    Break the data into topics, and discuss each topic separately. Each topic should flow smoothly into the next. If you have very little data, you should still divide the data into separate topics. Three or four separate topics are optimal. Recap each topic before you move on to the next. Transitions are vital to a good seminar. You must provide a bridge of logic between each topic, and from section to section of the seminar.

    Don't read your talk. Use your slides as cue cards to prompt you.

    Stay enthusiastic through the seminar. **Don't be negative** about your own data!

    Discuss any problems honestly, but not extensively. Don't beat yourself on the head. If possible, deal with any problems or difficulties with the interpretation of the data during the body of the talk. Describe the future experiments you will do to address the problems.

    Summarize your data, point by point, but briefly. Give your conclusions of your data in a slide. It is okay to read this slide.

    Remind the audience frequently what the data mean, why you are doing these experiments and where you are going.

    It is generally most comfortable to end with acknowledgments. The tradition is to show a slide with a list of people who contributed to the research and to give a one-sentence summary of each person's contribution: A variation on this is to show group or single pictures of each person as you discuss the contributions. Don't worry that thanking too many people will take away from your own glory. It won't. Thank everyone who helped you, including those who may have helped prepare your slides.

    If you haven't put in an acknowledgment slide, you must verbally acknowledge all contributions to the work.

    Don't leave people hanging. End with the feeling that there is no unfinished business.

- **Answering questions.** If there isn't a chairperson who will thank you and request questions, you should thank the audience and ask for questions. You don't have to tell all. If some data are not ready to be discussed, say so. Respond only to what is being asked. If you don't know the answer, say it. Listen to the question until the end. Clarify questions "Do you mean ..." or "Let me recap your question." Treat everyone respectfully, even those who are acting hostile. Avoid debates. If someone is argumentative, try to gracefully and tactfully defuse the situation. Suggest meeting after the seminar.

> ## Controlling the seminar
>
> You should control not only the data, but also the physical environment.
>
> 1. **Sound.** Request an around the neck or clip-on microphone—don't get stuck with a permanently fixed mike.
>
> 2. **Stage.** Choose where to stand. Move to keep the audience's attention.
>
> 3. **Podium.** Put your notes on it and move away! Don't be chained to one position.
>
> 4. **Lights.** Don't put the house lights out. Check whether there is a light at the podium if you briefly need one.
>
> 5. **Room.** Encourage people to sit near you.
>
> 6. **Visual aids requirements.** Don't let your visual aids become dominant. Keep yourself as the focus.
>
> 7. **Take back-ups.** If you take your own projector, have a bulb. Bring a pointer.
>
> 8. Be sure about your **time length.** If the seminar is going longer than planned, do what you can, including cutting a section from your talk, to be finished in time.
>
> 9. **Try it all out.** Arrive early and test your equipment, including lights, pointers, and slides.
>
> Hamlin, S. *How to Talk so People Listen,* p 185.

Ten-minute talks

Many talks you will give at meetings will be only 10 minutes. Arranging a good 10-minute talk is an art: Short talks are harder to organize than long ones. You must not describe all of your research. You must try to make one or two points only, and be extremely selective in what data you show. Polish that little talk like a jewel.

The *introduction* is 1 to 2 minutes of your precious allotment. It should be brief but thorough, for it sets the scene for data to be understood. One or two slides, especially of data, should be used.

Jump right in to the *data presentation.* Use three to six slides, and describe each very thoroughly. Don't use text slides for transitions, but make transitions orally.

A *conclusion slide* will help clarify the point of the seminar. Summarize your data, and avoid predictions and long descriptions of future plans.

There will be a brief *question and answer* period after the talk, with time for only two or three questions. Have with you extra slides describing data you had no time to show, but which may be used for answering questions.

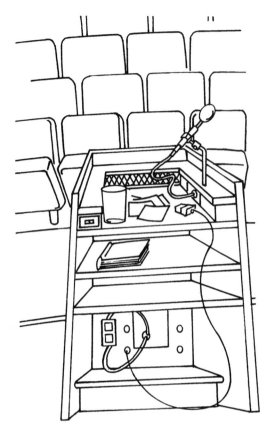

FIGURE 2.

Be sure you understand how to work the lights and pointer before the seminar starts.

Journal Clubs

People tend to think journal club presentations are a waste of time and have nothing to do with their own research (which is, of course, the only thing that is important). Wrong! First of all, you can learn a lot through journal clubs. And more importantly, make no mistake that your general science knowledge isn't being judged, and that that impression can imply something about your own research. If you are poorly prepared, can't explain the figures, and know nothing about the background of the work, it is very easy to imagine that your own research is being tackled as sloppily. But a sharp and brief presentation will leave the room with the impression that you are in control.

- **Format.** There are two common journal club formats: a very brief review of five or six current and unrelated papers, or a more in-depth review of one or two papers on the same topic. You will not have to do a journal club until you have sat through a few, so take note of the format and follow it for your first journal club.

- The tools of presentation are overheads, photocopies, blackboard, or nothing.

- The length of the journal club is usually 15 minutes to 30 minutes.

- You may share a journal club slot with someone else, or talk alone. If you are sharing time, you are usually expected to be more concise.

- There may or may not be handouts.

- The journal article or topic may be assigned, assumed, or left totally up to you.

- You may be expected to have the article distributed or, at least, the citation ready and posted a week or several days before the journal club.

Choice of Topic for Journal Club

Some departments expect each presenter to choose something close to that person's own research, and others expect that the choice should be on a different topic, for the sake of a learning experience. Follow the custom.

Pick something that the department, in general, will be interested in. Will be, not should be. Although all of science is connected, you'll have to work much harder to impress tired and harried animal physiology researchers with the importance of plant response to light than you would if you choose a more immediately relevant topic.

A combination of the known and unknown is usually best. Choose a topic that you are not totally unfamiliar with, since you will feel more comfortable with the presentation and will not have to do too much background reading. But don't, unless it is an amazingly splendid, controversial, or important paper, always pick a paper that is concerned exactly with your own research. You will appear (and well may be) one-dimensional. Use the journal club as an opportunity to learn something and show something of yourself.

Pick a current paper, one from the last month or so. The exception is a topic very important to the group, and a very good paper.

Pick a solid paper. Although you will point out the flaws of whichever paper you choose, a paper with too many problems will make everyone wonder what on earth you were thinking when you chose the paper. Don't assume that, because a paper is in *Nature, Science,* or *Cell,* it is a good paper. But picking a paper from a well-known journal does reduce journal club anxiety and defensiveness, and tends to make the audience assume that the time listening is a good investment.

Pick a simple paper. If the reasoning is too complicated, you will lose your audience unless you have a special gift for inspiring harried people to concentrate. And obviously, pick a paper that *you* understand!

Pick an interesting paper. Don't pick a paper that adds only incrementally to the great fund of knowledge. For example, don't pick papers that compare the effects of 15 agents on one protein—this is boring to listen to, and gives people no insight into their own work (actually, maybe it will! But they won't like it.) Papers that suggest a mechanism work the best for a group of people with mixed interests.

- **Length of presentation.** Rule number 1—Don't go over time! Journal clubs are traditionally held at lunchtime or at the end of the day: Experiments are brewing, time is tight, and most people go reluctantly. Keep it short, and keep their interest.

- **Organization of the presentation.** Introduce the paper: Title, authors, and brief discussion of the topic. Give the background, 10–20% of the total time. Introduce your paper and make clear its place in the background and why it is important or interesting. Say why you chose it.

  Explain the data, 50–80% of the total time. If necessary, briefly describe unusual methodology. Give the author's conclusion.

  Point out any flaws in the data, the paper itself, or the conclusions. Are the author's conclusions warranted by the data? Quickly (three sentences) summarize the conclusions and the importance of the paper.

  Have the paper picked out a week before your presentation. Plan on spending two whole evenings to prepare your first few journal clubs. As you read, anticipate questions. Buffer concentrations you can look up during the presentation: a description of a competing theory you cannot.

> *Know the background of the paper. Read at least three papers referenced in the paper you have chosen. You should know the experiments that led up to this paper, and you should know if and why the results are controversial. You must understand how the experiments were done, and how dependable the methodology is.*

Presentation Tools

Unless you are giving a 5-minute presentation, you will need some sort of visual aid to help people focus. Use visual aids only to *augment* your talk. A flowchart can show the logic for your experiments, and a picture can impress and awe in a way a verbal description can't approach. But *you* should be the dominant source of interest during the seminar.

An *overhead projector* is an excellent aid for presenting data and keeping the crowd alert for a journal club. You can cut and paste the important figures (unless it is a short paper, it is not necessary to show all figures) from the paper, and draw your own figures and summaries. You can draw on the sheet during the talk.

Write large and boldly, because tiny writing can't be seen. If your handwriting is not neat and clear, type the text using a minimum type size of 14 points. Assemble the master sheet figures in the order in which you will present them, with a piece of paper between each one.

You will need to get the plastic pages for making overheads. These are special, because they need to fit onto the photocopy machine. Check the office or a stationery store. If you are drawing all your figures, you can do it on any transparent plastic sheets.

Speak loudly, above the noise of the projector. Don't stand in the way of the projected image.

Photocopies are basically the same as using an overhead projector, as far as preparation goes. Try to minimize the number of photocopies. Don't forget to maintain contact with your audience. Eye contact sometimes gets lost if you have text in front of you. You may photocopy the entire article and distribute it, but this is usually a waste of effort and paper.

A few anchoring figures can be drawn on the *blackboard* before the journal club starts. In this case, the board is being used like an overhead projector. The best use of the blackboard is to quickly draw and write as you are speaking. You must be well organized and thoroughly versed in your topic to do this, so you know before you start just what you will draw.

Slides are the heart and mainstay of a formal seminar.

- Find out how your lab makes slides a month in advance of your talk. Figures may be sent away, or photographed and developed at the institutional media center: Figures may be sent directly via computer to the media center. The use of a presentation or graphics program will help greatly in making both text and graphic slides, but don't wait until the day before to try it unless you don't have a shred of panic in your body.
- Slides should be finished a week before your talk. This gives you time to add new slides, to check that all slides can be read from the back of the room, and to redo slides that can't be read.
- Many labs have Polaroid cameras, which can make slides in 30 minutes. These cameras are usually for black and white film only and are better for text than for pictures. Find out if you have access to such a camera, get some film, and learn how to use it: You may realize the night before that you need a slide.
- Use at least a 20-point size for text. Check your completed slides to be sure they can be read from the back of the room.
- Each slide should make one point. Don't overload slides with information.
- Figures should be well labeled, so that they are understandable without any explanation. Unlike tables and figures for manuscripts, tables and figures for slides should have all axes labeled and a title that summarizes the figure.
- Look at your slides, projected on a screen in a room approximately the same size as the room in which you will talk. Some slides look very good on paper, but don't project well.

- 20–40 slides is a good number to have for a 45–60-minute talk. Don't have more than 20 "hard" data slides: If you have more than 20 slides, they should include pictures, drawings, models, and text slides.
- Put a mark on the lower left of each slide. Slides are placed in a carousel upside down, with the dot on the upper right.
- To avoid fumbling and incorrect slide loading, have your slides loaded into a carousel before seminar time. Check the order and placement of the slides before the seminar.

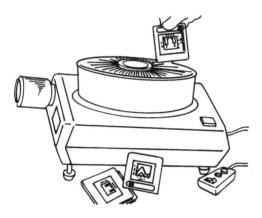

Computer slide shows that use presentation programs such as PowerPoint (Microsoft) are becoming increasingly common. These programs allow you to create as well as present your data, making it easy to customize and alter your presentations even when you are on the road. Resist the urge to add all the available whistles and bells, and keep the graphics and text simple. Follow the same rules for organization as for a "regular" slide show.

Checklist of slides
- A text introduction slide.
- Background slides. These can be borrowed from other investigators, or made from textbooks or the literature.
- Data slides.
- A text slide of one sentence for each section of the talk.
- A text summary or conclusions slide.
- An acknowledgment slide should be shown at the end of the talk. Include not only technical and theoretical research help, but also assistance with slide preparation and computer graphics, and people who contributed materials. No one will think you haven't done the work if you list many people, but forgetting to acknowledge someone is a breach of courtesy.

WRITTEN PRESENTATIONS

Manuscripts

The scientific, to say nothing of the political, machinations involved in getting a paper published are quite complicated. There are several books on the topic (some of which are listed in Resources), and plenty of good and practical advice from other scientists.

Some general tips

- Think of your experiments, from the beginning, as figures in a paper. Yes, it does sound as if mere ambition has supplanted scientific interest. But you must publish, and thinking about the publications can stop you from venturing too far down dead ends. It also helps you to always include the appropriate controls.

- Base the paper on the data, not the other way around. Prepare your figures before you do any writing.

- Your data must be reproducible before you can make a story out of it.

- Write your papers as soon as you can. Write them before you are ready. There will probably not be a pat answer to a story, so put an ending on, and wrap it up. If more needs to be done, it will become clear during the writing.

- Write up all papers before you switch projects or labs. No man or woman can serve two masters. Project carryover is very distressing, and you should have all writing finished before starting anew.

- Use spell and grammar checks. Spelling mistakes will cause you to lose credibility with readers.

- Be selective and thorough with the references and be sure, in your final draft, that the references are placed correctly. These sometimes get mixed up when running a bibliographic management program.

- Get at least three readers for your paper. Do this before you give the paper to the P.I. to read! Ask two people familiar with the field: They will point out omissions of background, suggest implications, etc. Ask someone, not necessarily in the field, who can read the manuscript for mistakes in logic, spelling, and grammar. Do this for every draft of the paper. Try to use the same readers. Don't get too many readers, because you will

If someone asks you to read a manuscript for comments, do it as soon as possible. Only quick feedback is useful. If you won't be able to read it for a few days, inform the person before you take the manuscript.

get in a complete muddle from conflicting suggestions. But do get good quality readers, people whom you know will be thorough, prompt, and honest.

- Assess the quality of the paper when choosing the journal to which you will submit it. If the choice of journal is your decision, ask the P.I. for advice. Journals tend to accept papers more readily from some labs than from others, and the P.I. will know the history of the submissions from your lab.

- Don't be discouraged by a negative review. Many reviews can be argued, and it is always worth a try. And actually, most papers are improved when revised in accordance with a review.

> *By the time the P.I. gets the paper, it should be in almost publishable form. It is not the job of the P.I. to correct your grammar and spelling mistakes.*

> *When you submit a manuscript to a journal, you must include a short introductory letter to the editor.*

When writing manuscript reviews

Be critical.
Be prompt.
Don't be pompous.
Don't be petty.

Research definitions

These abused research definitions have been circulating in laboratories for years. There is a painful truth to them, and most of the phrases should be avoided.

"IT HAS LONG BEEN KNOWN ..." I haven't bothered to look up the original reference.

"OF GREAT THEORETICAL AND PRACTICAL IMPORTANCE" Interesting to me.

"WHILE IT HAS NOT BEEN POSSIBLE TO PROVIDE DEFINITE ANSWERS TO THESE QUESTIONS ..." The experiments didn't work out, but I figure I could get publicity out of it.

"EXTREMELY HIGH PURITY, SUPERPURITY" Composition unknown except for the exaggerated claims of the supplier.

"THREE OF THE SAMPLES WERE CHOSEN FOR DETAILED STUDY" The results on the others didn't make sense and were ignored.

"ACCIDENTALLY STAINED DURING MOUNTING" Accidentally dropped on floor.

"HANDLED WITH EXTREME CARE DURING EXPERIMENTS" Not dropped on the floor.

"TYPICAL RESULTS ARE SHOWN" The best results are shown.

"PRESUMABLY AT LONGER TIMES ..." I didn't take the time to find out.

"THESE RESULTS WILL BE REPORTED AT A LATER DATE" I might get around to this sometime.

"THE MOST RELIABLE VALUES ARE THOSE OF JONES" He was a student of mine.

"IT IS BELIEVED THAT ..." I think.

"IT IS GENERALLY BELIEVED THAT ..." A couple of other guys think so too.

"IT MIGHT BE ARGUED THAT ..." I have such a good answer for this objection that I shall now raise it.

"IT IS CLEAR THAT MUCH ADDITIONAL WORK WILL BE REQUIRED BEFORE A COMPLETE UNDERSTANDING ..." I don't understand it.

"CORRECT WITHIN AN ORDER OF MAGNITUDE" Wrong.

"IT IS TO BE HOPED THAT THIS WORK WILL STIMULATE FURTHER WORK IN THE FIELD" This paper is not very good, but neither are any of the others on this miserable subject.

"THANKS ARE DUE TO JOE GLOTZ FOR ASSISTANCE WITH THE EXPERIMENT AND TO JOHN DOE FOR VALUABLE DISCUSSIONS" Glotz did the work and Doe explained it to me.

(Anonymous)

Grants

A grant is a much more complicated piece of writing than a manuscript because you must not only convince the audience of the validity of the work, you must also convince them that you are the person for the job. Grantsmanship is inseparable from politics.

Politics and practicalities of submission

- Stay in close touch with the grants office at your institution. These vary greatly in performance and responsibility. Some offices do nothing but sign the grants before they are submitted. Others actually critique the science as well as the financial and administrative sections, and give suggestions as to improvements. Try to keep to the grants office deadlines. They will understand, but you must give them as much time as possible to take advantage of the help they can offer. Cover pages—on disk—may be available at your grants office. If not, they may be available from the agency.

> *Many agencies solicit grants on particular topics throughout the year. These generally have higher funding percentages.*

- It makes sense to submit the same grant to as many agencies as possible. But make no mistake about the amount of time reworking a grant for another agency will take. It is usually at least a week.

- Be a perfectionist. The reviewers have a lot of good grants to go through for each study section and are often looking for a reason to eliminate a grant from consideration.

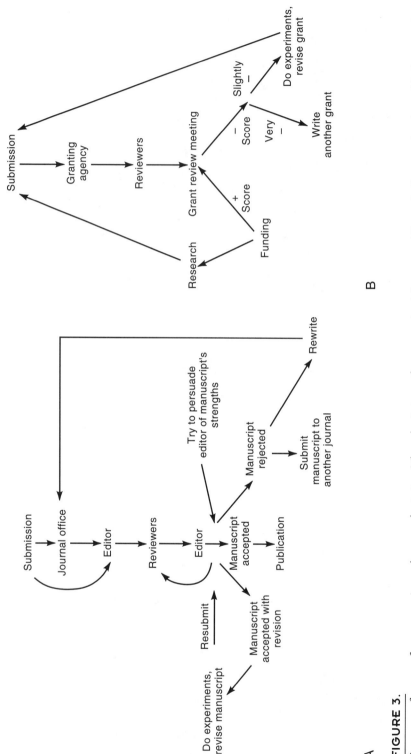

FIGURE 3.

Sequence of events after manuscript and grant submission. The submissions of a manuscript (*A*) or grant (*B*) are similar to each other, with the exception that more options are available for submission and maneuvers for manuscripts. Both sequences usually take approximately 3–6 months for funding or publication. Not all grant and manuscript submissions exactly follow the sequence shown here: For example, some editors do not send revised manuscripts back to reviewers, but accept or reject the manuscript personally. Revised grants are reviewed by the same people who reviewed the first submission in some granting agencies, and some agencies give an "accept" or "reject" without supplying a score or ranking or reason for the decision.

- The best way to get a grant is to already have published papers on the topic.

- You must have preliminary results before you submit the grant. This is especially important if you are doing something you haven't been trained in, or if you want to work on something controversial or new. The preliminary results don't necessarily have to be your own.

- Many agencies will allow you to submit additional data after the grant has been submitted, before review. Take advantage of this only if you have very clean, persuasive, and relevant data to add.

> *Avoid red flags! These are mistakes and omissions which, to a reviewer, are like waving a red flag at an angry bull. Anything that suggests sloppiness, for example, can put a reviewer in an extremely unreceptive mood. Examples are misspellings, incorrectly numbered references, and badly labeled figures.*

- Add collaborators who can supply expertise you don't (or don't appear to) have. Mention these collaborators in the grant. Most agencies will request that you also submit the proposed collaborator's C.V., as well as a copy of a letter to you from the collaborator, affirming the collaboration.

- Get at least three readers for your grant, as you would for a manuscript. Revise it and ask the same people to read it again.

RESOURCES

Alley M. 1996. *The craft of scientific writing*, 3rd ed. Springer, New York.

Bardwick J.M. 1995. *Danger in the comfort zone*. American Management Association, New York.

Barnes G.A. 1982. *Communication skills for the foreign-born professional*. ISI Press, Philadelphia.

Carter S.P. 1987. *Writing for your peers. The primary journal paper*. Praeger, New York.

Davis M. 1997. *Scientific papers and presentations*. Academic Press, San Diego.

Day R.A. 1997. *How to write and publish a scientific paper*, 4th ed. Oryx Press, Phoenix.

Gleeson K. 1994. *The personal efficiency program. How to get organized to do more work in less time*. John Wiley & Sons, New York.

Hamlin S. 1988. *How to talk so people listen*. Harper and Row, New York.

Mandell S. 1993. *Effective presentation skills. A practical guide for better speaking*. Crisp Publications, Menlo Park, California.

Matthews J.R., Bowen J.M., and Matthews R.W. 1996. *Successful scientific writing. A step-by-step guide for the biological and biomedical sciences*. Cambridge University Press, United Kingdom.

Pell A.R. 1995. *The complete idiot's guide to managing people*, Chap. 4. Alpha Book (Simon and Schuster MacMillan Company), New York.

Rosenberg A.D. 1997. *Career busters. 22 Things people do to mess up their careers and how to avoid them*, Chap 2. McGraw-Hill, New York.

Strunk W., Jr. and White E.B. 1979. *The elements of style*, 3rd ed. Macmillan Publishing, New York.

Tufte E.R. 1992. *The visual display of quantitative information*. Graphics Press, Cheshire, Connecticut.

Section 3
Navigating

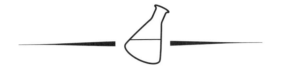

CHAPTER 7
Making Reagents and Buffers 129

CHAPTER 8
Storage and Disposal 163

CHAPTER 9
Working without Contamination 185

CHAPTER 10
Eukaryotic Cell Culture 205

CHAPTER 11
Bacteria 245

CHAPTER 12
DNA, RNA, and Protein 279

CHAPTER 13
Radioactivity 313

CHAPTER 14
Centrifugation 345

CHAPTER 15
Electrophoresis 373

CHAPTER 16
The Light Microscope 403

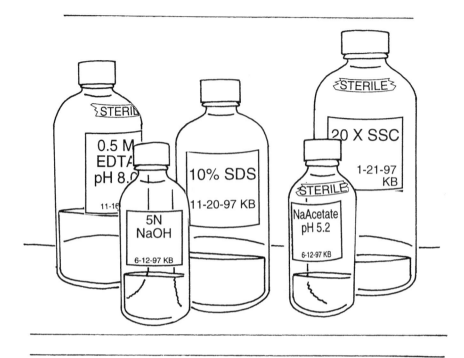

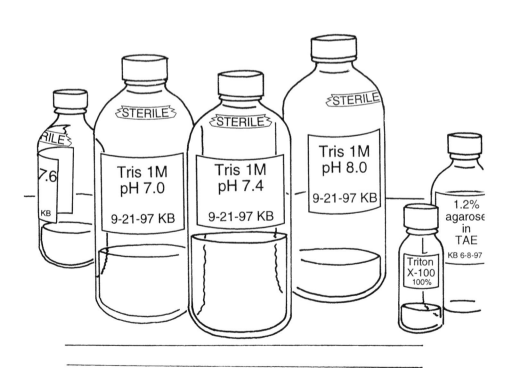

7

Making Reagents and Buffers

MUCH OF THE TIME spent in an experiment is not found in the experiment itself, but in preparation of the reagents and tools needed to do and analyze the experiment. The first thing a newcomer to the lab generally needs to do is to make a supply of buffers, so that the shelves above the lab bench won't look so newcomer-ishly empty, and you can start doing experiments. Buffer- and reagent-making is an activity that will continue throughout your time in the lab: Your experiments will depend on the quality of your reagents.

A *buffer* is a solution that does not change pH readily. Since each enzymatic reaction, each cell, and each extraction has a pH optimum, buffers have countless uses. They are used to wash cells, to cut DNA, to perform electrophoresis—any activity in which the structure and/or activity of biological material must be maintained. Some salt solutions, such as sodium chloride, do not need to be buffered, usually because they become part of a complex solution that will be buffered.

DETERMINING WHAT YOU NEED	130
Safety	131
Which water to use?	134
Plasticware and glassware	135
CALCULATING WHAT YOU NEED	136
Molar solutions	137
Percent solutions	139
Dilution of stock buffers	139
Recipes	142
Preparation of phenol and phenol chloroform	145
WEIGHING AND MIXING	146
Weighing	147
Mixing	149
MEASURING PH	150
Calibrating the pH meter	151
Determining pH	152
STERILIZING SOLUTIONS	155
Using the autoclave	156
Filter sterilization	157
STORING BUFFERS AND SOLUTIONS	158
When to discard buffers	159
RESOURCES	161

DETERMINING WHAT YOU NEED

If you are in any lab doing biomedical research, you will need certain reagents, no matter what your particular experiments will be. These are the first reagents you will make, and you can find out from other lab members exactly which ones to make before you start on experiments. Most of these chemicals and reagents will be stocked in the lab. Some of these reagents are listed in Chapter 3, and the recipes for some common reagents are listed later in this chapter.

After discussions with the P.I. and other lab members, and after your own readings and research, you will be given or will devise a protocol, a game plan detailing the logistics of the experiment. At least a day or so before the experiment you must ensure that all the buffers and reagents needed for the experiment will be made and autoclaved and ready for use. For more detail on following protocols, see Chapter 4.

Always work to a protocol!

1. **Go through the protocol for your experiment, and write down all the solutions that are used.** Record the name, the concentration (molarity or percentage), the pH, and the volume used in the experiment.

2. **Determine how much of each solution you should make.** If you know you won't do the experiment more than a couple of times (unlikely—most experiments are done multiple times), make the reasonable *minimum* volume. If the protocol calls for 10 ml of 1 M NaCl, plan on making 100 ml. And if 1–50 ml are used at a time, and you will do the experiment routinely, make 500 ml or a liter. However, if the material is expensive or unstable, make only what you require for one experiment.

3. **Decide whether you should make a "straight" solution or a concentrated solution.** Many complex buffers are made at a 5, 10, 20, or 50X concentration and are diluted to the desired concentration at the time of the experiment.

> For example, Tris/glycine SDS buffer (Laemmli running buffer), commonly used for protein gel electrophoresis, is often made at a **10X concentration.** Since the working concentration of 1X is 25 mM Tris, 192 mM glycine, and 0.1% SDS, 10X would be 250 mM Tris, 1.920 M glycine, and 1% SDS. At the time of the experiment, the 10X would be diluted 1:10 in water.

The limit in concentrated buffer stocks is the solubility of the buffer, for the salts will come out of solution if they are too concentrated. This isn't a disaster, but you aren't exactly saving time if you have to warm and mix the buffer until it is back in solution. Check with someone in the lab or with the manufacturer if you aren't sure how concentrated you can make a particular buffer, but you are probably safe with 5X. Concentrated buffers are usually stored at room temperature to avoid precipitation.

Other buffers commonly stored as concentrated stocks are **PBS** (10x), **SSC** (10 or 20x), and **TAE** (10x). Many companies also offer premade concentrated buffers, so check into the lab custom before you fire up the buffer factory. These are expensive, but they make life very easy.

> *Keep one or two bottles of autoclaved double-distilled water in the refrigerator, to be used to make buffers from concentrated stocks.*

4. **Find out if the chemicals you need are available in the lab.** Okay, let's say that your protocol calls for a 1 M NaCl solution. Before you get all geared up, find out if the lab has the NaCl, or if it will have to be borrowed or ordered. Commonly used materials such as NaCl are usually in stock in the lab, and generally, they are available for common use. *But actually open the bottle and check it first,* before getting out the glassware—someone may have left only half a gram, and neglected to order more ("But I didn't use it up! There was some left in the bottle!").

5. **Get what you need if it isn't in stock.** Check with the person who orders, or with the purchasing department or company, to see if the replacement has been ordered. If you are in a huge hurry, the NaCl is really gone, and the newly ordered NaCl will take 3 days to get to you, you have several options. You can go down the hall and borrow some NaCl, with the promise to return what you took when your delivery comes in. Politics will determine whether you actually should return it, and whether, in fact, you should borrow it from that particular lab in the first place!

An easier solution is to get some concentrated stock from a coworker. Researchers often have a bottle of 5 M NaCl on their shelf. NaCl is a component of many complex buffers used in molecular biology, and 5 M can be easily diluted to the molarity needed. Figure out the minimum you need to get by until you can make your own stock, and *ask* to "borrow" that amount. You probably won't need to return the 20 ml—most people won't even want to take a buffer from a new lab member. But make the offer.

Safety

Before you make up any reagent or buffer, *you* must check to see what, if any, hazards are associated with handling the material. No one else will do this for you. Some hazards are well known and well advertised: For example, no one in a lab would let you be too casual with ethidium bromide. **But because no one says anything to you, you cannot assume a material is safe to handle freely.**

- **Know the composition and associated hazards of every material you work with.**

    1. Check the Materials Safety Data Sheet (MSDS). The MSDS must be included with every chemical purchased and should be kept on file in the lab. It is a

description of the composition and properties of the chemical, and it lists the hazards of the chemical and the ways in which the hazard should be dealt with.

2. Look for a hazardous material classification label. These labels (which follow DOT and NFPA recommendations and are approved by OSHA) describe the health hazard, fire hazard, reactivity, and specific hazards of the material.

3. Read the bottle carefully for warnings. Not all materials will have the hazardous materials classification label, but may still carry warnings, sometimes in small print.

4. If you see no warnings, look the material up in the Merck Index.

5. If the label is in another language, or you can't find a listing for it, consult the manufacturer or your EHS Office.

• **Follow the recommendations for handling** that you find. Follow the precautions needed for the particular material you will be working with. Your lab should have a chart or a list of the safety precautions needed for classes of dangerous reagents. If not, call EHS.

1. **Gloves.** Be sure you are wearing the correct gloves for the job. Latex or polyvinylchloride gloves should always be worn when making up any reagent, and these are good protection against most powdered reagents. But these offer no protection against, for example, phenol. For organic solvents you will need chemical-resistant rubber or neoprene gloves. If you have an allergy to latex, speak with EHS.

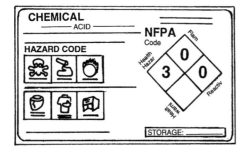

FIGURE 1.

Hazardous materials classification label. The specific hazard is listed in the lower left quadrant. Reactivity, health, and fire hazards are rated with increasing numbers, with 0 posing no hazard and 4 being very dangerous.

Some people have an allergy to the chemicals used to manufacture latex. This allergy usually shows itself as chronic dermatitis, and gets worse over time. If you develop a rash on your hands that is linked to the use of latex gloves, stop using latex gloves. Consult with EHS about a substitute kind of glove. The use of powder-free latex gloves may help prevent latex allergy.

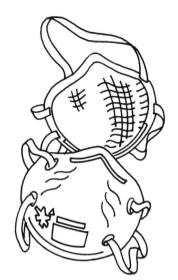

FIGURE 2.
Dust-mist mask.

2. **Eye protection.** For any potential splatters, aerosols, combustible, or breaking glass, wear plastic glasses or goggles.

3. **Hood.** Volatile substances should always be made up in a chemical hood. Be sure that the hood is certified for use.

4. **Mask.** Some powders, such as SDS, can cause damage to the nasal passages. A simple dust-mist mask or a surgical mask will protect you. But other substances, particularly if volatile, may require the use of respirator masks. Don't feel you are going overboard because no one else is taking precautions!

5. **Labels.** Label your bottle with the hazard associated with it. You may not remember, or it may be necessary for someone else to use your reagents.

Hazardous reagents

The following common reagents are potentially dangerous, and should be handled with more than the usual care. Wear gloves. Follow the cautions carefully—don't cut corners here!

Acrylamide. This neurotoxin is used for protein and sequencing gels. Wear a mask.

Ethidium bromide. EtBr, a mutagen, intercalates in DNA and is used to label nucleic acid. It is toxic, and the solid is irritating to skin and mucous membranes.

Phenol. Phenol is highly corrosive and can burn skin. Use a fume hood when doing extractions with or preparing phenol.

Phenylmethyl-sulfonate fluoride (PMSF). Used to inhibit proteinases during protein isolations, PMSF can be fatal if swallowed or absorbed through the skin.

Sodium dodecyl sulfate (SDS). This detergent is a burning powder and is extremely irritating, especially to nasal passages. It is light and fluffy; measure gently, and wear a mask.

- **Know how to operate the fume hood.**

  1. *Turn the fume hood on,* and be sure it is exhausting; you will be able to hear and feel it. No air conditioners or fans should be working near the fume hood, as this will interfere with the air currents within the hood.

  2. *The sash must be below chin level*! Lower the sash to the level indicated on the front of the hood. This level is determined by EHS when the hood is certified. The lower the sash, the more containment there is: If you are working with high-speed aerosols, the sash must be all the way down.

  3. *Work at least 6 inches within the hood.*

  4. *Secure papers and other lightweight materials.* They could become trapped in the exhaust system.

  5. *Do not block the rear exhaust slot* or the space between the tapered metal front lip and the work surface.

Which Water to Use?

Water is an important component of solutions; it is not merely something to dissolve things in. Water quality, composition, and pH can drastically affect experiments, and everyone knows stories of experiments that stopped working after the water source was changed.

> *Assume the solvent is water, unless it is stated otherwise.*

There are several broad classifications of water quality, in order of increasing purity:

1. **Tap water.** Tap water quality varies wildly, its mineral and impurity composition dependent on the geographical location, the pipes, or the amount of rainfall that spring. Some minerals can inhibit enzyme reactions, or prevent cell growth: At the very least, tap water is a nonreproducible variable in the experimental equation and should not be used. It is used only for washing glassware and other laboratory equipment.

2. **Laboratory grade water.** Laboratory grade water has been pretreated by reverse osmosis or distillation. It is adequate for making buffers.

3. **Reagent grade water.** Through distillation or deionization, laboratory grade water is further purified, and can be used for cell culture and biochemical reagents, as well as for buffers.

4. **Ultrapure reagent grade water.** Some labs have particular and stringent water requirements. For example, water treated by ultrafiltration to be sure it is endotoxin-free (endotoxin is a ubiquitous bacterial cell wall component) may be required for certain cell cultures.

Distillation is still the most commonly used method of water purification in labs. Reagent grade water is also made with a combination of units capable of *reverse osmosis* (the water is pushed through a semipermeable membrane through which impurities can't pass) and *deionization* (the removal of ions by passage through anion and/or cation removal resins). *Ultrafiltration, adsorption, and ultraviolet oxidation* are used in some facilities to further purify the water. Ultrapure reagent grade water can also be purchased from scientific and hospital vendors.

Many institutions have "house-distilled" water, which is distilled at a central location and is dispensed through a tap near the sink. This is laboratory grade water, and can be used for buffers: However, it should not be used for cell culture or buffers that will be used in enzymatic reactions. Its most common use is rinsing glassware after washing with tap water.

> *Always keep ready a liter or two of autoclaved, reagent grade water, to use for making diluted buffers from concentrated stock buffers.*

If reagent grade water is plentiful, use it for *all* of your buffers.

Plasticware and Glassware

To make reagents, you will need **graduated cylinders, beakers, volumetric and Erlenmeyer flasks.** These are reusable laboratory supplies and will be stored in a closed or sheltered cabinet to keep dust off.

Some labs use glass, some plastic; most use a mix. Glass is clear, but breaks during washing. Plastic is hardy, but some types, particularly after being autoclaved, become tinted or opaque, and no meniscus forms in some plastic graduated cylinders. Use whatever is there, as it all works.

Glassware to use for mixing

Beaker. Use for most solid-to-solvent mixing. Plastic or glass is fine.
Erlenmeyer flask. Use if a gas will be generated.
Test tube. Use for volumes less than 10 ml.
Volumetric flask. Use for two liquids, but mix by swirling, not with a stir bar.

Glassware not to use for mixing

Graduated cylinder. Resist the temptation to dump the solids directly into the cylinder. The base of the cylinder is usually too high for a magnetic stir plate to work, and covering the top with parafilm to shake the cylinder can turn into an extremely messy and potentially dangerous procedure.

Plasticware and glassware (both sometimes referred to as glassware) are usually **autoclaved** before being placed back on the shelves after washing: Foil closing may be the only indication that the item is sterile.

Don't hoard glassware at your bench. If the lab starts to run out of graduated cylinders in the afternoon, order more.

There is probably a motley selection of bottles for **reagent and buffer storage.** Some were bottles purchased just to hold buffers, but many are recycled bottles that had been purchased for their contents.

Glassware to use for buffer storage

Glass bottles with lined caps. Good for media.
Cell culture medium bottles. Premade culture medium and buffers are purchased in these bottles. They can be reused indefinitely.
Narrow mouth bottles. Excellent for buffers.

Glassware not to use for buffer storage

Wide-mouthed jars. The contents get contaminated easily.
Amber containers. Use these only if you have a light-sensitive reagent.
Poorly threaded capped bottles. Contamination will be a problem. Also, a bottle without a good-fitting cap probably wasn't made to last.
Any container that looks chipped, scratched, or damaged in any way. Damaged glass is much more susceptible to breakage during autoclaving or even changes in temperature.

CALCULATING WHAT YOU NEED

The protocol or recipe will describe each solution either as a molar solution or a percent solution.

Molar (M) Solutions

To make a solution of a particular molarity from scratch, you need to know what volume you require and the formula molecular weight of the substance.

To determine the formula molecular weight

- If the name is given, and you don't know the formula, check the *Merck Index* or one of the on-line chemistry dictionaries.

- You could determine the molecular weight (MW) from the periodic table (for example, for sodium chloride, Na is 22.98, Cl is 35.45, so the formula molecular weight of the substance is 58.43).

The Merck Index also contains information on solubility and stability.

• The best way to get the molecular weight is from the bottle from which you will take the substance. This way, you can be sure that the substance is exactly what you need. If the molecular weight is obscured on the label, check the catalog or call the technical services of the company that made the material.

Read the label carefully and be sure you are getting the formula weight of the substance you need. Be sure to look at the formula, not just the name, as there are differences that could be missed, and will make a difference. In particular, check for:

Salt or acid/base form. The major problem in using a salt vs the acid is in the difference in pH. For example, Tris, a common buffer, comes as Tris HCl, or as Tris base, and a 1 M solution will vary in pH by several units.

Anhydrous or hydrated. Extra water in the material won't usually be a problem, as long as the water is calculated as part of the formula weight.

To calculate molarity

> **There is only one calculation you need**
>
> **Gram molecular weight of known is to 1 M as unknown grams is to desired molarity.**
>
> MW: molarity as x : desired molarity

Multiply the MW by the desired molarity, and divide by the molarity of the known. This presumes a desired volume of 1000 ml. (Always think of 1 liter as 1000 ml.)

Example: 1 liter (1000 ml) of 1 molar NaCl
1 molar (or 1 M) is easy, since 1 mole equals the gram molecular weight of the substance. Thus, since the formula weight of NaCl is 58.43, you need 58.43 g in one liter of water. No calculations.

Example: 1 liter (1000 ml) of 5 M NaCl
58.43:1 as x :5
58.43 × 5 /1 = 292.15 g

Example: 300 ml of 1 molar NaCl
If you only need 300 ml of 1 M NaCl, reduce the grams the same proportion as you reduce the volume of water.
58.43 g :1000 ml as x : 300. (58.43 g is to 1000 ml as the unknown g are to 300 ml) Multiply 58.43 by 300, and divide the product by 1000. The answer, 17.5 g, should be dissolved in 300 ml to give 300 ml of 1 M NaCl.

Example: 400 ml of a 0.25 molar solution of NaCl
For different volumes and different molarities, it might be easiest to do the cal-

culations in multiple steps, rather than trying to figure out the grand calculation. So, for 400 ml of a 0.25 M solution of NaCl:

1. Figure out how many grams you need for a liter of a 0.25 M solution.
   58.43 g : 1000 ml as x g : 250
   58.43 × 250 = 14607.5, divided by 1000 = 14.6.
   For 1000 ml of a 0.25 M solution, you need 14.6 g of NaCl.

2. Calculate the grams needed for 400 ml of 0.25 M.
   14.6 : 1000 ml as x g : 400 ml
   400 × 14.6 = 5840, 5840 divided by 400 = 5.84.
   For 400 ml of a 0.25 M solution, you need 5.84 g of NaCl.

Example: 10 liters of a 5.0 M solution of NaCl
1. Figure out how many grams you need for a liter of a 5.0 M solution.
   58.43 :1000 as x : 5000
   58.43 × 5000 = 292150, divided by 1000 = 292.15
   For 1 liter of a 5.0 M solution, you need 292.15 g of NaCl.

2. Calculate the grams needed for 10 liters of 5.0 M.
   292.15 g: 1 liter as x g : 10 liters 292.15 g × 10, divided by 1 = 2921.5

The calculations will become instinctive: For 10 liters of a 5.0 M solution of NaCl, it will be fairly obvious that you only need to multiply 58.43 × 50 to arrive at the grams needed. But work through the entire calculation until you have a feel for the numbers.

> *Record your calculations in your notebook. Even for experienced lab personnel, most mistakes in buffer making occur at this step, and it is much easier to track down the reasons for nonworking experiments if you record everything.*

Normal (N) solutions

Molarity is defined as the number of gram molecular weights (moles) per liter of solvent. Normality is defined as *a gram molecular weight of a dissolved substance divided by the hydrogen equivalents per liter of solution.* Molarity sees the world as bases and their salts; normality sees the world in terms of acids.

What does this mean? For most chemicals, the value is the same for molarity and normality. 1 M HCl is the same as 1 N HCl. But when working with any divalent or trivalent species (sulfate, phosphate, carbonate, etc.), it will make a difference. For example, for concentrated sulfuric acid (H_2SO_4), there are two equivalents of H^+ per molecule: the concentration of sulfuric acid is 18 M but 36 N. If you multiply the molarity of a solution by the number of moles of that substance that occur in a chemical equation, you have the normality.

Percent Solutions

Percent solutions are based on 100 ml (or, occasionally, 100 grams). Almost all the percent solutions you will calculate will be (w/v) solutions, in which the weight in grams of the powder is mixed with the volume in milliliters of the water.

Three ways of expressing concentration in the form of a percent

- *Percent weight by volume (w/v). Grams of solute per 100 ml of solvent.* Generally, a percent solution is considered to be weight/volume (w/v) and w/v is assumed if not designated otherwise.

  Example: 20% NaCl. For a 20% NaCl solution, dissolve 20 g of NaCl in 70 ml of water, and bring the volume up to 100 ml.

- *Percent by volume (v/v). ml of solute per 100 ml of solution.* This is commonly used when diluting a concentrated stock.

  Example: 1% SDS solution. Everyone has a 10% SDS solution (w/v) on his or her shelf. Dilute 1:10 by adding 10 ml of 10% SDS to 90 ml of water, top up to 100 ml.

- *Percent by weight (w/w). Grams of solute per 100 g of solvent.* This is never used in making standard buffer or salt solutions, but is found in protocols for making gradient solutions.

  Example: 10% (w/w) sucrose solution. Weigh 10 g of sucrose, and add to 90 g of water. Theoretically, a ml of water equals a gram, so add 90 ml of water to the beaker in which you are weighing the water.

Dilution of Stock Buffers

Once you have really set your roots down, most of your working lab buffers will be made by simply diluting your stock buffers.

Do all manipulations as cleanly as possible. It is not necessary to flame the bottles, if they are not used for cell maintenance. Use sterile pipets, and replace caps immediately.

When you are diluting sterile buffers, use aseptic technique (Chapter 9). Use only sterile pipets, and replace all caps immediately.

> *To dilute the stock buffers:*
> $$C1 \times V1 = C2 \times V2$$
> $C1$ = *the concentration before dilution*
> $V1$ = *the volume before dilution*
> $C2$ = *the concentration after dilution*
> $V2$ = *the volume after dilution*

> For example, if you need 100 ml of 1.0 M and have a 5 M stock of NaCl:
> 5.0 M **x** V1 = 1.0 M **x** 100 ml
> V1 = 20 ml
> Add 20 ml of 5.0 M to 80 ml of distilled water for a volume of 100 ml.
> Either use sterile 5 M and sterile distilled water, or sterilize the final 100 ml by autoclaving or filtration through a 0.2 micron filter.

> Dilutions are denoted differently from lab to lab. Generally, adding 1 ml of concentrate to 9 ml of diluent is written 1:10. This notation is confusing, as adding 1 ml of concentrate to 1 ml of diluent is written either as 1:1 or 1:2. It would be better to use 1/10 for 1 in 10 and 1:10 as 1 and 10.

Serial dilutions

Serial dilutions are the easiest way to **reduce the concentration** of a reagent, bacterial or cell sample, standard, or anything you want to use to test increasing or decreasing concentrations. Progressive dilutions are made, yielding concentrations differing from successive dilutions by the same factor.

Stock solution. The stock solution is the concentrated solution.

Dilution factor. Before setting up the dilutions, you must consult a protocol or the literature to decide on the dilutions you will need. 1:10 or 1:2 dilutions are the most commonly done. The serial dilution you choose will be based on how close in concentration you need your working dilutions to be. To survey for an effect, the dilutions will generally be spread, and you might use a factor of 1:10 or 1:100. To pinpoint the effectiveness of a particular concentration, a 1:2 dilution series would be more useful.

When considering the concentrations you will need, don't forget to take into account the dilution that occurs when you add the substance from the dilutions into the experimental containers.

Diluting medium. Do your dilutions in the medium or buffer you will actually be using in the final experiment. Don't just use water or the same solvent the stock solution is made of, unless they are what you require.

Volume. The volume you use for dilutions and the size of the tubes are dependent on how concentrated you need your final volumes. Don't do dilutions in microfuge tubes if you will need to add 3 ml of the

Oftentimes, the stock solution is made up in a solvent in which the substance could be dissolved but which is harmful for cells or for an enzymatic reaction. Dilution of the substance also serves to dilute the solvent to a nonharmful concentration.

dilutions to arrive at your final concentrations. Likewise, don't use 15-ml tubes if you are diluting 1-ml volumes.

Tubes. Set the tubes up, and add the diluting medium. Write the dilution on each tube, and/or record all dilutions in your lab notebook. Orient the test tube rack in the same way, every time, so you know which way you are working. Always pipet from left to right, to achieve decreasing concentrations. Set the tubes up to facilitate this.

> *The carryover from high to low concentration tubes can erratically make the actual concentration higher than you have calculated it to be. This is not the time to conserve pipets.*

Pipets. Use a pipet or pipettor appropriate for the volume being transferred. Discard pipets and tips after you pipet into each tube!

Adding the dilutions to the working container. Add the required volume to your experiment or assay tubes in increasing concentrations. You may use the same pipet only if you are adding samples from increasing concentration dilution tubes, where the carryover effect will be negligible.

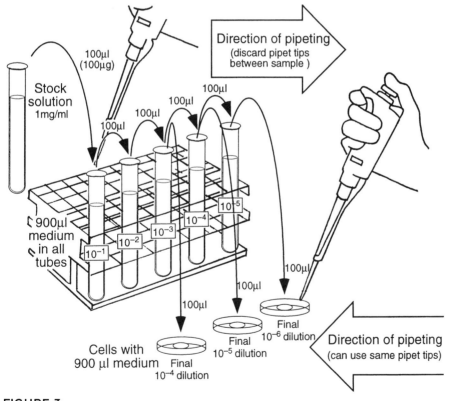

FIGURE 3.

An example of a serial dilution used to dilute a 1 mg/ml stock solution to achieve final concentrations of 100, 10, and 1 ng.

Recipes

TABLE 1. Concentrations of Acids and Bases: Common Commercial Strengths

Substance	Formula	Molecular weight	Moles/ liter	Grams/ liter	Percentage by wieght	Milliliters/liter to prepare 1 M solution
Acetic acid, glacial	CH_3COOH	60.05	17.4	1045	99.5	57.5
Acetic acid		60.05	6.27	376	36	159.5
Formic acid	HCOOH	46.02	23.4	1080	90	42.7
Hydrochloric acid	HCl	36.5	11.6	424	36	86.2
			2.9	105	10	344.8
Nitric acid	HNO_3	63.02	15.99	1008	71	62.5
			14.9	938	67	67.1
			13.3	837	61	75.2
Perchloric acid	$HClO_4$	100.5	11.65	1172	70	85.8
			9.2	923	60	108.7
Phosphoric acid	H_3PO_4	80.0	18.1	1445	85	55.2
Sulfuric acid	H_2SO_4	98.1	18.0	1766	96	55.6
Ammonium hydroxide	NH_4OH	35.0	14.8	251	28	67.6
Potassium hydroxide	KOH	56.1	13.5	757	50	74.1
			1.94	109	10	515.5
Sodium hydroxide	NaOH	40.0	19.1	763	50	52.4
			2.75	111	10	363.6

(Reprinted, with permission, from Sambrook et al. 1989.)

TABLE 2. Approximate pH Values for Various Concentrations of Stock Solutions

Substance	1 N	0.1 N	0.01 N	0.001 N
Acetic acid	2.4	2.9	3.4	3.9
Hydrochloric acid	0.10	1.07	2.02	3.01
Sulfuric acid	0.3	1.2	2.1	
Citric acid		2.1	2.6	
Ammonium hydroxide	11.8	11.3	10.8	10.3
Sodium hydroxide	14.05	13.07	12.12	11.13
Sodium bicarbonate		8.4		
Sodium carbonate		11.5	11.0	

(Reprinted, with permission, from Sambrook et al. 1989.)

TABLE 3. pK$_a$ Values of Commonly Used Buffers

Buffer	Molecular weight	pK$_a$	Buffering range
Tris[a]	121.1	8.08	7.1–8.9
HEPES[b]	238.3	7.47	7.2–8.2
MOPS[c]	209.3	7.15	6.6–7.8
PIPES[d]	304.3	6.76	6.2–7.3
MES[e]	195.2	6.09	5.4–6.8

(Reprinted, with permission, from Sambrook et al. 1989.)
[a]Tris(hydroxymethyl)aminomethane
[b]*N*-2-hydroxyethylpiperazine-*N'*-2-ethanesulfonic acid
[c]3-(*N*-morpholino)propanesulfonic acid
[d]Piperazine-*N,N'*-bis(2-ethanesulfonic acid)
[e](*N*-morpholino)ethanesulfonic acid

TABLE 4. Preparation of Stock Solutions

Solution	Method of preparation
10 M Ammonium acetate	Dissolve 770 g of ammonium acetate in 800 ml of H_2O. Adjust the volume to 1 liter with H_2O. Sterilize by filtration.
10% Ammonium persulfate	To 1 g of ammonium persulfate, add H_2O to 10 ml. The solution may be stored for several weeks at 4°C.
1 M $CaCl_2$	Dissolve 44 g of $CaCl_2 \cdot 6H_2O$ in 200 ml of pure H_2O (Milli-Q or equivalent). Sterile the solution by passage through a 0.22-micron filter.
1 M Dithiothreitol (DTT)	Dissolve 3.09 g of DTT in 20 ml of 0.01 M sodium acetate (pH 5.2). Sterile by filtration. Dispense into 1-ml aliquots and store at −20°C.
0.5 M EDTA (pH 8.0)	Add 186.1 g of disodium ethylenediamintetra-acetate•$2H_2O$ to 800 ml of H_2O. Stir vigorously on a magnetic stirrer. Adjust the pH to 8.0 with NaOH (~20 g of NaOH pellets). Dispense into aliquots and sterilize by autoclaving.
Ethidium bromide (10 mg/ml)	Add 1 g of ethidium bromide to 100 ml of H_2O. Stir on a magnetic stirrer for several hours to ensure that the dye has dissolved. Wrap the container in aluminum foil or transfer the solution to a dark bottle and store at room temperature. **Caution:** Ethidium bromide is a powerful mutagen and is moderately toxic. Gloves should be worn when working with solutions that contain this dye, and a mask should be worn when weighing it out.
1 M $MgCl_2$	Dissolve 203.3 g of $MgCl_2 \cdot 6H_2O$ in 800 ml of H_2O. Adjust the volume to 1 liter with H_2O. Dispense into aliquots and sterilize by autoclaving. $MgCl_2$ is extremely hygroscopic. Buy small bottles (e.g., 100 g) and do not store opened bottles for long periods of time.
β-Mercaptoethanol (BME)	Usually obtained as a 14.4 M solution. Store in a dark bottle at 4°C.
Phenol chloroform	Mix equal amounts of phenol and chloroform. Equilibrate the mixture by extracting several times with 0.1 M Tris•HCl (pH 7.6). Store the equilibrated mixture under an equal volume of 0.01 M Tris•HCl (pH 7.6) at 4°C in dark glass bottles. **Caution:** Phenol is highly corrosive and can cause severe burns. Wear gloves, protective clothing, and safety glasses when handling phenol. All manipulations should be carried out in a chemical hood. Any areas of skin that come into contact with phenol should be rinsed with a large volume of water and washed with soap and water. Do *not* use ethanol.
10 mM Phenylmethyl-sulfonyl fluoride (PMSF)	Dissolve PMSF in isopropanol at a concentration of 1.74 mg/ml (10 mM). Divide the solution into aliquots and store at −20°C. If necessary, stock solutions can be prepared in concentrations as high as 17.4 mg/ml (100 mM). **Caution:** PMSF is extremely destructive to the mucous membranes of the respiratory tract, the eyes, and skin. It may be fatal if inhaled, swallowed, or absorbed through the skin. In case of contact, immediately flush eyes or skin with copious amounts of water. Discard contaminated clothing.
Phosphate-buffered saline (PBS)	Dissolve 8 g of NaCl, 0.2 g of KCl, 1.44 g of Na_2HPO_4, and 0.24 g of KH_2PO_4 in 800 ml of distilled H_2O. Adjust the pH to 7.4 with HCl. Add H_2O to 1 liter. Dispense the solution into aliquots and sterilize them by autoclaving for 20 minutes at 15 lb/sq. in. on liquid cycle.
1 M Potassium acetate (pH 7.5)	Dissolve 9.82 g of potassium acetate in 90 ml of pure H_2O (Milli-Q or equivalent). Adjust the pH to 7.5 with 2 M acetic acid. Add pure H_2O to 100 ml. Divide the solution into aliquots and store them at −20°C.

(*continued on following page*)

TABLE 4. (*continued*)

Solution	Method of preparation
Potassium acetate (for alkaline lysis)	To 60 ml of 5 M potassium acetate, add 11.5 ml of glacial acetic acid and 28.5 ml of H_2O. The resulting solution is 3 M with respect to potassium and 5 M with respect to acetate.
3 M Sodium acetate (pH 5.2 and pH 7.0)	Dissolve 408.1 g of sodium acetate•H_2O in 800 ml of H_2O. Adjust the pH to 5.2 with glacial acetic acid or adjust the pH to 7.0 with dilute acetic acid. Adjust the volume to 1 liter with H_2O. Dispense into aliquots and sterilize by autoclaving.
5 M NaCl	Dissolve 292.2 g of NaCl in 800 ml of H_2O. Adjust the volume to 1 liter with H_2O. Dispense into aliquots and sterilize by autoclaving.
10% Sodium dodecyl sulfate (SDS) (also called sodium lauryl sulfate)	Dissolve 100 g of electrophoresis-grade SDS in 900 ml of H_2O. Heat to 68°C to assist dissolution. Adjust the pH to 7.2 by adding a few drops of concentrated HCl. Adjust the volume to 1 liter with H_2O. Dispense into aliquots.
	Wear a mask when weighing SDS and wipe down the weighing area and balance after use because the fine crystals of SDS disperse easily. There is to need to sterilize 10% SDS.
20x SSC (3.0 M Nacl and 0.3 M sodium citrate)	Dissolve 175.3 g of NaCl and 88.2 g of sodium citrate in 800 ml of H_2O. Adjust the pH to 7.0 with a few drops of a 10 N solution of NaOH. Adjust the volume to 1 liter with H_2O. Dispense into aliquots. Sterilize by autoclaving.
20x SSPE	Dissolve 175.3 g of NaCl, 27.6 g of NaH_2PO_4•H_2O and 7.4 g of EDTA in 800 ml of H_2O. Adjust the pH to 7.4 with NaOH (~6.5 ml of a 10 N solution). Adjust the volume to 1 liter with H_2O. Dispense into aliquots. Sterilize by autoclaving.
Trichloroacetic acid (TCA) 100% solution	To a bottle containing 500 g of TCA, add 227 ml of H_2O. The resulting solution will contain 100% (w/v) TCA.
1 M Tris	Dissolve 121.1 g of Tris base in 800 ml of H_2O. Adjust the pH to the desired value by adding concentrated HCl

pH	HCl
7.4	70 ml
7.6	60 ml
8.0	42 ml

If the 1 M solution has a yellow color, discard it and obtain better quality Tris.

Allow the solution to cool to room temperature before making final adjustments to the pH. Adjust the volume of the solution to 1 liter with H_2O. Dispense into aliquots and sterilize by autoclaving.

The pH of Tris solutions is temperature-dependent and decreases approximately 0.03 pH units for each 1°C increase in temperature. For example, a 0.05 M solution has pH values of 9.5, 8.9, and 8.6 at 5°C, 25°C, and 37°C, respectively.

Solution	Method of preparation
50x Tris-Acetate-EDTA buffer	Dissolve 242 g of Tris base in 500 ml of H_2O. Add 100 ml of 0.5 M EDTA (pH 8.0). Add 57.1 ml of glacial acetic acid. Adjust volume to 1 liter with H_2O and sterilize by autoclaving.
Tris-buffered saline (TBS) (25 mM Tris)	Dissolve 8 g of NaCl, 0.2 g of KCl, and 3 g of Tris base in 800 ml of distilled H_2O. Add 0.015 g of phenol red and adjust the pH to 7.4 with HCl. Add distilled H_2O to 1 liter. Dispense the solution into aliquots and sterilize them by autoclaving for 20 minutes at 15 lb/sq. in. on liquid cycle. Store at room temperature.

(Modified, with permission, from Maniatis et al. 1982.)

PROTOCOL

Preparation of Phenol and Phenol Chloroform (Reprinted, with permission, from Sambrook et al. 1989)

Phenol

Most batches of commercial liquified phenol are clear and colorless and can be used in molecular cloning without redistillation. Occasionally, batches of liquified phenol are pink or yellow, and these should be rejected and returned to the manufacturer. Crystalline phenol is not recommended because it must be redistilled at 160°C to remove oxidation products, such as quinones, that cause the breakdown of phospho-diester bonds or cause cross-linking of RNA and DNA.

Caution: Phenol is highly corrosive and can cause severe burns. Wear gloves, protective clothing, and safety glasses when handling phenol. All manipulations should be carried out in a chemical hood. Any areas of skin that come into contact with phenol should be rinsed with a large volume of water and washed with soap and water. Do *not* use ethanol.

Procedure

Equilibration of phenol

Before use, phenol must be equilibrated to a pH >7.8 because DNA will partition into the organic phase at acid pH.

1. Liquified phenol should be stored at −20°C. As needed, remove the phenol from the freezer, allow it to warm to room temperature, and then melt it at 68°C. Add hydroxyquinoline to a final concentration of 0.1%. This compound is an antioxidant, a partial inhibitor of RNase, and a weak chelator of metal ions (Kirby 1956). In addition, its yellow color provides a convenient way to identify the organic phase.

2. To the melted phenol, add an equal volume of buffer (usually 0.5 M Tris•HCl [pH 8.0] at room temperature). Stir the mixture on a magnetic stirrer for 15 minutes, and then turn off the stirrer. When the two phases have separated, aspirate as much as possible of the upper (aqueous) phase using a glass pipet attached to a vacuum line equipped with traps.

3. Add an equal volume of 0.1 M Tris•HCl (pH 8.0) to the phenol. Stir the mixture on a magnetic stirrer for 15 minutes, and then turn off the stirrer. Remove the upper aqueous phase as described in step 2. Repeat the extractions until the pH of the phenolic phase is >7.8 (as measured with pH paper).

4. After the phenol is equilibrated and the final aqueous phase has been removed, add 0.1 volume of 0.1 M Tris•HCl (pH 8.0) containing 0.2% β-mercaptoethanol. The phenol solution may be stored in this form under 100 mM Tris•HCl (pH 8.0) in a light-tight bottle at 4ºC for periods of up to 1 month.

Phenol:Chloroform:Isoamyl Alcohol (25:24:1)

A mixture consisting of equal parts of equilibrated phenol and chloroform isoamyl alcohol (24:1) is frequently used to remove proteins from preparations of nucleic acids. The chloroform denatures proteins and facilitates the separation of the aqueous and organic phases, and the isoamyl alcohol reduces foaming during extraction.

Neither chloroform nor isoamyl alcohol requires treatment before use. The phenol:chloroform:isoamyl alcohol mixture may be stored under 100 mM Tris•HCl (pH 8.0) in a light-tight bottle at 4ºC for periods of up to 1 month.

WEIGHING AND MIXING

Weighing out ingredients to make a buffer isn't one of the hardest things you will do, but it is one of the most important. Gather *everything* you need before you start, so you don't have to leave your powder uncovered on the balance while you frantically search for a clean beaker.

Never weigh a sample directly on the balance pan.

You will need

Weighing paper (for solids under a gram and smaller than a golf ball) or

Weighing boats. These come in several sizes, so take one larger than you need. A *small beaker* can be used for liquids or a large amount of powder.

Spatulas. Spatulas also come in several sizes, in reusable metal and disposable plastic, and you should use a large one for large amounts, small ones for small amounts. You can't make a mistake, you can only have a slightly awkward time.

A clean graduated cylinder of a volume as close to the target volume as you can get. Err on the side of a cylinder larger than the desired volume, rather than measuring multiple times from a too small cylinder.

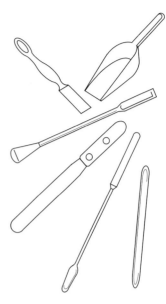

FIGURE 4.

Weighing utensils are known by various names in different labs and companies. Spatula, microspatula, scoop, and spoon are some of the contenders. Most labs have one name for all the utensils, but you will be understood with any one term.

Beaker or Erlenmeyer flask, whatever you will make the buffer in. Choose a size that will allow room for mixing, and for pH-ing: For a 500-ml volume of solution, use a 1-liter beaker.

Magnetic stir plate and stir bar. The magnetic stir plate does not need to have a heater. The stir bar should be the largest that will rotate freely in the beaker or Erlenmeyer flask.

Don't use a plastic beaker or flask on a hot plate!

Place to dispose of spatulas, magnetic stir bars. This is lab dependent—just look to see whether they are washed immediately, or placed somewhere for washing.

Kimwipes. This is lab tissue paper, used for delicate wiping and blotting.

Distilled water. Your solvent is assumed to be water. Use filter-purified or glass-distilled water. Do not use tap water.

Weighing

1. Put on surgical gloves. In general, this protects you and protects the contents of the jars you are dipping into. Gloves are expensive, and if you must limit glove use, put them on to protect yourself from potentially harmful substances.

2. Read the bottle, and see if you need to wear a mask or heavyweight gloves. Many substances are, at the least, powdery, and no matter how careful you are, may form

a little duststorm and fly into your nasal passages. Others are blatantly toxic.

3. Turn on the balance. Depending on the balance, and the lab, some balances are left on all day, perhaps on standby. Most are not. If the balance isn't clean, clean it before you weigh anything.

4. Tare the weigh paper/boat. Place it on the balance, and push the tare or weigh button. The scale should then read zero.

5. Weigh your material. With the spatula, remove a small amount of material from the tilted open jar, and place it on the weigh boat/paper. Once you have a feel for

> *Some balances may not have an automatic tare feature. If not, you must tare the weighing vessel manually.*
> *1. Weigh the beaker or weigh boat.*
> *2. Record the weight.*
> *3. Add the boat/beaker weight to the target weight of the material.*
> *4. Weigh the material and adjust to the weight calculated in step 3.*

what amount weighs how much, you can move a bit faster. As you get closer to the desired weight, add less material. Resist the temptation to pour from the jar, until you know the feel and properties of an inert substance and what will or will not make a mess.

If you put too much on the paper/boat, you can put it back in the jar *if* (1) The material is not hydroscopic. Hydroscopic material absorbs water, and might have done so in the time it has been out of the jar. (2) The material has not touched anything but a clean spatula or weigh paper/boat.

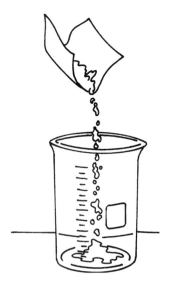

6. When you have the correct amount of material, pour it into the beaker or flask. To do this, grasp the boat or paper by opposite ends, gently bending the ends toward each other to make a funnel-like opening through which you can pour. Pour slowly. If any material sticks to the paper/boat, knock it off on the side of the beaker.

7. Close the lid of the stock jar. The longer it is open, the more dust can get in, the more likely that someone might knock it over or spill something in it. **Replace the jar** as soon as possible, even if you are still weighing other things. The more clutter you can remove, the less chance of a mistake or a mess.

8. Clean the balance when you are finished. There may be a brush there that you can use to sweep any stray bits off the pan. Otherwise, use a Kimwipe or a paper towel. Wipe any liquid drops

with a Kimwipe. If you spilled something, remove the pan, wash it with distilled water and dry it, and replace it on the balance. Make sure the entire weighing area is clean—no weighing papers, beakers, bottles, paper towels, or Kimwipes should be left, and the surrounding counter space should be wiped if necessary.

> *Label, label, label! Any container with any substance (even water) in it should be labeled. Even if you are putting it on the bench for "one minute." Post-Its are handy for temporary labels.*

If you can't add water immediately, cover the top of the beaker with foil or plastic wrap, LABEL IT, and place it on your lab bench.

Mixing

Theoretically, all you have to do now is to add the water, but there are several schools of thought on this simple procedure. For example, there are those who will add the material to the water in the graduated cylinder, cover it with plastic wrap, and shake. Don't do it! Even if you don't break the cylinder or spray the lab with water, you probably will not get a very well mixed solution. Others add the powder and the water directly into a beaker, and use the beaker as a cylinder, to measure the amount of water added. Don't do that, either: It just isn't accurate enough.

> *Remember the old chem lab adage when mixing acids and water:*
> > *Do as you oughta.*
> > *Add acid (and base) to watah.*

For most solutions

1. Add 80% of the total final volume of water to the beaker, and then add the solid. For a liter, add 800 ml of water, measured with a graduated cylinder. *Note:* For concentrated solutions—say, over 3 M or 5X—there will be too much powder to get the stir bar moving. In these cases, pour the powder slowly into a beaker, in which there already is 80% of the desired volume of water and a spinning stir bar. Pour slowly, around 2 tablespoons worth at a time, making sure all powder has dissolved before you add more. If you are having considerable trouble getting things to go into solution, find a stir plate with a heater and warm the solution mildly (a setting of 2–3, or a one-quarter turn of the dial) while stirring. *The solution must be cooled to room temperature before you pH it* or you may get an erroneous pH.

2. Gently drop in a magnetic stir bar, as large as will spin freely.

3. Put the beaker on the magnetic stir plate first, and turn on the stirrer very slowly. If you do it too fast, or turn on the stirrer before you put the beaker on the plate or the stir bar in, the stir bar will jump wildly enough to break the beaker.

If the stir bar loses its rhythm, turn off the stirrer, wait until the stir bar settles, and turn the stirrer on slowly.

4. Stir until the powder is completely in solution.

5. Pour the solution into the graduated cylinder or volumetric flask to check the volume and bring the volume up to 90% of the desired final volume.

6. Pour the solution back into the beaker or Erlenmeyer flask for pH-ing.

7. Label the contents of the beaker. Label with tape only. Never write directly on a bottle, cylinder, or flask.

> *If you don't need to pH the mixture, bring the volume to 100% and pour it immediately into a container suitable for autoclaving or prepare for filter sterilization.*

> *After pH-ing the solution, pour it into a graduated cylinder or volumetric flask and bring the solution to the desired volume with water.*

MEASURING PH

It is critical that all buffers and solutions used in biology be at the appropriate pH. Solutions are pH-ed before autoclaving, with the use of a pH meter.

pH tips

- The pH meter has a sensitive electrode that measures the H^+ concentration in a solution. The electrode is protected by a plastic sleeve, but be very careful not to bang the electrode on the glassware or with the stir bar. When not in use, the electrode is left in a small beaker or medicine cup containing a neutral buffer (the soak buffer). The pH meter, especially if it is fairly new, will have many buttons for functions you don't need to know about to determine a pH. The only buttons you will probably need to use are the standby, standardize, and pH buttons.

- There are several kinds of electrodes; some filled with a gel or liquid, some not; some requiring maintenance, some not. In many labs, no one even knows what kind of electrode they have until there is a problem and they must search through the drawers for the package literature to figure out what to do. Check with a knowledgeable lab member or with the manufacturer before you have problems.

- The pH meter should be calibrated daily, using two buffers of known pH. From these calibrations are derived the pH determinations, so don't scrimp (and render your pH reading inaccurate) by standardizing only to one buffer of pH 7. There is a lot of inertia and worry about calibrating the pH meter, but it is necessary, it does make a difference, and it is ridiculous to go through the trouble of pH-ing at all if it isn't done correctly.

- If you are pH-ing a series of solutions, you don't need to recalibrate between solutions. Do recalibrate if someone known to be sloppy calibrated the meter.

> *Don't use the pH paper you may find in the drawer to routinely pH your solutions. It is used to check the pH of small volumes, or to do a quick pH check before use of the pH meter. Always remove a drop from the solution to add to the paper; never dip the pH paper into the solution.*

- pH will affect solubility. An example of this is 0.5 M EDTA, a common molecular biology reagent. It is usually made at a pH of 8.0, and won't even go into solution until that pH is approached.

- pH is dependent on temperature. Be sure the buffer you are pH-ing is the same temperature as the buffer standards you use to calibrate the pH meter. And be sure the buffer and the standards are at the temperature at which the buffer will be used.

Calibrating the pH Meter

You will need:

At least two pH standard solutions. Near the pH meter you should find standards of 4, 7, and 10. In most labs these are purchased ready-made and are stored in 500-ml bottles. Generally, using standards of 4 and 10 is sufficient.

3 or 4 50-ml beakers or medicine cups, glass or plastic.

Kimwipes.

1. Raise the electrode out of the soak (or storage) buffer, and rinse it with distilled water from the wash bottle. Rinse the electrode over a beaker used only for washes. Do not rinse the electrode into the soak beaker. The pH meter should still be set on standby. Touch electrode gently with a Kimwipe, to remove excess fluid.

> *Choose your standards according to what you will be pH-ing. If you will be pH-ing a solution of extreme pH (that is, above 10 or below 4) you should standardize with buffers closer to the target pH. For example, if you will be pH-ing a buffer to 3, it would be better to standardize to buffers of pH 2 and 4, or 2 and 7. After, recalibrate to pH values of 4 and 10.*

Calibration with one buffer

If you are going to measure buffers of approximately the same pH, you could standardize the pH meter with just one buffer.
- Use a standard of 7.0 for neutral buffers, 10 for basic buffers, or 4 for acidic buffers.
- Calibrate the pH meter and measure the pH as described for 2-buffer standardization.

Should you need to pH a buffer of a different pH, you will have to restandardize the pH meter.

---

2. Pour approximately 1.5 inches of standard pH 4 (it could be 10; there is no order necessary) into a small beaker or medicine cup. Recap the bottle of standard 4, and then immerse the tip of the electrode into the beaker.

3. Press "standardize" and wait until the display reading has stabilized at pH 4.

4. Press "standby," raise electrode, and rinse and dry it as in step 1.

5. Pour the standard pH 10 into a fresh beaker, immerse the electrode, and press "standardize." Wait until the display reading has stabilized at a pH of 10.

6. Press standby, rinse and dry electrode, and leave it immersed in a beaker of storage buffer.

7. Read the pH of the standardization buffers. If the pH is not as it should be, repeat the calibration until the pH reads as it should. The pH meter is now standardized for most buffers and solutions.

Determining pH

Have ready the same materials needed for calibration, as well as a magnetic stir plate, stir bars, and pasteur pipets. You will also need acids and bases to actually determine pH: concentrated HCl (12.1 M) and 1 M HCl, and NaOH (5 or 10 M) and/or 0.1 M NaOH should be found next to the pH meter.

1. Stir the solution to be pH-ed on a magnetic stir plate. The stir bar should be stirring as slowly as possible, to lessen the chance of electrode damage should the electrode mistakenly come in contact with the bottom of the flask or beaker.

2. Raise the electrode out of the soak beaker, rinse it with distilled water from the wash bottle, and blot dry gently with a Kimwipe. The pH meter should still be set on "standby." Do not rinse the electrode into the soak beaker.

3. Immerse the tip of the electrode into the solution you want to measure. Make sure the bar clears the electrode before you turn on the magnetic stirrer.

What should I use to pH buffers?

Most labs use **HCl and NaOH** to adjust the pH on the acid or basic form of routine buffers. (Other strong acids or bases could also be used.) It is true that using HCl or NaOH to pH a buffer adds anions (Cl^-) or cations (Na^+) to your buffer, and that these could interfere with certain experiments. But it usually doesn't, and it is often assumed that you will do it that way. A Tris-Cl buffer means that after dissolving the base form of Tris, the pH was adjusted with HCl. A Tris-acetate buffer means that the pH was adjusted with acetic acid.

One could also add the acid and base forms of a buffer separately to obtain the desired pH. Phosphate and acetate buffers are often made this way. If you know the pKa, you can calculate the ratio you need of base form to acid form of the acid-base pair for a particular pH. You will probably never have to do this. The protocol or recipe will specify the amounts of acid and base you must add to achieve the desired pH, or you can consult one of the many tables found in catalogs.

4. If the pH meter has a function switch, change it from standby to pH. (If you need to take the electrode out of the beaker to mix by swirling, turn the function switch to standby first.)

5. Wait for the readings to stabilize. Read the pH, and adjust it by adding NaOH if the pH is too low, and HCl if the pH is too high. Use a pasteur pipet and bulb, or a transfer pipet, to add the pH-ing solutions: Use a separate pipet for each solution. Start with one drop at a time: Add a drop to the stirring solution and wait until the pH has changed and stabilized before adding another drop.

    If the pH is off by more than a unit, use concentrated HCl (12.1 M) or NaOH (5 or 10 M). Otherwise, use 1 M HCl or 0.1 M NaOH.

    Continue to add acid or base, dropwise, until you have reached the target pH. You will need more drops as you approach the pH at which a solution is buffered. If the pH isn't budging, use a more concentrated solution to pH it, but be very, very careful to do so slowly and dropwise.

6. Turn function switch back to standby.

7. Raise the electrode out of the solution, rinse the electrode with distilled water, and wipe it gently with a Kimwipe.

8. Leave the electrode immersed in storage buffer.

9. Pour the solution into a graduated cylinder or volumetric flask and bring the volume up to 100%.

Be sure the stir bar is not autoclaved with the solution in the bottle. Few things infuriate lab personnel more than seeing a row of autoclaved reagents, complete with stir bars inside; most labs don't have unlimited numbers of stir bars. Should you accidentally pour the stir bar into the bottle, retrieve it before autoclaving with the long, magnetized rod that you should find near the sink.

10. Pour the solution into a glass or plastic bottle with a cap (see below for auto-clavable plastic.) Do not store buffers in flasks, beakers, or cylinders, covered with parafilm.

11. Label the bottle. Use a piece of tape and a Sharpie or other marking pen. Write the date (including the year), the components, the concentration, the pH, and your initials.

12. Put a piece of autoclave tape on the bottle. It is heat sensitive and will darken visibly only after being autoclaved. If you are unable to autoclave immediately, store the buffer at 4ºC to reduce the chance of contamination.

If readings are erratic, check

- **The electrode.** Some electrodes contain a buffer, which must be maintained. If so, fill it with the correct buffer (check the manual) and close. The electrode may also be cracked or broken, and need to be replaced.

- **The standards.** People often pour the standards back into the stock bottle after use, arguing that it was used so little that it is as good as new. Not true, and this practice will have a negative effect. Try a new bottle of standard buffer.

- **The temperature** of the buffer. Since pH is dependent on temperature, be sure all buffers are at room temperature before reading the pH. Common culprits are freshly distilled (too warm) or refrigerated water (too cold), just-made exo- or endothermic buffers, or the heat of the hot plate stirrer.

- **The storage solution.** If the storage solution in the beaker has dried up, salt may be encrusted around the tip of the electrode. Rinse the electrode well with water, and store the electrode in a beaker of fresh storage buffer.

> **Tris buffers** can be difficult to pH, giving unstable readings. A few electrodes give spurious readings for Tris-containing solutions. In particular, silver/silver chloride reference electrodes used with Tris solutions containing protein can be inaccurate.
>
> After you pH your Tris solution, wait 10 minutes and pH it again. If your readings are different, call the electrode or pH meter manufacturer to find out whether that electrode is compatible with Tris buffers. If not, Tris-compatible electrodes are available, of course.
>
> Most of the Tris solutions you will make will not contain protein, and there should be no problem pH-ing those buffers.

- **Your technique.** Rinse electrodes well between buffers. Always stir moderately while pH-ing.

STERILIZING SOLUTIONS

 Autoclaving or filtration? Most buffers are sterilized before use and storage, to prevent bacterial and fungal growth. And most buffers are autoclaved: Although filtration would be as effective, the large volumes in which buffers are usually made would make filtration extremely tedious.

> *Even if you require the buffer for a nonsterile application, it should still be sterilized, because microbial growth can cause changes in pH and in the nature and function of the buffer.*

Be sure the solution can be autoclaved: Heat-labile ingredients cannot be heated, and a solution containing such an ingredient must either be filter-sterilized or autoclaved without the ingredient (which can be filtered and added later to the autoclaved material).

Autoclave

- Most buffers.

- Undefined bacterial and yeast media.

Do not autoclave

> *If a heat-labile or otherwise non-autoclavable ingredient must be added to an autoclavable buffer, autoclave the buffer first. When the buffer has cooled to room temperature, add the filter-sterilized ingredient.*

- Buffers with detergent, such as 10% SDS, because they will boil over.

- Organic solvents, including phenol.

- Heat-labile ingredients such as serum and vitamins, antibiotics, and proteins (BSA).

- Mammalian, plant, and insect media.

- HEPES-containing solutions.

- Dithiothreitol (DTT)- or β-mercaptoethanol (BME)-containing solutions.

Using the Autoclave

Autoclaves work by subjecting the material to high heat (121°F) and pressure. If you are unfamiliar with the autoclave, ask someone to demonstrate its use. This is not a machine to experiment with, although it is quite safe when used correctly.

   Be sure the flask or bottle is borosilicate glass or autoclavable plastic. Glass will generally be used for buffers, because repeated autoclaving is rough on most plastics. A rough rule of thumb is that the more brittle-feeling plastics aren't suitable, but you will have to check the catalog or ask someone about a particular item.

1. Leave at least a quarter of the total flask or bottle volume as free space. This leaves plenty of room for boiling liquids.

2. Place containers in a shallow metal or autoclavable plastic pan to catch anything that might break. Traditionally, a couple of inches of water are placed in the pan to reduce the chance of glass breaking with a sudden pressure change: This is not necessary, but you may be considered to be crazy for not doing it.

3. Be sure caps are loose to prevent buildup of pressure. If you are using tin foil as a cap, tape one side of the foil to the flask to prevent the top from getting knocked off.

4. Stick a small piece of autoclave tape on each item to be autoclaved. This is pressure-sensitive tape, which will show a design or color change only after autoclaving. On the cap or just above the identification label are logical places to put it. Write the date on the tape.

5. Close and tighten the autoclave door. It should be tight, but not so tight that it will be a strain to open. If it is a two-door autoclave, be sure both doors are closed.

6. Adjust appropriate settings and turn on. Most autoclaves are automatic, and will have a minimum of a liquid (solutions in glass containers require a controlled rate of cooling and slow release of pressure) and a dry setting (which requires no cool-down period). The newer programmable autoclaves may have numbered programs, as well as manual settings. If you have large volumes, the cycle will take longer than for small volumes.

    > *For a 2-liter Erlenmeyer flask containing 1 liter of medium, set 30 minutes of sterilization time.*

7. Be sure the autoclave has returned to ambient pressure before opening. Open very slowly, standing back from the door, to avoid contact with any escaping steam.

8. Put on heat-resistant gloves. The gloves should be large, heavyweight gloves. Don't use potholders or oven gloves.

> **To avoid precipitates, browning, and substrate breakdown**
> • Autoclave glucose separately from amino acids/peptones or phosphate components.
> • Autoclave phosphates separately from amino acids/peptones or other mineral salt components.
> • Autoclave mineral salt components separately from agar.
> • Avoid autoclaving media at a pH greater than 7.5. Autoclave at neutral pH and adjust to the desired pH with a sterile base solution after cooling.
> • Avoid autoclaving agar solutions at less than pH 6.0.
>
> (Reprinted, with permission, from Cote and Gherna 1994.)

9. Tighten caps before taking the bottles out of the autoclave. The liquid may boil over as you remove them.

10. Let the bottles sit at room temperature until cool. If you put the bottles immediately into the cold, the glass may crack. It usually works out well to leave the bottles on the bench overnight.

Filter Sterilization

If a liquid is heat-labile or volatile, or less than 20 ml in volume, it should be sterilized by filtration. The solution is passed (aided by gravity, force, or vacuum) through a filter of a pore size small enough (0.2 or 0.1 µm) to exclude most microorganisms. Note that viruses are not removed by filter sterilization. Use 0.4-µm filters only as a prefilter for a viscous solution: A passage through 0.4 µm will not sterilize a solution, and so must be followed by passage through a 0.2-µm filter.

> *0.2 µm is typically used for buffer sterilization and most medium sterilization. 0.1 µm is used for some tissue culture media.*

 There are many reusable and disposable filtration systems commercially available. Some labs or departments make their own media and have large-scale, pump-driven filtration units. There are several kinds commonly used at the bench for individual filtration needs:

- Non-disposable filtration apparatus, vacuum driven: volumes 20 ml–1000 ml.

- Disposable filter cup units, vacuum driven: volumes 15 ml–1000 ml.

- Disposable filtration units with storage bottle, vacuum-driven: volumes 15 ml–1000 ml.

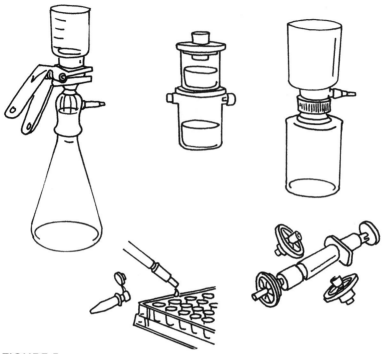

FIGURE 5.

Clockwise, from left: A nondisposable unit; a disposable cup unit; a disposable filtration unit with storage bottle; syringe and micro-syringe filter units; and a microfuge tube filter unit.

- Syringe filters: volumes 1 ml–20 ml.

- Micro-syringe filters: volumes less than 1 ml.

- Spin filters, microfuge tube filters: volumes less than 1 ml.

Work aseptically. Doing the filtration in a biosafety cabinet adds an extra measure of security. See Chapter 9, Working without Contamination, for filter-sterilizing techniques.

STORING BUFFERS AND SOLUTIONS

 Store media at 4°C.

 Buffers can be stored at 4°C or at room temperature. Some buffers, especially concentrated ones, will precipitate in the cold: This is usually not a problem, as heating at 37°C for a few minutes will redissolve the precipitate. Storage in the cold will dampen the growth of contaminants that might be introduced during use. There is a psychological component as well, for people tend to be more careful with things stored in the refrigerator rather than on the bench. In general, store buffers for culture in the cold, buffers for biochemical assays at room temperature.

 Store concentrated solutions at room temperature.

 Light-sensitive reagents should be stored at the appropriate temperature in a brown bottle, or in a bottle kept in a box or covered with foil and tape. See Chapter 8 for more details on the storage of solutions.

When to Discard Buffers

Many buffers can be used for years, especially if they have been sterilized and kept in the cold. But there are several reasons to throw the bottle away.

- **Discoloration.** If a buffer looks discolored—that is, if it has acquired a tinge of *yellow*—discard it. It is probably okay, but using it will always leave a feeling of unease that isn't worth saving the effort of making another bottle. Make sure it isn't a buffer that is normally colored. For example, MOPS, one of the Friend zwitterionic buffers, is always yellowish above a 1 molar concentration.

- **Contamination.** A sure reason to immediately discard a buffer is contamination. This is usually *mold*, and will appear as a discrete, ball-shaped item, sometimes furry, often white or blue-greenish. If a clear, colorless bottle becomes cloudy, discard it. Desperate people have filtered the mold away and used the buffer, but it isn't worth it: Even if the solution is now sterile, it might have been changed by metabolic by-products.

    Bacterial contamination is less likely, and will either settle on the bottom of the container or will make the solution appear cloudy. Get into the habit of swirling your bottles and eyeballing them as you get ready to use them, to check for contamination.

  > *When in doubt, throw it out. There is too much resting on the quality of your reagents to try to save time and money here.*

- **Precipitation.** It is sometimes difficult to tell bacterial contamination from precipitated salts. If you are in doubt, place the buffer in a 37°C water bath for 20 minutes and see if the cloudiness dissolves. If it does, storage in the cold is causing some salt to precipitate, and you can warm it up before use. (But you should plan on replacing it soon.) If the cloudiness remains, you don't know whether it is a stubborn precipitate or contamination, but it doesn't matter—throw it away immediately.

If you really need to know whether it is precipitate or contamination, put a drop of it on a slide with a coverslip, and look at it on a microscope at 100X. A precipitate will appear as large *crystals,* contamination as tiny and uniform shapes.

RESOURCES

A.L.E.R.T. (Allergy to Latex Education and Resource Team). 1997.
http://www.execpc.com/~alert/news.html/

Bateman R. and Evans J. 1996. *Biochemistry laboratory manual.* I. Solution preparation.
http://www-chem.st.usm.edu/biochem/lab_manual/lab.html/

Bateman R. and Evans J. 1996. *Biochemistry laboratory manual.* II. Buffer preparation and testing.
http://www-chem.st.usm.edu/biochem/lab _manual/lab_manual.html/

Cote R.J. and Gherna R.L. 1994. Nutrition and media. In *Methods for general and molecular bacteriology* (ed. Gerhardt P. et al.), pp. 155–178. American Society for Microbiology, Washington, D.C.

Gershey E.L., Party E., and Wilkerson A. 1991. *Laboratory safety in practice: A comprehensive compliance program and safety manual.* Van Nostrand Reinhold, New York.

Heidcamp W.H. 1995. *Cell biology laboratory manual.* Gustavus Adolphus College, St. Peter, Minnesota.
http://www.gac.edu/cgi-bin/user/~cellab/phpl?index-1.html/

Lenga R.E. 1988. *The Sigma-Aldrich library of chemical safety data,* edition II, vol. I and II. Sigma-Aldrich Corporation, Milwaukee.

Lide D.R., ed. 1997–1998. *CRC Handbook of Chemistry and Physics,* 78th edition. CRC Press, Boca Raton, Florida.

Maniatis T., Fritsch E.F., and Sambrook J. 1982. *Molecular cloning: A laboratory manual.* Cold Spring Harbor Laboratory, Cold Spring Harbor, New York.

Sambrook J., Fritsch E.F., and Maniatis T. 1989. *Molecular cloning. A laboratory manual.* 2nd edition. Cold Spring Harbor Laboratory Press, Cold Spring Harbor, New York.

Sigma Chemical Company. 1996. *TRIZMA. Tris(hydroxymethyl)aminomethane; Tris. Technical Bulletin no. 106B.* St. Louis, Missouri.

UW GenChem Pages. 1996. Department of Chemistry, University of Wisconsin-Madison.
http://genchem.chem.msg.edu/labdocs/

Windholz M., ed. 1976. *Merck index,* 9th edition. Merck and Co., Inc. Rahway, New Jersey.

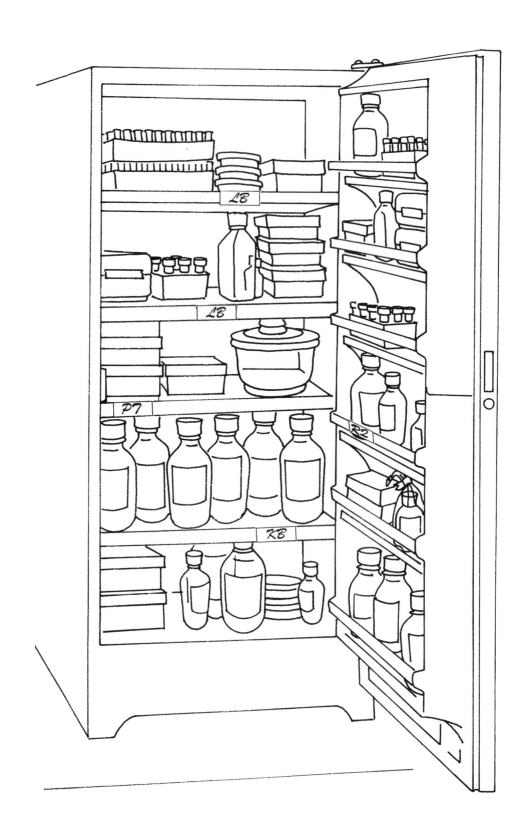

8

Storage and Disposal

AFTER YOU MAKE IT, after you use it, when you are done with it, you have to put it somewhere! *Everything in a lab must be accounted for and placed in an appropriate place at all times.* For the storage of experimental materials, this is obvious. Incorrect storage can ruin reagents and organisms. But it is less obvious for trash. Here the issues are of safety and expediency, and not necessarily your own safety and expediency, so people are more casual. Improper

EMERGENCY STORAGE	163
STORING REAGENTS	165
ALIQUOTING	170
REFRIGERATORS AND FREEZERS	172
DISCARDING LAB WASTE	175
What you need to know to dispose of	
material as waste	175
Order of priority for disposal	182
RESOURCES	183

disposal of material can be a health hazard to those responsible for removing it. It can be harmful to the environment. It is illegal in many places. And it can be grounds to have the entire lab shut down.

EMERGENCY STORAGE

Where should I put it??? It is 1 A.M., your experiment took 3 hours longer than you expected, everyone else has gone home, and you forgot to ask where to put your tubes. There are certain assumptions you can make about where things should go. In the morning, find out about long-term storage for the material and move it.

> *When in doubt, the general rule for emergency short-term storage is: COLD IS BEST.*

- **Acids or bases.** Leave on your bench until the morning. Store acids and bases separately, in polyethylene trays that could contain the spill if a bottle breaks.

- **Antibodies, monoclonal and polyclonal.** 4°C. Most purified antibodies are stored long term at 4°C, but some are stored at –20°C.

163

- **Assay tubes.** You can try 4ºC, but assay stability is extremely variable. Most colorimetric assays will not be readable the next day.

- **Bacteria.**
   Plate or stab cultures, 4ºC.
   Liquid cultures, 4ºC.
   Lyophilized cultures, 4ºC.
   Frozen cultures, –70ºC.

- **Buffers.** 4ºC.

- **Cells.** Back where they came from, or discard: *Never* put living cells where you don't KNOW they belong.

- **Detergents.** Room temperature.

- **DNA.** 4ºC.

- **Enzymes.** Most restriction enzymes are stored at –20ºC, but read the tube to check, as some can't be frozen. Most other enzymes should also be stored at –20ºC.

- **Ethanol.** Room temperature.

- **Growth factors and cytokines.** –20ºC.

- **Hazardous chemicals.** You cannot compromise with even the overnight storage of hazardous chemicals. Before you begin work with such a substance, you must find out all relevant storage and disposal information.

- **Lipids.** –20ºC. Many lipids are unstable and are sensitive to oxygen or light, or to changes in temperature.

- **Media.** 4ºC.

- **PCR reactions.** 4ºC. You may find the previous user's tubes in the cycler.

- **Radioisotopes.**
   ^{32}P: nucleotides at –20ºC, phosphate at 4ºC.
   ^{33}P: 4ºC.
   ^{35}S: methionine at –70ºC.
   ^{125}I: protein A at 4ºC, iodine in a fume hood at room temperature.
   ^{3}H: 4ºC.
   ^{14}C: 4ºC.

Ethanol is a fire and explosion hazard. Large volumes are stored at room temperature, in a high-density polyethylene or steel (terne plate, galvanized, or type 316 stainless) safety can. However, some protocols call for cold ethanol: Two common uses of cold ethanol are cell and tissue fixation and nucleic acid precipitations. Investigators often try to keep a small bottle of 100% ethanol in the refrigerator, but EHS teams always remove it during inspections. If it is stored cold, it should be kept in an explosion-proof refrigerator. Otherwise, remove some and keep it on ice before the experiment to cool it.

- **RNA.** –20ºC with ethanol, –70ºC in water.

- **Serum.** 4ºC.

STORING REAGENTS

For long-term storage, you want a situation for each chemical in which the biological and chemical activity of the material is preserved as best as it can be, in as safe a location as possible for all lab personnel. These requirements are specific to *each* chemical and reagent, and you must check the situation for the individual reagent, and not merely for the class or type of reagent.

What you need to know to store material

> *Reagents must be stored with all storage requirements satisfied. For example, if a substance is radioactive and oxygen-sensitive and requires cold storage, it must be stored under nitrogen and placed in an area of a freezer in which radioactive material is permitted to be stored.*

- **Temperature requirement.** Must it be stored in an oven, at room temperature, refrigerated, frozen, deeply frozen, or in liquid nitrogen?

- **Gas requirements.** Is the material sensitive to oxygen? Does it require another gas?

- **Moisture sensitivity.** If water vapor would harm the material, it needs to be desiccated. Must it also be under vacuum?

- **Associated hazards.** Is the material radioactive, flammable, extremely toxic, or volatile? If it is a solution, is the solvent organic?

How to find storage and disposal information

- **The Materials Safety Data Sheet (MSDS),** which comes with every chemical, describes the composition and properties, toxicology, and instructions for handling, spill control, and waste disposal. If you cannot locate one, call the manufacturer and ask them to fax one to you.

- **The Merck Index.**

- **EHS department.** The EHS (Environmental Health and Safety) department probably keeps the data sheet on file for every chemical used by the department. Even if you have this information, you should be in frequent contact with EHS to find out the storage and disposal rules for your institution. EHS can offer advice on storage and disposal containers, and sometimes can supply some or all of the needed containers.

On the WWW. There are many universities, distributors, and manufacturers with web sites detailing storage of chemicals. See Kowahl (1996) as an example of such a site.

 How to store reagents that need to be desiccated

Many reagents are adversely affected by water vapor, and lose structural and biological activity. These reagents should be stored in an airtight jar that contains desiccant, a material that will absorb water vapor and reduce the humidity in the jar. Sometimes the jar is placed under vacuum to further reduce the amount of water vapor.

- **Containers**

    The container must be able to close tightly, and must have room in it for desiccant.

    > *Don't use an aluminum container, because you must open it to check the desiccant.*

    For a few reagents, a large-mouth jar will be fine.

    For larger bottles, a glass or plastic desiccator will be needed. These come in various shapes and sizes and materials. Size is your primary concern.

    > *Don't glob on the vacuum grease, or the seal won't be effective and you might get grease inside the container.*

    Fussy reagents require vacuum. Vacuum containers have a spout or opening to which a tube is attached from the container to the vacuum source. Glass jars are available with O-rings and grooves on the top and bottom, or with smooth edges. These do not require vacuum grease. Glass jars with smooth tops and bottoms require just a bit of vacuum grease to keep a seal. Any container used for anaerobic culture of bacteria can also be used.

- **Desiccant**

    Desiccant is usually found as blue or purple rough pellets of calcium carbonate, resembling pebbles. It may also come in bags, cartridges, or perforated cans.

    Desiccant is blue when it is dry, pink when moist. It can be regenerated by being dried in an oven for 1–3 hours at approximately 200°C (the

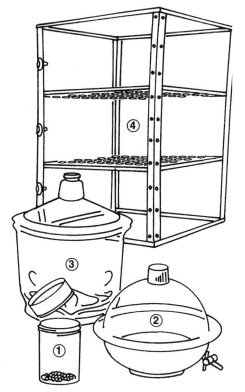

FIGURE 1.

Various styles of desiccators. There is room for desiccant at the bottom of all containers. With the exception of the screw-top jar, most models can be purchased with or without a stopcock for use with vacuum. **Key:** (1) *Screw-top jar.* Good for desiccation of small reagent bottles at room temperature or in the refrigerator. (2) *Plastic desiccator.* Can be obtained in solvent-resistant and unbreakable plastic, and can hold medium-size bottles. (3) *Glass desiccator.* The larger sizes can accommodate bacterial plates as well as reagent bottles. These containers are heavy, and are best used on the bench at room temperature. (4) *Desiccator cabinets.* Cabinets hold filters and plates as well as bottles and tubes.

actual temperature depends on the amount and type of desiccant), until the blue color is restored.

Desiccant can also be dried by gas, but most labs are not set up for this.

Drierite (registered trademark of W.A. Hammond Drierite Company) is often used synonymously with desiccant.

To put the container under vacuum

1. Slide the lid into place, with or without grease, as needed.

2. Turn the vacuum spout or stopcock so the container is open to the air.

3. Attach vacuum tubing from the container to the vacuum source.

4. Turn on the vacuum. House vacuum, which is fairly weak, may take a couple of minutes to evacuate a large container. A pump takes less time. You will know you have a vacuum when you can't slide the lid.

5. Close the container and quickly turn off the vacuum.

6. Wait a few minutes to take the tubing from the container.

To open a vacuum-sealed desiccator

1. Slowly open the stopcock to release the vacuum.

2. Try to slide the lid off.

3. If it won't slide, release the vacuum by slowly prying and wiggling a flat-edged weighing spatula between the top and bottom. A razor will also work, but you must be careful.

4. Once you hear the hiss of the releasing vacuum, slide the top off while holding the bottom firmly. Never try to lift the top off.

To open a desiccator that is kept in the cold

The standard wisdom says that the desiccator must be brought to room temperature before it is opened, in order to avoid condensation inside the container. The problem is that the reagents inside react adversely not only to water, but also to warmth.

For non-vacuum desiccators and grease-free desiccators, it is fine to open the jar immediately, remove the reagent you need, and quickly replace the lid and the jar in the refrigerator. If it makes you feel better, quickly wipe the inside of the container with a Kimwipe before you put the lid on, but it probably won't matter.

Let vacuum desiccators come to room temperature before you open them. Cold grease won't seal well, so you can't return greased desiccators to the cold immediately, anyway. You might as well avoid any chance of condensation and open the desiccator only when it is warmed.

 How to store reagents that are light-sensitive

If something arrives from the manufacturer in a brown bottle, assume that it is light-sensitive. If possible, store the reagent in this container. When you make a solution of the material, you will have to store that solution away from light, also. Either obtain a brown or amber reagent bottle, or cover a clear bottle with aluminum foil and tape. Once you have capped the bottle, cover the cap and the top of the bottle with a square of foil.

Small tubes of the reagent can be kept in a box. A freezer box is good for this, or the shipping box. Label the box with the usual information, as well as with a label saying "Light-sensitive material inside!" But the light-sensitive material should be the only material in the box: You don't want to be rifling through the box for tubes and bottles.

Straight-edge razors are a hazard in the lab. Either discard razors and scalpels immediately after use, or keep only one active at a time. Store it by inserting the sharp edge into a piece of styrofoam or into a styrofoam tube rack, so you can't inadvertently grab the sharp edge. Dispose of razors in a sharps container.

Some common light-sensitive reagents are actinomycin D, mitomycin C, nitroblue tetrazolium, phenol, Rifampicin, and tetracycline.

Don't rely on the fact that the freezer or refrigerator door is usually closed to store your reagent in a clear bottle.

 How to store reagents that are sensitive to oxygen

Gaseous nitrogen is usually used to drive off the oxygen in oxygen-sensitive reagents: This is what the phrase "under nitrogen" means.

1. A cylinder of nitrogen must be set up next to a fume hood, as it is usually solutions with organic solvents that require nitrogen. Turn the hood on.

    The use of aseptic technique (Chapter 9) will prevent the introduction of contaminants into the tube while you gas the tube.

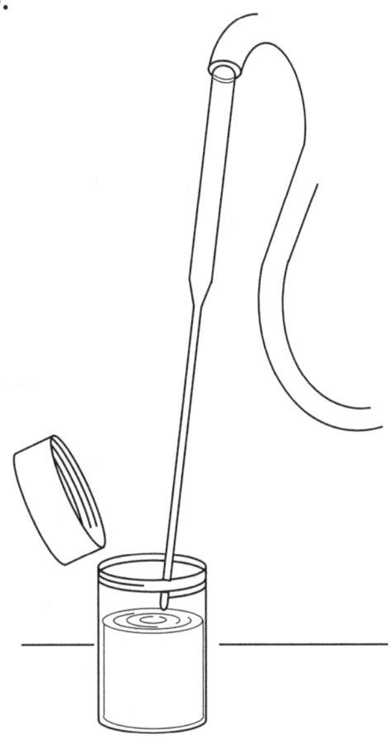

2. Be sure the cylinder is strapped into place. (See Chapter 10 for the use of gas cylinders and pressure regulators.)

3. Insert a pasteur pipet into the tubing connected to the regulator.

4. Turn on the nitrogen. Adjust the flow until you can barely feel it when applied closely to the back of your hand.

5. Open your tube or bottle in the hood. It should be held firmly in a rack.

6. Lower the pipet tip into the mouth of the container until you can just see the surface liquid ripple. Leave it there for 5–10 seconds for tubes, longer for containers with a higher liquid-to-air ratio.

FIGURE 2.

Control the flow of the nitrogen so the surface of the fluid ripples gently.

7. Cap the container quickly.

8. Turn off the nitrogen.

9. Store the vial. It usually must be at –20°C, and may also be put under vacuum.

ALIQUOTING

Many substances in the lab are stored in small volumes.

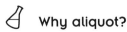 **Why aliquot?**

> *The stock solution is the concentrated solution that will be aliquoted. The working solution is the final concentration of the material after the aliquot has been diluted at the time of use.*

• **To prevent breakdown of the stock solution by repeated freeze-thawing.** Many materials are unstable to freeze-thawing, and small aliquots can be used once or twice and discarded, or held for a short time at 4°C. Examples of this are *serum* and *antibodies.*

• **To prevent contamination by multiple users.** The more people that use a stock solution, the greater the chance of introducing a contaminant. This is true even if the stock is used at the same temperature at which it is stored. Examples are *enzymes* and *media.*

Commonly aliquoted material

Antibiotics. 1:100 or 1:50 is a typical and useful dilution. See Chapters 10 and 11 for concentrations of tissue culture and bacterial culture antibiotics.

Antibodies. Most antibodies react unfavorably to repeated freezing and thawing.

Bacteria. The most common use for aliquoted bacteria is for transformations. Competent bacteria are stored at a concentration that enables the investigator to remove a tube and immediately perform the transformation.

Cells. Cells must be stored, in liquid nitrogen or in deep freeze, at a concentration that buffers the inevitable cell death but doesn't allow a freshly started culture to overgrow.

Enzymes. Generally, it is best to buy in small volumes, even if it is more expensive. Only a very large lab, with a dedicated person in charge, can spare the time and effort to aliquot enzymes without costly mistakes.

Serum. Serum is cheaper if purchased in large volumes, but it retains activity best if stored at –20°C, without being frozen and thawed.

- **For physical convenience.** It is much easier to manipulate a 10-ml tube than a 500-ml bottle!

- **To save time.** Instead of weighing out a powder and dissolving it every time, this can be done once and an aliquot merely tipped into place.

Don't aliquot when

- The diluted substance has little stability.

- You will only use a substance infrequently.

- You will be using varying and wide-ranging concentrations of the substance.

> *Stock and working solutions are given either in w/v or molarity. Keep your stock and working solutions in the same units.*

How to aliquot

1. To make a stock solution, you need to know:

    - The working concentration of the substance. Working concentration is also given as the final concentration. It may be given as w/ml or in molar concentration.

      > For example, the working concentration of chloramphenicol to use for amplification of plasmids is 170 µg/ml, and for selection of resistant bacteria, 10 to 30 µg/ml.

    - *What to dissolve the substance in.* Not everything can be dissolved in water. Some substances must be dissolved in another solvent at the stock solution concentration, but can then be dissolved in water at the working concentration.

      > *You will find the working concentration of a substance in a protocol, a manual, or a paper, or from a colleague. Be sure you get the working concentration for your particular application.*

      > Chloramphenicol can be dissolved in methanol or absolute alcohol, or in warm water at low concentrations. Since methanol is more poisonous to cells and bacteria than ethanol, the concentrated stock solution is made in ethanol.

- *The volumes you will be dissolving the aliquots in.* The volume of the aliquot should be appropriate to the volume of the final diluent.

2. Decide how many aliquots to make. This is a compromise between *convenience and need.* It is difficult to weigh out very small amounts, so you may have to make more aliquots than you will ever need. 10–100 is usually a good amount.

3. Set up sterile tubes. Label well. Keep the tubes on ice if the aliquots must be frozen or refrigerated (as they usually must be). Loosen the caps.

> *To find the solubility of a substance in water or other solvent, check the substance container or its data sheet, the catalog, or call the manufacturer. Manuals and other sources of protocols often describe how to make a stock solution of the substance.*

> *Make aliquots so they must be used at convenient ratios such as 1:1000 or 1:100 to arrive at the desired final concentration.*

> You want a 20 mg/ml stock solution of chloramphenicol, to make a final 1:1000 dilution for 20 µg/ml.
> If you will be making 1 liter (1000 ml) of medium, you need 1-ml aliquots.
> If you will be making 100 ml of medium, you need 100-µl aliquots.

4. Make the stock solution and filter it, if necessary. Work in a laminar flow hood or a place without drafts.

5. Dispense the sterile solution into the tubes. Place in a freezer box or rack at the appropriate temperature.

6. Record the aliquot information in your lab book.

> *Label each tube. The label should include the name and concentration of the substance, the date the solution was made, and your initials. Your name and the contents must be clearly identifiable by anybody in the lab or by safety personnel. If you will have a rack or a box of only one type of aliquot, you can label the rack or box and put only an identifying mark on the lid of each tube.*

REFRIGERATORS AND FREEZERS

- *Use the appropriate refrigerator or freezer.* If radioactive or biohazard materials are stored within, no food is permitted, and there will be a sign on the door to this effect. Flammable materials (such as ethanol) must be stored in an explosion-proof refrigerator, which has an enclosed motor to eliminate sparking.

- *Only open the door when you need to.* If you must manipulate, remove the box or rack and put it on ice while you search for a certain tube.

- *All containers in the refrigerator or freezer must be completely labeled and securely capped.* No loose tubes in styrofoam cups, or tucked into the egg rack! Every tube must be able to withstand shaking and moving (such as you would find if a frantic investigator were pawing wildly through a refrigerator to search for a lost tube) without falling from a rack.

> *If the stock solution needs to be filter-sterilized, make more (10%) than you need. Check the dry material, for it may be sterile: If you use the entire amount and dissolve it in sterile water or ethanol, you won't need to filter-sterilize it.*

- *Periodically discard material you no longer need.* Bottles with only 10 ml of medium left, petri dishes of bacterial medium, and duplicate sample retained "just in case" can take up a lot of room and make it difficult to find anything.

- *Keep a record of the location of all of your reagents.* It is very easy to quickly slip a tube in a box, with the intention of moving it later to a labeled box. Have a system set up so it is effortless to record the placement of any reagent.

> *Frost-free freezers. It is often recommended that enzymes and growth factors, which are sensitive to changes in temperature, not be kept in a frost-free freezer. This is because the frost-free freezer cycles slightly in temperature to prevent frost buildup.*
>
> *Frost-free refrigerators. Refrigerators should be frost-free to prevent water damage.*

- *Respect private space.* Space in refrigerators is frequently allocated to investigators, with everyone given a shelf or rack. Don't spill over onto someone else's space. If, after throwing away or rearranging everything you can, you still need space, speak with the czar of the freezers and refrigerators and request more space.

How to defrost a freezer

Defrosting a laboratory freezer is a laboratory job, and requires the cooperation and assistance of all lab members. It is a 1- to 3-day job: The contents must be moved, the defrosting actually done, the freezer washed and brought back to temperature, and the contents repacked.

- *The defrosting must be planned a week in advance.* All workers should be notified of the

> *Finding a place for the contents of a low-temperature freezer is a formidable task, because that freezer and every other one is usually completely filled. EHS departments can sometimes arrange a "loaner" low-temperature freezer for emergencies and for short-term storage. You should know where to find another freezer before an emergency occurs.*

date and time by which they must remove all of their reagents from the freezer. Ideally, an empty freezer is available for temporary storage; otherwise, everyone must find a bit of cold space somewhere.

- *The pre-defrosting cleanup is a good time to unload unnecessary reagents.* Each investigator should discard expired reagents and ones that will never be used. Go through the tubes, and update your records.

- *Pack all tubes carefully for the move, no matter how short a distance you are going.* There should be no microfuge racks or any holders from which a tube can spill. Every box and container must be labeled with the contents and your name. Do not rely on location to recognize your reagents!

- *Start the defrosting as early as possible in the morning.* Do not do it overnight—huge amounts of water can be generated, and someone must be there at all times. Pull the plug, and open the door.

- *Wear gloves for all fiddling and removal of the ice.* Medium-weight rubber gloves (such as used for washing dishes) are excellent for protecting your hands against the cold and whatever nasty material might have spilled into the ice. Beware of broken tubes embedded in the ice.

- *Have ready:* Mop and bucket, newspaper, paper towels, bench diapers, anything that will absorb the water. Also useful are basins into which the sodden material can be thrown.

- *Help the defrosting along,* but be careful. Everyone says not to chip at the ice, but everyone does: If you do, be sure the ice is partially melted, and that it is thick enough that you are in no danger of puncturing the freezer. Try to pry, rather than chop.

Ice buildup on inner doors and gaskets of −70ºC freezers is a chronic problem and may prevent the doors from closing tightly. This, in turn, leads to condensation and more ice accumulation. Once a week, scrape the ice free with a plastic windshield ice scraper.

- *Hairdryers are used for small freezers,* but the danger of electrocution is high, and this should not be done. Buckets filled with hot water are a good compromise. Fill a bucket with as hot water as you can, and place the bucket inside the freezer and shut the door. Replace the bucket in 20 minutes. You can also spill almost-boiling water inside the freezer; this will speed up the defrosting but add to the amount of water you must clean up.

- *Remove all water as you go along.* This is relatively easy but tedious for upright freezers, as most of the water will go on the floor or in the bottom of the freezer, where it can be collected and mopped. In horizontal freezers, the water is difficult to reach on the bottom. The water can be siphoned or pumped out, or mopped. There are also inexpensive, disposable plastic pumps that can be used for this.

- *Keep the area surrounded by dry material, so the floor stays dry.* A wet lab floor is a death trap.

- *Clean the defrosted freezer.* Once the freezer has been thoroughly defrosted, wipe it down with a mild disinfectant.

- *Only when the freezer is completely dry can you plug it back in.* It will take hours, certainly overnight, before the freezer will be back down to temperature. Make sure the temperature is stable before you reintroduce tubes.

- *Record the placement of all material.* Space may be allocated by one worker as a laboratory job, but each investigator should know and record the contents of his or her own boxes.

DISCARDING LAB WASTE

Every paper, cell, chemical, pipet, or tube has its own place to be discarded—nothing can be casually thrown away. Consult your institution's safety office for the specifics of trash disposal at your institution. Be very careful, and not only for safety reasons: *Throwing garbage in the wrong place is an easy way to tick off everyone in the lab.*

What You Need to Know to Dispose of Material as Waste

- The chemical composition.

- If it is hazardous or nonhazardous.

- If it is radioactive.

- If it is a biohazard.

> *You must check with the EHS department of your own institution for the rules regarding storage and disposal.*

- **If it can be recycled.** Newspaper and other paper can be recycled. So can some reagent containers, dry ice shipping containers, and shielded casings for radioactive material. Each is disposed of in a separate place.

NEVER

- put radioactive waste anywhere but in the designated radioactive waste area, not even for a minute.
- put sharp items, such as needles, pasteur pipets, or scalpels, in regular or regular biohazard trash. They must be placed in a special sharps disposal box and are usually treated as biohazard material.
- put broken glass anywhere but in a box or container dedicated to that purpose. If the glass contained biohazard material, it must be autoclaved first.

Acids. Small amounts (<100 ml) may be neutralized (check with pH paper) and slowly poured down the drain with large amounts of water. Larger amounts are handled as hazardous chemical waste.

Acids and bases should not be mixed.

Aluminum foil. Recycle: look for a bin in the hall or department.

Antibodies. Biohazard waste.

Bacteria. Biohazard waste. Plates and slants go into solid biohazard waste. Reusable flasks and bottles are autoclaved or rinsed with 10% Clorox. Liquid cultures are either brought to 10% bleach by the addition of Clorox, or autoclaved, before being poured down the sink. Supernatants from bacteria should be treated as a liquid culture (yes, even for regular old *E. coli*) and should be autoclaved or bleached before disposal down the sink.

Do not autoclave solutions containing Clorox!

Bases. Small amounts (<100 ml) may be neutralized (check with pH paper) and slowly poured down the drain with large amounts of water. Larger amounts are handled as hazardous chemical waste.

Biohazard waste is anything derived from a living thing or that comes in contact with living things. Both liquid and dry waste will be generated.

Don't put acidic or basic waste (pH less than 3 or greater than 9) in metal cans, which can corrode.

- Liquid (over 1 ml) biohazard waste should have Clorox added to 10%, be allowed to sit for 30 minutes, and be poured down the sink.
- Dry biohazard waste is discarded in bins lined with biohazard bags.

Buffers. Most buffers can be poured down the sink. See "Chemical waste–hazardous" for exceptions.

Cells. Biohazard waste. Liquid cultures are either brought to 10% bleach by the addition of Clorox, or autoclaved, before being poured down the sink. Aspirate liquid from disposable plates, dishes, tubes, bottles, and flasks before throwing the containers into solid biohazard waste. Reusable flasks and bottles (unusual for cells) are either rinsed with 10% bleach or are autoclaved.

Chemical waste–hazardous. Generally, you should not mix chemicals. When mixing is done, it is for small vol-

Keep organic waste separate from aqueous waste.

umes of solvents from the same category; for example, all halogenated solvents. Check first with EHS. Of course, it is also done if mixtures are part of a process, such as from a DNA synthesis machine, or from extractions (phenol-chloroform).

All bottles must be labeled and/or tagged. The full chemical name, the percentage of the mixture, if any, the waste volume, the location, and your name must be on the tag or label, which is often provided by EHS.

Use the correct bottles. You cannot just pick up any spare bottle in the lab and pour hazardous waste into it: There may be the danger of an explosion or fire or a leak. Ask EHS for the correct bottle and cap to use for disposal for every single chemical you will dispose of.

Hold the waste bottles in the appropriate holding area until pickup (or dropoff) by EHS. Some waste must be neutralized before it is picked up. It is a good idea to check the pH of all waste—now you get to use all that pH paper!

Do not flush flammable, water immiscible, water reactive, or highly toxic materials down the sink.

Record the pH on the label. Check with EHS about safe neutralization instructions.

- Examples of hazardous chemical waste

Acetonitrile	Hydrofluoric acid
Acrylamide	Hydrogen cyanide
Benzene	Mercury
Chloroform	Methylene chloride
Chromic acid	Methylmercuric hydroxide
Cyanogen bromide	Osmium tetroxide
Diisopropyl fluorophosphate (DFP)	Peracetic acid
Hydrogen peroxide	Perchloric acid
Diethyl ether	Phenol and phenol solutions
Dimethyl formamide (DMF)	Picric acid
Dimethyl sulfoxide (DMSO)	Pyridine
Ethidium bromide	Trichloroethylene
Formaldehyde	Xylene
Hydrazine	

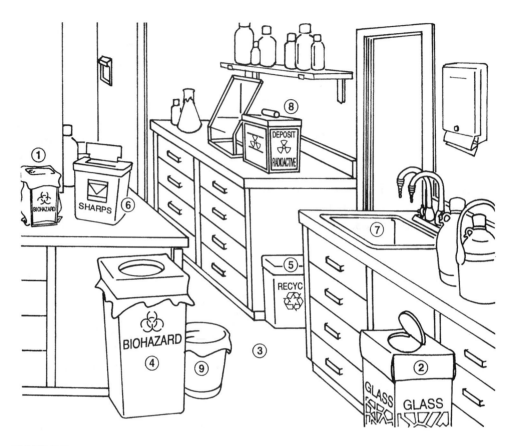

FIGURE 3.

Waste disposal areas are found throughout the laboratory. **Key:** (1) *Benchtop biohazard bag.* (2) *Glass disposal box.* (3) *Hazardous waste pick-up area.* (4) *Large biohazard trash bag.* (5) *Paper to be recycled.* (6) *Sharps disposal.* (7) *Sink.* (8) *Radioactive waste.* (9) *Trash.*

Chemical waste–nonhazardous. Dispose of as trash if solid. Liquids should be flushed down the drain in the laboratory sink, followed by large amounts of water.

- Organic chemicals
  Acetates: Ca, Na, NH_4, and K
  Amino acids and their salts
  Citric acid and salts of Na, K, Mg, Ca, and NH_4
  Lactic acid and salts of Na, K, Mg, Ca, and NH_4

- Inorganic chemicals
  Bicarbonates: Na, K
  Borates: Na, K, Mg, Ca
  Bromides: Na, K

Carbonates: Na, K, Mg, Ca
Chlorides: Na, K, Mg, Ca
Fluorides: Ca
Iodides: Na, K
Oxides: B, Mg, Ca, Al, Si, Fe
Phosphates: Na, K, Mg, Ca, NH_4
Silicates: Na, K, Mg, Ca
Sulfates: Na, K, Mg, Ca, NH_4

> *Nonflammable, noncorrosive, nonmetallic, nontoxic, odorless, water-soluble substances may be discarded down the sink. Most buffers can be discarded in this way.*

DNA. Biohazard waste.

Dry ice. Let the dry ice evaporate in the ice bucket or container. Do not dispose of it down the sink, even while running the water, because the pipes can freeze and crack.

Gels. Biohazard waste.

Glass. Dispose of in a sealed and clearly labeled box. Autoclave. Many labs have a dedicated glass disposal box.

Gloves. If gloves are used for work with biohazard material, dispose of them in the solid biohazard waste. Otherwise, gloves can go in regular trash (but check, because some institutions require that anything that has the appearance of biohazard material should go into biohazard trash).

Needles. Sharps disposal box.

Paper. Recyclable paper is put in a dedicated lab area, bin or box. Non-recyclable paper, such as paper towels, goes into trash.

> *Never remove a needle from a syringe. Never recap a needle—this is where most needle accidents happen! Throw the syringe with attached needle directly into the sharps disposal box!*

Phenol and phenol-containing solutions. Dispose of as hazardous chemical waste. Keep a working bottle at your bench, and dispose of appropriately when it is filled, noting on the label the concentration of phenol and other solvents such as chloroform and isoamyl alcohol. Obtain a waste bottle with advice from EHS: Don't use ordinary lab bottles.

Photographic fixer, developer, stop bath. Diluted material may be discarded down the sink, or they may be collected by EHS. If they are, keep fixer, developer, and stop bath separate from each other.

Pipets. Disposable pipets are usually discarded directly into biohazard trash. However, pipets can pierce the biohazard bag, so double-bag to prevent leaks or injury to personnel. Your lab may use a biohazard bag-lined box, dedicated to pipets. Reusable pipets are usually placed in a pipet bucket that can be put into a pipet washer. Since this causes an aerosol, it is preferable to use cotton-plugged pipets and place them in a horizontal container.

Protein, cell extracts. Biohazard waste.

Radioactive waste. Radioactive waste includes all paper towels, absorbent paper, pipet tips, and everything used during the experiment.

> *Do not dispose of volatile chemical waste, such as chloroform or ether, by allowing it to evaporate in a fume hood or on the bench. Treat volatile material as hazardous chemical waste.*

RNA. Biohazard waste.

Serum. Biohazard.

Sharps. (Pasteur pipets, needles, syringes with needles attached, automatic pipet tips, glass slides and coverslips, razor blades and scalpels) in a sharps disposal box. Depending on the kind of lab, there may be separate "regular" and biohazard sharps disposal boxes, or a biohazard sharps box into which all sharps, biohazard or not, are placed. Radioactively contaminated sharps must be collected in a separate sharps disposal box.

Solvents. Hazardous chemical waste—do not pour down the sink! Use a waste container with a volume as close to that of the waste as possible. Do not combine different solvents: Of course, some waste is already a mixture and should be labeled accordingly.

> For disposal of the products of manual synthesis or of other processes generating complex wastes, separate the solvents into:
> * Halogenated (e.g., dichloromethane, dichloroethane, chloroform)
> * Flammable (e.g., toluene, xylene, benzene)
> * Aqueous (e.g., HPLC waste, amino acid analysis waste)
> * Phenol-chloroform

Supernatants. Supernatants from centrifugation spins of cells, viruses, and bacteria are liquid biohazard waste. Autoclave or bring to 10% Clorox before pouring it down the sink. While centrifuging, keep a bottle for pouring or aspiration of supernatants: Do not pour supernatants down the sink directly.

Syringes. With attached needle, in biohazard sharps disposal. Syringe alone, in solid biohazard waste (for appearance sake) or sharps container. Check with EHS for local regulations.

Thermometers. Mercury thermometers must *not* be discarded with glass waste. Most mercury thermometers are encased with plastic or resin to contain the mercury in case of breakage: If the integrity of the seal has not been broken, pick up the thermometer (with gloves), place in a sealed box or beaker, and contact EHS for pickup. If mercury has been spilled you should call EHS immediately. Thermometers filled with alcohol or mineral spirits can be discarded with glass waste.

Tips. Sharps disposal box.

Trash. Nonrecyclable, nonradioactive, nonbiohazard, nonsharp, nonhazardous: There won't be very much of this! This will contain mostly paper towels. Usually disposed of in a bin, either unlined or lined with a plain (not biohazard) black or green bag. Remember—you aren't supposed to be eating in the lab, so there shouldn't be food items in the trash! This is a red flag to EHS personnel, so get rid of soda cans and sandwich wrappings outside of the laboratory.

Volatile chemicals. Dispose of volatile materials according to their chemical composition (hazardous, organic, etc.). Do not dispose of volatile chemicals by allowing them to evaporate in a fume hood.

Never remove a needle from a syringe. Throw the syringe with attached needle directly into the sharps disposal box!

Don't throw pipet tips in the solid biohazard disposal or in the trash. Pipet tips are considered sharps because they can pierce through plastic biohazard bags, exposing lab and custodial personnel to the contents of the bag.

WATCH FOR YOUR TURN IN REMOVING THE WASTE. Every lab has its own policy on removal of waste from the lab, and custodians are seldom responsible for anything other than "trash." It will fall to the lab members to do everything else (and new lab members are probably not exempted!). This may be done by a rotating task list, by honor, or by assignment: Take this very seriously, and don't miss your turn.

Order of Priority for Disposal

Much of the waste in the lab falls under several categories at once. It may be only biohazard, or it may be biohazard and radioactive, or it may be biohazard and radioactive and an organic solvent. Dispose of the waste according to its highest numbered priority:

1. Radioactive, solid.

2. Radioactive, liquid.

3. Hazardous chemical.

4. Biohazard.

5. Sharp.

6. Nonhazardous chemical.

RESOURCES

Collins C.H., Lyne P.M., and Grange J.M. 1991. *Microbiological methods,* 6th edition. Butterworth-Heinemann, Oxford.

Fisher Safety Products Reference Manual. 1993. Fisher Scientific, Pittsburgh.

Gershey E.L., Party E., and Wilkerson A. 1991. *Laboratory safety in practice: A comprehensive compliance program and safety manual.* Van Nostrand Reinhold, New York.

Harlow E. and Lane D. 1988. *Antibodies. A laboratory manual.* Cold Spring Harbor Laboratory, Cold Spring Harbor, New York.

Kowahl V.C. 1996. *Laboratory survival manual.* Environmental Health and Safety, University of Virginia at:

http://www.virginia.edu/~enhealth/A-D/waste-seg.html

Lenga R.E., ed. 1988. *The Sigma-Aldrich library of chemical safety data,* edition II, vol. I and II. Sigma-Aldrich Corporation, Milwaukee.

Windholz M., ed. 1976. *Merck index,* 9th edition. Merck and Co., Inc. Rahway, New Jersey.

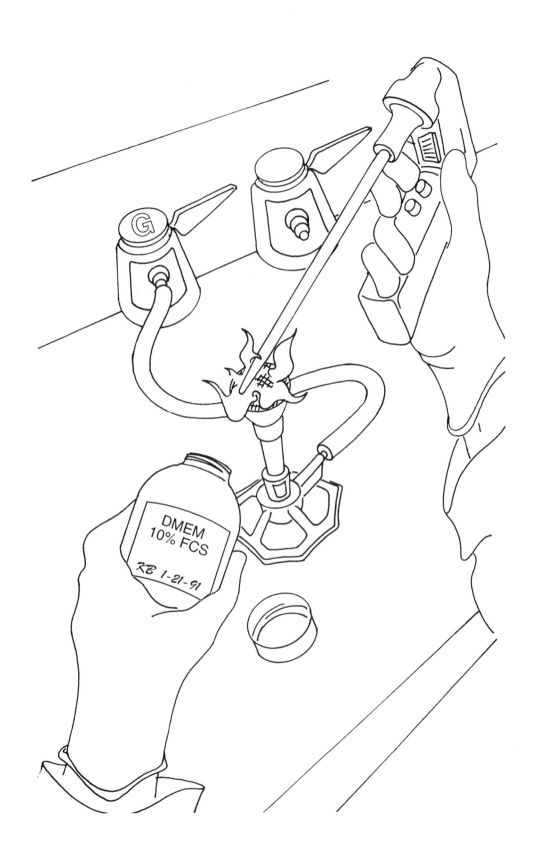

9

Working without Contamination

ASEPTIC (OR STERILE) technique is a way of working that maintains sterility. Before the advent of hoods, it is the way all benchwork in a lab was done. In many labs today, aseptic technique is no longer rigorously practiced; in fact, in some molecular biology labs, there is not even an attempt at maintaining sterility.

Big mistake! Although the need for aseptic practice is not as clear in a biochemistry lab as in, say, a cell biology or infectious disease lab, its use can

WHEN TO USE STERILE TECHNIQUE   186

STERILE TECHNIQUE   187
  Rules   187
  Technique tips   189

PROTECTING THE INVESTIGATOR   197
  Biosafety level requirements   197
  Biosafety cabinets   198

STERILE TECHNIQUE IN THE
  CLASS II BIOSAFETY CABINET   198

RESOURCES   203

avoid many problems that would be impossible to diagnose. Also, the demarcations between different kinds of fields of study are not so well defined, with molecular biology generally now considered to be a technique, not a field, and everyone may need to grow his own cells or freeze his own bacteria.

Aseptic technique should be to you not merely a way to open your cultures sterilely, but a way of thinking and acting *always* in the lab. There is no aspect of lab work that won't profit by extra care. Use it to prepare RNA buffers, to set up restriction enzyme digestions, to prepare membrane proteins. When you are used to working aseptically, following the rules for using radioactivity or hazardous material will seem very familiar.

All procedures are described for right-handed workers.

WHEN TO USE STERILE TECHNIQUE

 When you must use sterile technique. You **must** use sterile technique whenever you are working with living organisms, or with any media, buffers, or culture containers used for living organisms. For example:

- Setting up a culture of *E. coli* for a transformation
- Making LB plates
- Splitting cells
- Filtering serum for media
- Opening and rehydrating a vial of lyophilized bacteria

 When it helps to use sterile technique. You **should** use sterile technique whenever you don't want the contents of one container or area to enter another container or area. Yes, this is true of just about anything you do in the lab. Even when you are working with buffers with a high salt and/or detergent content, in which it is unlikely that any organism would grow, you must be careful not to introduce oils from your hands or dust from a greasy pipet.

You **should** also use sterile techniques when working with any hazardous agents, such as radioactivity or toxic chemicals. Of course, protecting yourself is of primary concern, and you must sometimes modify your procedures. Fortunately, protecting your material and protecting yourself both involve creating barriers between you and the material, and so involve the same means and the same end. For example:

- **Setting up restriction digests.** Contamination of restriction enzymes can be a huge disaster. Although most enzymes are packaged in glycerol, and glycerol concentrations over 50% are bacteriostatic, diluted enzymes and others without glycerol are susceptible to bacterial contamination. In addition, traces of common elements can inhibit enzyme reactions.

- **Setting up PCR reactions.** PCR reactions are notoriously plagued with contamination by other DNAs. By working aseptically, and setting up reactions in a room away from the PCR machine and the place where the analysis of the PCR products is done, the introduction of stray DNA can be avoided.

- **Labeling cells with [^{32}P] phosphate.** In this case, working aseptically is for your protection, and not for the protection of the cells. When you think aseptically, you will not leave open caps, generate aerosols, or accidentally reuse a radioactive pipet.

STERILE TECHNIQUE

The bottom line is this: The air is dotted and filled with dust and spores and germs, and you don't want them in your bottles or cells. Unless air currents blow them away from the working area, these potential contaminants will descend to the working surface, into open bottles, and onto pipet tips. Microorganisms will "fall" from hands and sleeves, and descend to the surface. Arm motions, rapid pipeting, and passersby will stir up unpredictable currents that can't be guarded against.

The use of sterile technique will *minimize* the exposure of your material to contaminants. It cannot completely protect in all conditions and, thus, can't completely prevent all contamination. But the better your technique is, the better your record on contamination will be.

> *Keep surfaces clean, bottles closed, and movements minimized.*

Rules

- **The working area should be as far away from drafts and traffic as possible.** No windows should be open, and you should try not to be near an active doorway. The use of a biosafety cabinet makes aseptic technique easier to maintain, but is not at all necessary.

- **Be sure there is a clear working area.** Remove all supplies and equipment you won't be using. Old flasks and containers must not be nearby. When you are finished, remove or put away all supplies and equipment, and wipe down the area again.

- **Wipe down the working area with an antiseptic or cleaning agent before use.** 70% ethanol is fine for most labs. (But use whatever the laboratory uses, since alcohols may not be effective against a particular lab's nemesis.) Keep a squirt bottle of 70% ethanol next to every working area, and use it liberally. Wipe the work surface down at the end of the day, before the start of an experiment, and after a spill.

- **All pipets and bottles should be sterile.** If you don't KNOW something is sterile, don't use it. Reusable bottles and pipet canisters should have autoclave tape that indicates sterility, or a written note on the tape that the container has been sterilized. Disposable pipets, if opened, must be in a bag in which the sterility of the tips has clearly not been disturbed. If the bag is old, torn, or found left completely opened, do not use the pipets.

- **Set the working area up to minimize hand movements.** Have the tools you will use with the right hand placed to the right of the open space, the ones you will use with the left hand placed to the left of an open space. For example, for the removal of a small volume from a jar by a right-hander, pipet aids, pipets, and pipettors should be to the right, the jar to the left.

- **Have ready everything you will need,** so you don't have to leave the working area to retrieve something. The more you rustle around, the more the air will be disturbed. Leaving the working area also breaks your concentration.

- **Wear latex gloves, and change them frequently.** Gloves protect the working material and the investigator. If gloves are not available, needed, or desired, wash hands before and after working. You may prefer to work without gloves, and for nontoxic material and nonpathogenic materials, that is fine. But you will need gloves for many procedures, and it is just as well to get used to working with them.

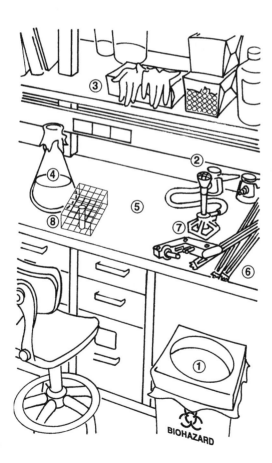

FIGURE 1.

Lab bench setup for aseptic work. **Task:** To transfer 5 ml of growing bacterial culture from a tube into 100 ml of culture medium. The supplies needed are arranged for a right-handed investigator, so that things to be manipulated with the right hand are set up to the right of the working area, and things to be manipulated with the left hand are set up to the left of the working area. **Key:** (1) *Biohazard disposal.* (2) *Bunsen burner.* (3) *Box of gloves.* (4) *Flask of culture medium.* (5) *Clear area.* (6) *Individually wrapped pipets.* (7) *Pipet aid.* (8) *Test tube with bacterial culture, in a test tube rack.*

Technique Tips

Every task you will do will be a bit different. This is why it is necessary to think carefully about your actions: it is not possible to describe every action one will perform.

Generally, what you will be trying to do is to minimize the encounter of your material with potential contaminants. To do this, minimize all actions.

- **Minimize:**

    Distance. The closer all supplies are to you and to each other, the less movement you will make.

    Exposure. The more you move something through the air, the more airborne particles it will encounter. The longer a bottle is left open, the more airborne particles can enter the jar. Flaming a bottle or pipet fixes particles to the surface and creates an upward flow that minimizes exposure to airborne particles.

    > *Flaming is not done to sterilize. 1–3 seconds through a flame is sufficient.*

    Motion. Motions create air currents. Faster motions create faster air currents. Make all movements necessary, and make them gentle. Don't wave pipets in the air, or cross your hands over your open working area.

    Pouring. Pouring creates aerosols, which disturb the air and can carry contamination to unwanted areas. Also, the fluid left on the lip of a bottle after pouring is one of the greatest sources of contamination to the contents of the bottle, as it creates a bridge from the outside to the inside (Freshney, p 56). Use a pipet to transfer liquids whenever possible.

    > *Pipets are available that can pipet up to 50 ml. If you use one, be sure the pipet is set firmly into the pipet aid. 50-ml pipets are larger, and if they are not set in squarely during use, the vacuum will be lost and the fluid will drip out.*

- **Open all bottles with the bottle pointed at approximately a 45° angle.** This minimizes airborne contamination and the creation of aerosols when pipeting.

- **If you must put a cap or lid down, place it face down on a clean surface.** Try not to do this. With a face-up lid, there is more chance of contamination by hands and bottles moving above it.

- **Flame glass pipets and open bottles before manipulation.** Position the Bunsen burner between your working hand and the bottles, etc. you will be working on.

- **Do not flame plastic bottles or pipets!** Work quickly, minimize open bottles, and tilt all bottles at a 45° angle when pipeting, whether you flame the opening or not.

> *There are two schools of thought on the placement of the cap, face up, or face down. Both are right: Choose one method, and stick to it. If you leave the caps up, avoid moving your hands over it. If you leave the caps down, be sure the surface below has been well disinfected.*

- **Pipet gently and don't swirl bottles.** This minimizes aerosols. Also, be careful when opening centrifuge bottles.

- **Don't leave any bottle open.** When you place an open bottle down, cover it immediately with the cap or lid. Do not leave bottles with pipets in, and the cap off.

- **Stop what you are doing.** There is a great deal of overkill in working aseptically, so things usually work out fine. Relax and stay aware. But there are a few *common mistakes* that should result in immediate termination of whatever action you are performing.

Mistakes that break sterility

1. Pipeting up too far in the pipet. Discard the pipet and check the pipettor: You may need to change filters.
2. Touching the tip of the pipet against a bottle, the ground, the outside of the pipet container, or anywhere solid. Discard the pipet.
3. Dropping an opened container or tube to the ground. Discard it.
4. Touching anything, including a gloved hand, to either the HEPA filter that prevents the suction of particulates through the vacuum system, or to the filter used in a flask vacuum system. This is a major source of contamination in hoods. Discard whatever touches the filter.
5. Reusing pipets while working. Once a pipet has been wetted, it is much more likely to pick up airborne contaminants.

Pipeting

 Pipeting with reusable glass pipets. Reusable pipets are stored usually in metal canisters, or cans. For work with cells or bacteria, the pipet should be plugged with cotton.

> *A small canister top could be held in the last two fingers of the left hand.*

1. Loosen the top of the canister.

2. Hold the canister in the left hand, and remove the top of the canister with the right hand.

3. Flame the top and the open end of the canister. Place the top down, on its side.

4. Hold the canister horizontally in your left hand and gently shake and tip the canister so the tops of one or two pipets stick out of the top of the canister about an inch and can be easily grasped.

5. Lay down the canister top on its side, or hold it in your left hand, and remove a pipet. Slide it out, holding it with your thumb and index finger about 2 inches from the top, without touching the pipet to the side of the canister.

6. Pass the bottom third of the pipet through the flame for 1–3 seconds. Rotate the pipet 180° as you pass it through the flame.

7. Insert the pipet into the pipet aid.

8. Hold the bottle from which you will pipet at a 45° angle with your left hand. While holding the pipet aid in the right hand, open the donor bottle with the last two fingers of the right hand. Retain the cap in those fingers.

9. With the left hand, pass the opening of the bottle through the flame.

10. Pass the pipet through the flame again.

11. Place the tip of the pipet into the container from which you are removing liquid. Don't touch the tip to the inside at all, but place it straight into the liquid. Pipet the volume you require and carefully withdraw the pipet.

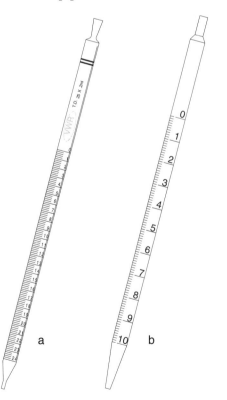

a   b

FIGURE 2.

Note carefully the type of measurement on the pipet. Most pipets are made to deliver (marked T.D., to deliver, on the top of the pipet) the chosen volume when the fluid is released entirely from the pipet (*a*). Other pipets (marked T.C., to contain) are made to release the chosen volume only when the fluid is released to a measured point (*b*).

12. Flame the donor bottle and recap it. Place it to the side.

13. While holding the pipet as still as possible, open the receptacle bottle as in steps 7–9.

14. Place the pipet into the receptacle bottle carefully, as in step 10, and dispense the liquid.

15. Withdraw the pipet and place in the appropriate place to the side. This may be a beaker for temporary storage. Afterward, all pipets will generally go into a soaking basin.

16. Flame the receptacle bottle, recap, and put down.

All other pipeting will be similar. In fact, all other manipulations will be variations of the ones described above.

 Pipeting with disposable pipets

1. Be sure the top of the plastic package has been opened (or, if taped, the tape has been removed) so it will be easier to quickly take a pipet.

2. Hold the pipet package in the left hand while you remove a pipet with the thumb and index finger of the right hand. Try not to touch the inside of the bag or the other pipets with the tip of the chosen pipet. Gently squeezing the bag to make a tube helps to create an open area in the bag through which you can withdraw the pipet.

> *Contamination tends to occur when withdrawing the final inch of pipet from the package. Fingers may touch the tops of the pipets in the package, and a touch of the tip of the pipet against the top of the packaged pipets can contaminate the pipet and anything else it touches.*

3. Lay the package of pipets to the left.

4. Do all steps except flaming, as described for reusable pipets.

How to open an individually wrapped pipet

1. Hold the pipet in your left hand, about 3/4 to the top. Point the tip toward the left.
2. Tighten your left hand, so that the plastic wrapping cannot slip.
3. Grab the top of the plastic wrapping with your right hand.
4. While holding firmly to the pipet with the left hand, use the right hand to pull the wrapping against the top of the pipet, puncturing the top.
5. Continue pulling the wrapper down, folding 2 inches or so over the outside of the wrapper and pipet. Now you have a sterile tunnel through which the pipet can be withdrawn.
6. Withdraw the pipet from the wrapper, being careful not to touch the pipet to any surface. Put the wrapper to the left side, and dispose of it when you are through pipeting.

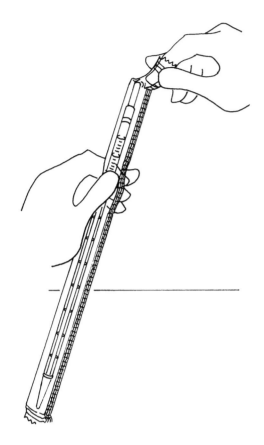

FIGURE 3.

Opening a disposable pipet.

Pouring

Hold the recipient container in the left hand, the donor in the right.

1. Flame the recipient container, with the flask pointed at an angle. Move in toward the left, keeping the container angled.

2. Flame the donor container. Wait 1–2 seconds (so the fluid in the container doesn't get scorched).

3. Maintain the recipient container at an angle, and hold it steady. Put the donor container, angled toward the recipient, approximately 2 inches above the recipient.

4. Tilt the donor and pour.

5. Flame the open mouth of both containers.

Since the chance of contamination is much greater when pouring than when pipeting, pour only when the volume is too large to be easily pipeted.

Filter Sterilizing

 Filtration of a small volume with a syringe filter

Materials

- A disposable 0.2 μm syringe filter
- A syringe of the volume of the solution. (1, 2, 5, 10, or 20 ml. 50-ml syringes are awkward to handle.) Use a sterile, disposable syringe to ensure cleanliness.
- A sterile tube as a receptacle
- Tube holder

1. Unwrap only the top of the syringe filter. This is the wider end, which will be twisted onto the end of the syringe.

2. Remove the wrapping from the syringe, and take out the plunger. Place the plunger on a clean surface.

3. Remove the protective cap from the tip of the syringe, and immediately twist the filter onto the syringe. Keep the wrapping on the exit tip of the filter, and lay the setup down.

4. Remove the cap from the sterile tube and place the tube in a holder.

5. Remove the wrapping from the exit end of the filter. Place the exit end in the tube, and hold the syringe upright.

You can directly draw up into the syringe the solution to be sterilized, before putting on the filter. But the syringe often won't fit the tube the solution is in.

6. Pour the solution into the syringe, replace the plunger, and push gently and firmly until the entire solution has passed through the filter into the tube.

7. Cap the tube, label it, and dispose of the syringe in biohazard/sharps waste.

 Filtration of a large volume with a disposable cup filter

Materials

- A disposable 0.2 μm filter
- A holder or stand for filter
- A sterile bottle as a receptacle

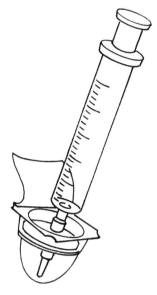

FIGURE 4.

Keep the filter in the wrapper until you are ready to dispense the contents.

- Vacuum source with attached tubing. House vacuum, found on lab benches, is the best and most common. The vacuum can also be water driven, or provided by a gentle pump.

1. Attach the vacuum hose to the filter. Place the filter in a stand where it will remain stable during manipulations.

2. Pour the solution into the filter. Don't worry if you have a bit more solution than will fit in the filter; you can add more after some of the solution has been filtered.

3. Put the lid on the filter and slowly turn on the vacuum. The solution will be pulled through the filter into a sterile receptacle. For some filters, this receptacle is actually a sterile bottle that can be used to store the buffer.

4. Turn off the vacuum and wait a minute.

5. Twist off the vacuum hose. Immediately pour the filtered solution into a sterile bottle and cap it. If the sterile bottle is part of the filter apparatus, just cap it.

6. Label the bottle. Be sure to note that the contents have been filter-sterilized (FS). Discard the filter.

There are also reusable filter apparatuses, with disposable filters, which can be used to sterilize large volumes of solutions. Attach the filter setup with a 0.2-μm filter to a sterile sidearm flask (to which the vacuum hose is attached). Turn on the vacuum, pour in the solution, and continue to pour until the entire solution has passed through the filter into the flask. Remove the vacuum hose, flame the opening, and pour the solution into a sterile bottle.

Aspirating

The motions involved in removing fluid with an aspirator are very similar to those used in transferring liquid with a pipet. Set your working area up as if you were pipeting from one container to another. Just add a test tube or beaker that can be used to place the used pipet and tubing temporarily.

> *A pipettor tip can be inserted on the end of a pasteur pipet, making flaming unnecessary. Gently stab the pipet into the tip in the tip box.*

1. Open a package of pipets or pasteur pipets. One will be attached to the aspirator.

2. Holding the pipet in the left hand, insert it into the tubing that is held in the right hand.

3. Hold the pipet near the place it enters the tubing.

4. If you are using a glass pipet, flame it lightly.

5. Turn on the vacuum.

> *The tilt of the tube not only helps prevent airborne contamination, but also protects the integrity of pellets while removing supernatants.*

6. Open the container or tube from which you will be removing fluid. Hold the cap in the last two fingers of the right hand. Maintain the tube at a 45° angle.

7. Flame the open container.

8. Insert the tip of the pipet just below the surface of the liquid. As the level of the liquid goes down, follow it with the pipet tip.

9. As you near the bottom, gently lift and move the pipet around the surface of the pellet, gently testing the strength of the pellet without touching it.

10. Remove the pipet and insert it into the tube or beaker until you have a chance to deal with it.

11. Flame the container, cap it, and put it down.

12. Hold the tubing and pipet pointing upward, to be sure all the fluid is drained from it.

13. Turn off the vacuum. Remove the pipet and discard it.

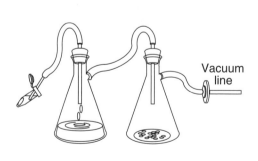

Vacuum line

An aspirator used for potentially infectious material must be equipped with a hydrophobic filter between the flasks and the vacuum supply. This prevents the uptake of material into the vacuum system. If the vacuum suddenly is reduced, it is usually because the filter has become wetted and must be replaced. Be sure you know where the replacements are.

PROTECTING THE INVESTIGATOR

Biomedical investigators work with a host of potentially infectious elements. These include virus-infected cells, human blood and waste products, and pathogenic bacteria. Organisms are classified according to the risk of transmitting disease. Several health organizations have established guidelines to be followed when working with different kinds of biohazard (potentially infectious) material: Your own institution may have additional rules. *Following the guidelines protects not only the immediate investigator, but also the other people in the laboratory.*

> *"However, he would then review the protocol... It was in this manner that I was introduced to Avery's extraordinary rigorous bacteriological technique ...he... had agreed that they would treat all bacterial cultures as if they contained the plague bacillus. They realized that it was a common failing to become sloppy in handling nonpathogenic organisms which in turn led to some relaxation of acceptable techniques when dealing with more infectious agents." McCarty, p 125.*

TABLE 1. Systems for Classifying Microorganisms on the Basis of Hazards to Laboratory Workers and the Community

	Hazard			
USPHS (1974)	Class 1 none or minimal	Class 2 ordinary potential	Class 3 special, to individual	Class 4 high, to individual
WHO (1979)	Risk Group I low individual low community	Risk Group II moderate individual low community	Risk Group III high individual low community	Risk Group IV high, to individual and community
ACDP (1990)	Hazard Group 1 unlikely to cause human disease	Hazard Group 2 possibly to laboratory workers, unlikely to community	Hazard Group 3 some hazard to laboratory workers, may spread to community	Hazard Group 4 serious hazard to laboratory workers, high risk to community

Several organizations have established guidelines to follow when working with each level of biohazard. The system of the U.S. Department of Health and Human Services (USPHS), a branch of the NIH, is used in the majority of descriptions in the United States.

Biosafety Level Requirements

In the USA, containment facilities are referred to as BL1, BL2, BL3, and BL4, BL standing for *B*iosafety *L*evel protection. They are sometimes also called P1, P2, P3, and P4, the "P" being an abbreviation for protection. The USPHS hazard classification for microorganisms corresponds to the Biosafety 1 containment level requirements. In other words, the Class III organism would require BL3 containment.

    Most of the guidelines concern the containment of the hazard. Containment is effected by the use of different levels of biosafety cabinets, which provide a closed environment with control of airflow and exhaust.

> *The procedure performed can also influence the actual hazard of the organism. Disruptive actions, such as sonication, that can cause aerosols increase the potential hazard and the protection needed is greater.*

TABLE 2. Summary of Biosafety/Containment Level Requirements

Level	Facilities	Laboratory practice	Safety equipment
1	Basic	GMT[a]	None. Work on open bench
2	Basic	GMT plus protective clothing, biohazard signs	Open bench plus safety cabinet for aerosol potential
3	Containment	Level 2 plus special clothing, controlled access	Safety cabinet for all activities
4	Maximum containment	Level 3 plus air lock entry, shower exit, special waste disposal	Class III safety cabinet, pressure gradient, double-ended autoclave

[a]GMT = Good microbiological technique.

Biosafety Cabinets

Biological safety cabinets are divided into three classes, I, II, and III, based on the amount of protection provided (see Table 3).

STERILE TECHNIQUE IN THE CLASS II BIOSAFETY CABINET

The highest level of biohazard most investigators routinely deal with is with class 2. The class II vertical flow cabinet is sufficient to deal with this.

    The *biosafety hood*, also known as the *laminar flow hood* or *class II vertical flow cabinet* provides filtered and recirculated airflow within the workspace. The airflow makes a curtain that stops passage of the outside air into the hood, and the air into the room. This protects the working investigator from the contents of the hood and makes the hood

> *Infected human blood and pathogenic organisms require BL3 (and sometimes BL4) containment, which is provided by a negative pressure room, a facility not found in many institutions.*

a good place to deal with potentially dangerous organisms. The exhaust air is filtered through a HEPA (high efficiency particle air) filter, so that biohazard material isn't released into the room or building.

    However, most hoods are used to *protect the experiment*, not the experimenter. Their most common use in labs is with routine tissue culture, to prevent contamina-

TABLE 3. The Use of Biological Safety Cabinets

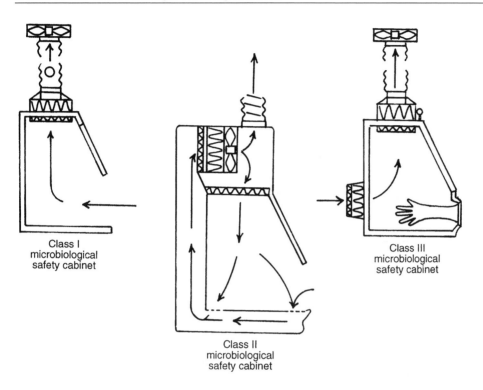

Class I
microbiological
safety cabinet

Class II
microbiological
safety cabinet

Class III
microbiological
safety cabinet

Class	Investigator protected?	Experimental materials protected?	Suitable for
I	Partially Circulating air barrier; HEPA-filtered exhaust	No No sterile work surface; unfiltered room air is drawn across the work area.	Low-risk oncogenic viruses Routine lab operations such as sonicating. Provides personnel protection for work with chemical carcinogens, low-level radioactive materials, volatile solvents. Similar to fume hood, filtration not as effective.
II	Partially Circulating air barrier; HEPA-filtered exhaust	Yes All intake air is filtered.	Low- to moderate-risk oncogenic viruses CDC class 1–3 agents, anything requiring BL2 containment. Cell culture *or* bacterial culture.
III	Yes Physical barrier (glove box); HEPA-filtered exhaust	Yes All intake air is filtered. Poorer air circulation than in class II; material not as protected	Used for CDC class 4 agents requiring BL4 containment. Highly toxic chemicals and carcinogens (provided that effluents are treated)

The Biosafety 1 containment levels of the hazard classification for microorganisms do not correspond to the classes of biosafety cabinets.

tion of the cells during splitting and experimental manipulations. Because of the design of the laminar flow hood, there will be fewer particles or microorganisms floating in the air, waiting to leap into your opened bottles. Thus, you can relax *somewhat* on your benchtop aseptic technique.

People who have first learned aseptic technique in a biosafety cabinet tend to be sloppier about their technique than a bench-trained person. They assume the hood will take care of all lapses. This isn't true! Vigilance is still necessary to prevent contamination. *The major cause of contamination is movement of the arms in and out of the cabinet, which breaks the air curtain and disturbs the flow.*

> *Work with **radiolabeled iodine**, often done sterilely, must **not** be done in a class II biosafety cabinet. Iodine is volatile, and must be used in a fume hood equipped with a TEDA charcoal filter. Be sure your fume hood is certified to do ^{125}I work before you think about an experiment.*

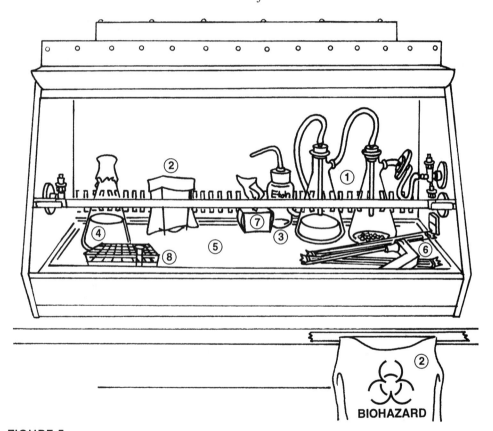

FIGURE 5.

Biosafety cabinet set up for aseptic work. **Task:** To transfer 5 ml of cell culture from a tube into 40 ml of culture medium. The supplies needed are arranged for a right-handed investigator, so that things to be manipulated with the right hand are set up to the right of the working area, and things to be manipulated with the left hand are set up to the left of the working area. **Key:** (1) *Aspirator with filter.* (2) *Biohazard disposal.* (3) *70% ethanol in squirt bottle.* (4) *Flask of culture medium.* (5) *Clear area.* (6) *Individually wrapped pipets and pipet aid.* (7) *Kimwipes.* (8) *Test tube with cell culture, in a test tube rack.*

⚗ Working sterilely in a biosafety cabinet

1. **Verify that the hood is on and air is circulating (on/off switch, sound, and dials).** The hood should be left on continuously, 24 hours a day. It sometimes is not, because of noise and heating issues: In this case, turn it on 5 minutes before use to allow the airflow to establish itself.

2. **Lower the sash to the calibration mark.** If there is no mark, lower sash either to the 100 ± 10-ft/min level (the readout is on the front of the hood) or to 12–14 inches. The sash must be below chin level. If you are creating aerosols, lower sash as far down as you can.

3. **Do not block airflow.**

   a. Don't cover the space between tapered metal front lip and the work surface, e.g., with spill paper.

   b. Do not block the rear exhaust slot. Place bulky items to rear and sides on a supporting mesh; elevate at least 2 inches.

   c. Don't block the face of the hood with shielding or large equipment.

   d. Locate work at least 6 inches inside the hood.

   e. Don't sit with your body flush against the cabinet.

4. **Secure papers and other lightweight material to prevent their entrapment in the exhaust line.** Don't write yourself notes on stray pieces of paper.

5. **Wipe down the surface with 70% ethanol or isopropanol or another disinfectant before each use of the hood.**

6. **If you must put a sterile cap down, put it face down on a clean surface.**

7. **Minimize hand movement in and out of the hood.** Bringing arms in and out of the hood disturbs the airflow. Before you start work, put everything you need inside the hood, including a receptacle to hold trash.

8. **Do NOT use a flame in a biosafety cabinet.** It interferes with the control of the airflow patterns.

> *Although it is no longer recommended that biosafety cabinets have UV lights installed (because they have been deemed to be ineffective against contaminants, and, therefore, to give a false sense of security), older hoods do have them and labs do use them. Just be sure the UV light is off before you work in the hood.*

Maintaining hood function

Get into the habit of checking the magnehelic dial on the outside of the hood whenever you sit down to work. If the reading changes, it indicates a problem with the airflow, and the cleanliness and protection afforded by the hood will be compromised.

The door must be closed to a level marked on the hood, in order to be effective. Lifting the hood sounds an alarm, indicating that the airflow has been perturbed. Every now and again, lift the door and be sure the alarm sounds. If it doesn't, notify EHS.

Biosafety cabinets are inspected regularly and certified for safety and integrity of airflow. The date of the previous and next inspection should be posted on the cabinet. Be sure the cabinet is inspected on time by the EHS department. At this time, the HEPA filters (which trap the particles in the hood) are usually changed, and the cabinet may need to be decontaminated with formaldehyde or another agent to permit the EHS representative to work safely. This takes at least a day, and the recertification of hoods in the lab should be coordinated so everyone always has access to at least one hood.

 Working courteously in a biosafety cabinet. There are seldom enough biosafety cabinets in a laboratory to satisfy all the investigators that require one. To ensure the safety of all investigators who use the hood, the rules of courtesy must be followed meticulously.

- Use and obey any sign-up sheet.

- Get in and out of the hood as quickly as you can. Be well organized before you start.

- Replenish supplies such as bleach and 70% ethanol as soon as they run out.

- Empty sharps containers and biohazard disposal when they near being full. Don't wait until they spill.

- Remove all of your supplies when you are finished. Clean the hood well.

RESOURCES

Collins C.H., Lyne P.M., and Grange J.M. 1991. *Microbiological methods,* 6th edition. Butterworth-Heinemann, Oxford, England.

Freshney R.I. 1994. *Culture of animal cells. A manual of basic technique,* 3rd edition, pp. 51–59. Wiley-Liss, New York.

Gershey E.L., Party E., and Wilkerson A. *1991. Laboratory safety in practice: A comprehensive compliance program and safety manual.* Van Nostrand Reinhold, New York.

Heidcamp W.H. 1995. *Cell biology laboratory manual.* Gustavus Adolphus College, St. Peter, Minnesota.
http://www.gac.edu/cgi-bin/user/~cellab/phpl?index-1.html

McCarty M. 1985. *The transforming principle. Discovering that genes are made of DNA.* W.W. Norton & Company, New York.

U.S. Department of Health and Human Services. 1988. *Biosafety in microbiological and bio-medical laboratories.* Public Health Services. Centers for Disease Control. HHS Publication No. (NIH) 88-88395. 2nd edition.

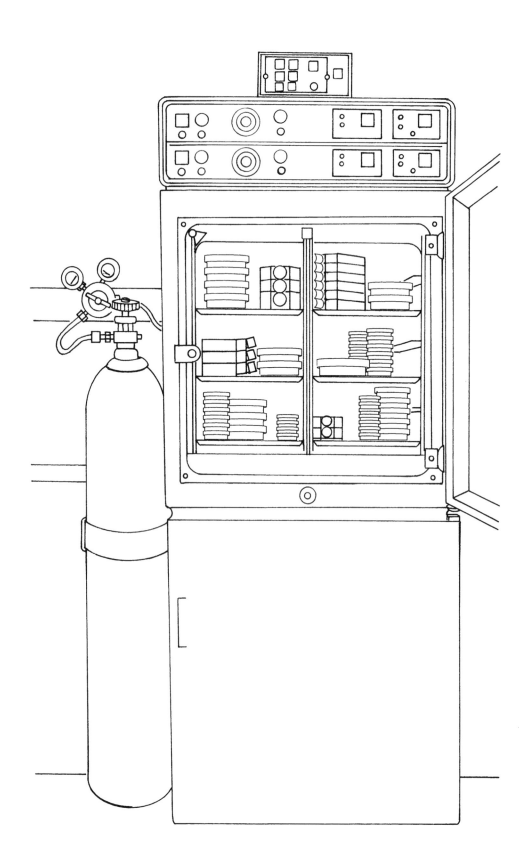

10

Eukaryotic Cell Culture

KNOW YOUR CELLS. When you start a series of experiments, someone in the lab may provide you with a tube or flask of cells, with brief instructions about the care of the cells. It isn't as simple as that. The cells may be easy to maintain, but the more you know about the cells, the more finely attuned you are to the cells' quirks, the quicker and more clear the interpretation of results will be. Look up the references for the cells. Speak to people who have used the cells, and ask for advice. Most importantly, monitor the cells constantly, until *you* are the expert on their growth.

TYPES OF CULTURES AND CELL LINES

Cell cultures are described in two ways:

- Origin of the cells.

- Manner of growth.

TYPES OF CULTURES AND CELL LINES	205
Classification by origin	206
Classification by manner of growth	208
OBSERVING CELLS	209
OBTAINING CELLS	211
Primary cells	211
Continuous cell lines	212
Culturing frozen cells	213
CELL MAINTENANCE	215
Routine maintenance of cell lines	215
Feeding and passaging	215
Splitting adherent cells	222
Splitting suspension cells	224
Microscopic count of viable cells	225
FREEZING AND STORAGE OF CELLS	228
Freezing cells	229
CONTAMINATION	231
How to recognize contamination	231
Mycoplasma contamination	234
Cross contamination	235
CO_2 INCUBATORS AND TANKS	236
CO_2 incubators	236
CO_2 tanks	239
RESOURCES	243

Classification by Origin

TABLE 1. Categories of Cell Cultures Based on Origin

	Origin	Similarity to original tissue	Ease of maintenance	Doublings
Primary cells	Animal tissue, fetal or adult	Representative	Difficult	0–1
Finite cell lines	Animal tissue, usually fetal	Representative	Difficult	Fetal: 20–80; adult tissue: very limited
Continuous cell lines	Spontaneous transformation of primary or finite cell lines	Not very representative; cells are less differentiated	Easy	Indefinite, with selection for higher growth rate
Transformed cell lines	Tumor tissue, spontaneous transformation in vitro of continuous cell line, or in vitro transformation with whole virus or virus DNA	Not very representative; less differentiated than parent	Easy	Indefinite, with selection for higher growth rate
Hybridomas	Fusion of antibody-secreting B cells and malignant myeloma cells	Not representative of either cell type, but not intended to be!	Difficult	Limited

 Primary cells are cells isolated from animal or plant tissue and cultured.

Once a cell has divided it becomes a finite cell line, with the potential to become immortalized.

Repeated passage of a *finite cell line* derived from normal cells is done in a way to select for faster-growing variants that might become a *continuous cell line*. This is considered to be spontaneous transformation.

The origin of the primary cell or finite cell line will influence the growth pattern. If a cell is a fibroblast, it will have the adherent growth typical of fibroblasts. However, once the cell has been transformed, the growth pattern may no longer be typical of the original primary cell.

 Continuous cell lines have a higher growth rate, a higher cloning efficiency, increased tumorigenicity, and more variable chromosome complement than finite cell lines.

Continuous cell lines are often manipulated to become transformed cell lines expressing a particular and needed phenotype.

> *The more differentiated the cell line, the slower it will grow.*

Some commonly used cell lines

Cell line	Cell type and origin	Adherent or suspension growth
3T3	Fibroblast (mouse, embryo)	Adherent
BHK21	Fibroblast (Syrian hamster, kidney)	Suspension
MDCK	Epithelial cell (dog, kidney)	Adherent
HeLa	Epithelial cell (human, adenocarcinoma)	Suspension or adherent
PtK1	Epithelial cell (rat kangaroo, kidney)	Adherent
L6	Myoblast (rat, skeletal muscle)	Adherent
PC12	Chromaffin cell (rat, adrenal pheochromocytoma) Neural cell studies	Adherent
Sf9	(Ovary, fall armyworm) Baculovirus infection	Suspension
SP2	Plasma cell (mouse, myeloma) Fusion for hybridoma	Suspension

 Transformed cells have been changed from normal cells to cells with many of the properties of cancer cells.

Some of these cell lines have actually been derived from tumors, or are transformed spontaneously in culture, by mutation. Cells can be deliberately transformed by a chemical or by a tumor-inducing virus. Such a virus carries a gene which induces either the errant or overproduction of a cell protein needed for growth, or the production of an aberrant protein needed for growth. No matter how transformation occurred, the result is a cell with altered functional, morphological, and growth characteristics, some of which are listed here:

- Growth to high cell density

- Lower requirement for growth factors and serum

- More anchorage independence

- Ability to proliferate indefinitely

Adherently cultured transformed cells are usually highly anchorage independent, and adhere lightly even to tissue culture dishes. Wash the cells very carefully, as the loose monolayer can be inadvertently aspirated away.

 Hybridomas secrete monoclonal antibody into the media, often at a high enough concentration that the cell supernatant can be used directly for hybridizations.

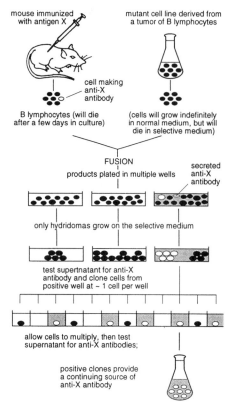

mouse immunized with antigen X

mutant cell line derived from a tumor of B lymphocytes

cell making anti-X antibody

B lymphocytes (will die after a few days in culture)

(cells will grow indefinitely in normal medium, but will die in selective medium)

FUSION
products plated in multiple wells

secreted anti-X antibody

only hybridomas grow on the selective medium

test supernatant for anti-X antibody and clone cells from positive well at ~ 1 cell per well

allow cells to multiply, then test supernatant for anti-X antibodies;

positive clones provide a continuing source of anti-X antibody

FIGURE 1.

Preparation of hybridomas that secrete monoclonal antibodies against a particular antigen (X). The selective growth medium used contains an inhibitor (aminopterin) that blocks the nonbiosynthetic pathways by which nucleotides are made. The cells must therefore use a bypass pathway to synthesize their nucleic acids, and this pathway is defective in the mutant cell line to which the non-B lymphocytes are fused. Because neither cell type used for initial fusion can grow on its own, only hybrid cells survive. (Modified, with permission, from Alberts et al. 1994.)

Classification by Manner of Growth

Cells are classified by the way they grow in liquid culture, or in semisolid medium. Growth characteristics are functional descriptions only, and are dependent on the origin of the cells.

> *Suspension and adherent growth are properties of the cell as well as of the culture conditions. Some cells can be manipulated to grow either way.*

 Suspension or adherent growth.
The first and most practical way cell growth is described is in terms of how the cells do in liquid culture. This information is always given with the cell line and, with origin of the cells, constitutes the major definition of the cell line.

- **Suspension cells** grow suspended in the growth medium. They are able to survive and proliferate without attachment to the culture vessel. Cells cultured from *blood, spleen,* or *bone marrow,* especially *immature* cells, tend to grow in suspension. Cells in suspension look like little balls. The *advantages* of suspension growth are the *large numbers* of cells that can be achieved, and the *ease of harvesting.*

- **Adherent cells** grow in a monolayer, attached to the surfaces of the culture vessel. Cells that derive from *ectodermal* or *endodermal* embryonic cell layers tend to grow adherently. This includes fibroblasts and epithelial cells. Cells grown adherently have various shapes, but are, generally, flattened: The same cells grown in suspension would then become rounded. The advantage of adherent growth is the ability of the cells to adhere and spread on surfaces such as coverslips, making *microscopy, hybridizations,* and *functional assays* more easily performed.

Anchorage-dependent and anchorage-independent growth.

A subdivision of adherent growth is anchorage-dependent versus anchorage-independent growth. Although anchorage independence is measured in soft agar (in which the cells are imbedded/suspended), it can also have an effect on culture in tissue culture dishes. Anchorage dependence and independence are properties of the cell and cannot be altered by growth conditions.

- **Anchorage-dependent cells** require attachment to the surface for cell proliferation.

- **Anchorage-independent cells** do not require attachment for cell proliferation. This is often a property of transformed cells. Growth of anchorage-independent cells in tissue culture dishes looks more haphazard than the growth of anchorage-dependent cells, with the cells only loosely applied to the surface.

OBSERVING CELLS

It must become second nature to you to look at every culture of cells, macroscopically and microscopically, whenever you take out a flask to subculture or use for an experiment. If your cells aren't healthy, your experiments won't work reproducibly.

As you remove the culture vessel from the incubator, note:

- The color of the medium. There is a pH indicator in most media (see below, under "Medium") that turns yellow if it is acid or purplish if it is alkaline. Medium too basic or acidic can indicate contamination, an overgrown culture, a dead culture, or faulty CO_2 measurement or delivery.

- Any cloudiness in the medium, which could indicate contamination or a grossly overgrown culture.

- Clumped cells (suspension culture) or peeling cells (adherent culture).

If you have a flask or dish of cells, look at it with an inverted microscope under 40X power, before you even put it in the hood. Make it your routine to place any flask from the incubator directly on the microscope.

 Adherent cells.

You should see a fairly regular arrangement of cells that appear to be relatively flat on the surface of the plate. Each type of cell has a characteristic shape in culture: round, triangular, squarish, elongated. The pattern of growth may be like a cobblestone street, or in swirls, or there may be random growth, with some cells seemingly growing on top of each other.

Within the individual cells you may see a darker round shadow of the nucleus, with the even darker nucleoli present. Sometimes the nucleus is so large that very little cytoplasm can be seen. Cells in cell division may appear as spheres, sometimes in pairs: Hourglass shaped (mitotic) cells with obvious alignment of the condensed chromosomes might even be seen.

 Suspension cells.

Suspension cells are spheres. Even in a suspension culture, some cells may adhere lightly to the flask: These may not move when the flask is gently moved and may appear to be slightly flattened or triangular. On top of those cells you can see the round, apparently floating cells. They may appear granular, but you will not be able to see the nucleus or other organelles, even under 100X.

You must learn to recognize what is normal for your cells. When you have a new cell line, look at as many cultures as you can, so you will be able to define for yourself the look of a "normal" culture. Consult with someone in the lab for even minor questions about the cells.

Most inverted microscopes only have a 40X lens as the highest power lens. If you want to observe your cells at higher magnification (if, for example, you want to check for bacterial contamination) you can remove a sample, and either fix and stain it or make a wet mount, and observe it under oil at 100X on an upright compound microscope (See Chapter 16).

OBTAINING CELLS

Have a **hepatitis B vaccine** if you are working in a lab that deals with primary human cells, and especially, with blood cells. Even if you are not isolating the cells yourself, any spill or aerosol could be a risk.

Primary Cells

Primary cells are difficult to obtain. An animal must usually be killed and dissected, the cells isolated and cultivated. It is time consuming and fraught with possible mistakes. For many cell types, the numbers obtained are small, and the cells are short-lived. But primary cells are the closest approximation to the "real" thing, and if you really need them (and think hard about that), the trouble is worth the results.

You cannot assume someone will give primary cells to you. Often a lab won't have enough for their own experiments. Request primary cells with consideration of the difficulty of obtaining them, and do not be offended if you are refused.

- **Ask someone in the lab or department** who works on the cells. For a first experiment, ask whether you could get any extra cells from the next isolation he performs. Offer to help in any way.

- **Ask another investigator** who works on the cells. Unless this is someone you already have a good relationship with, this can be tricky. If the primary cells are vital to the experiments and are particularly difficult to obtain, you may want to officially *collaborate* with the procurer of the cells. Check with the head of the lab first, because a collaboration can have undesirable political ramifications.

A request letter should

Introduce yourself and your lab (briefly!)
Introduce your project (briefly!)
Say how you heard of the investigator's cells (briefly)
Say what you will do with the cells (briefly but honestly)
Give your address and phone number
End with mucho thanks

A request letter can

Offer a collaboration

If you do not hear from the investigator in a few weeks, follow up with an E-mail or phone call. Requests for cells are generally pretty low priority, and such letters often stay on the bottom of the pile, so don't take a lack of answer personally.

- Even if someone else provides you with the cells, **observe the procedure** at least once. Things change, and you may have to do it yourself in a hurry one day. It is also good to know as much about the cells as possible, and to show interest and appreciation to the provider of the cells.

- **Hospitals and medical schools** are a good source for certain human tissue and cells, but you will have to find a contact to help you obtain the samples. Many **blood banks** may provide partially isolated blood cells for a fee.

- Most likely, you will have to **isolate the cells yourself.** Don't just get a protocol and try: If possible, ask someone who has done the isolation to show you.

- There are several **companies** that can provide primary cells, at a fairly steep price: This is worth it for a one-time experiment, when it doesn't make sense to lay out a huge expenditure on the isolation of a difficult or new cell type. Call your purchasing department for the numbers of those companies and, if possible, ask the company for the names of scientists who have used the cells and would be willing to talk to you.

> *A collaborator has a responsibility to supply the cells, but she then becomes a part of the project and an author on any publications resulting from experiments with the cells.*

> *Obtain as much information as you can about the maintenance of the cells.*

> *Watch the isolation by the provider of the protocol with your protocol in hand, noting down anything that isn't clear to you or wouldn't be remembered if you were alone. Cell isolations are notoriously dependent on the trivial details—such as how long you shake the tube, which centrifuge was used, how high to fill the plate—and you want to get as much of that detail as possible.*

Continuous Cell Lines

If a cell line grows well, it is usually simple to obtain cells. If it doesn't grow well, you may have the same difficulty getting the cells as you would obtaining primary cells.

- Never forget that cell lines experience **phenotypic drift** with continued culture, and that the same cell line cultured in two different labs could well have different characteristics. If you are obtaining cells for particular experiments, get the cells from the people doing those experiments.

> *Treat cells as infectious agents. Cells may harbor a variety of viruses and other organisms. Observe the same precautions you would for infectious agents. No mouth pipeting! Wear gloves! Be careful!*

- If you are using the same cells as the rest of the lab members, **ask someone for a frozen vial.** This is preferable to cells obtained after a split, as the passage number will be smaller, and the cells more likely to run to type. If you take cells from a split for a quickie experiment, the likelihood is that you will never get an earlier batch, and will regret it down the line.

- One of the most common and dependable sources for cell lines is the **American Type Culture Collection** (**ATCC**). This is a private, nonprofit organization that collects, preserves, and distributes (for a small fee) cultures of human and animal cells, as well as microorganisms, viruses, DNA probes, and plants. The cultures are guaranteed to be viable and contamination-free, and will be replaced if there is any problem in culturing them. The catalog contains not only the lists and descriptions of the cell lines, with references, media and freezing media formulations, and useful notes, but also has useful general information and tips.

> *You must reference the source of the cells in all publications and seminars.*

- There are other **service organizations,** usually dealing with more limited cell types, who will provide cells free or cheaply. Some investigators have NIH grants to maintain certain strains and to provide those cells to others for research.

- Look in the **Materials and Methods** section of the best papers dealing with the cells you want, and find the source of the cells used for the experiments. Note any particulars given, such as passage number or media used, as you will want to replicate conditions as much as possible. If the cells originated with that investigator, contact him for the cells.

> *If the investigator obtained his own cells from ATTC or another commercial source, you should not bother him for the cells, but should get them from ATCC yourself. The only exceptions are if money is really scarce for you, or if the investigator has derived his own cell line or subgroup from the ATCC line.*

PROTOCOL

Culturing Frozen Cells

Background

Eukaryotic cells are usually frozen in medium with serum and a freezing additive, and are stored in liquid nitrogen at $-196^{\circ}C$. If ordered commercially, they will arrive in a vial or ampoule on dry ice. Frozen cells must be thawed rapidly and cultured immediately to maximize viability. To remove the freezing additive the medium is changed after 24 hours.

> *If you go to a lab to pick up the cells yourself, bring some dry ice in an ice bucket in which to transport the cells.*

> *Frozen cells should be cultured as soon as possible. If you cannot culture the cells immediately, store them in liquid nitrogen.*

Materials

- Culture medium, warmed to 37°C

- Culture vessel

- 70% ethanol in a small beaker

- 1-ml and 10-ml pipet, pipettor and tips

Procedure

1. Hold the vial in a 37°C water bath and agitate it rapidly. It will thaw in about 1 minute.

2. Drop the thawed vial in a beaker containing 70% ethanol and place it in a laminar flow hood for all manipulations.

3. Open the ampoule or tube. Do not allow ethanol to drip inside the vial.

4. Transfer contents of ampoule to culture vessel and immediately add warmed medium.

5. Replace cap and incubate for 24 hours.

6. Replace medium with fresh medium.

7. Incubate for 2–3 days or as indicated in the directions for those cells.

> *Cells are usually frozen in 1 ml volume, and are added to 10 ml of fresh medium.*

> *The freezing medium can also be removed **before** culture by spinning down the thawed cells and resuspending them in fresh medium. This is only necessary if the cells are particularly sensitive to the freezing additive or if you won't be there the next day to change the medium.*

> *Ampoules are made of glass and are under pressure, and there is a very real chance that the ampoules can explode. Always open ampoules in a biosafety cabinet: If none is available, wear eye and face protection. You should wear eye and face protection whenever you are manipulating samples in liquid nitrogen.*

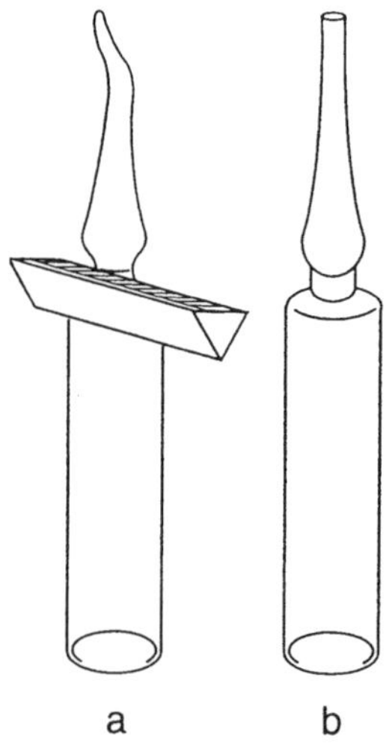

a   b

FIGURE 2.

Types of ampoules. Standard ampoules (*a*) must be nicked on the neck with a glass file that has been dipped in ethanol: After making a 1/8th score on one side, wrap the ampoule in gauze or a paper towel, hold the base firmly in the left hand and snap the top off with the right hand. Prescored ampoules (*b*) usually have a band around the neck, and can be wrapped and snapped open directly.

CELL MAINTENANCE

Routine Maintenance of Cell Lines

In order to maintain the cells, they must be:

- **Fed** (supplied with fresh medium). During growth, the medium will be depleted of needed factors and must be replaced.

  > *Feeding and passaging are accomplished at the same time: It would be difficult to do one without the other.*

- **Split** (passaged, the cell number reduced). During growth, the number of cells in the culture will increase beyond the capacity of the vessel and medium to sustain them.

- **Frozen.** Whenever you obtain or generate a cell line, aliquots of it must be frozen away. These aliquots are a backup for you should the cells phenotypically drift or all become contaminated.

> **Rule 1. Look at your cells!** Never split, experiment with, or freeze cells without looking at the culture macroscopically, and on an inverted microscope. By constant observation, you will not only find contamination before it becomes a major problem, and be aware when a cell line has started to drift by noting morphological alterations, but you will "know" the cells, know when to split, when to experiment, and when to dump the experiment.

Feeding and Passaging

The faster the cells grow, the more often they must be fed and split. When you obtain the cells, find out:

- Are antibiotics used?
- How are they grown?
- What medium works best?
- Do the cells require serum?
- How often should the cells be fed and split?

Antibiotics

Antibiotics are used standardly in many labs but should not be needed if aseptic technique is being properly done. The half-life of many antibiotics is quite short at 37ºC (see Table 2), so there often isn't as much antibiotic as the investigator believes.

With valuable cells or cells prone to contamination because of a lot of manipulation, it is sometimes too nerve-wracking for some investigators not to include antibiotics in the medium.

Antibiotics for cell culture are usually obtained as a dehydrated powder in a sterile vial. Rehydrate with sterile water or solvent. It is not necessary to filter-sterilize such a packaged antibiotic.

> *Antifungal agents amphotericin B (Fungizone) and Mycostatin (Nystatin) are not recommended for routine use, because they can affect the membrane permeability of all eukaryotic cells.*

Two standard antibiotics for cell culture

Gentamicin 5–10 mg/ml stock, final 50 µg/ml
Penicillin (10,000 units)/**Streptomycin** (10 mg/ml) stock, final 100 units/ml and 100 µg/ml

Aliquot in 1-ml tubes and store at –20°C. Add 1 ml of either solution to 99 ml of medium. If you use large quantities of media, make up 5-ml aliquots to add to 500-ml bottles of medium.

Culture Vessels

The type of vessel you use will depend on the kind of cells and the volume of cells you need. Most labs employ flasks and dishes that can be adapted to both adherent and suspension cultures, but there are a variety of containers for large-scale and specialized cell culture.

Most tissue culture containers are disposable, made of polystyrene, and have been radiation-sterilized. Glass containers are occasionally used, but the ease of use of disposable containers has made them the universal choice.

Untreated plastic is usually fine for suspension cells, but most adherent cells grow better on treated plastic. Labware companies sell "treated" dishes and flasks for tissue culture: The treatment (a permanent modification of the polystyrene surface with, for example, plasma or amino functional groups) varies from company to company. Cells may prefer the plates from a particular company, so it is not a trivial act to switch culture dish sources.

Plates may be treated with a protein that works nonspecifically, perhaps by supplying a positive charge. An example of this is poly-D-lysine.

Some cells require adherence to a particular substrate for differentiation or the expression of certain functions. This is usually a component or a mixture of components of the extracellular matrix, such as collagen, fibronectin, and laminin.

Dishes can be treated in the lab by adding a suspension of the material in solution to the dish to cover the surface, incubating the dish to promote attachment, pouring off the excess solution, and washing the surface with buffer or medium.

TABLE 2. Antibiotics Used in Cell Culture Medium

Antibiotic	Effective against	Working[a] concentration	Stock solution	Half-life in media (37°C)	Structural class	Mechanism of action
Benzylpenicillin (Penicillin G)	Gram-positive bacteria	100 units/ml (~100 µg/ml)	10,000 units/ml	2 days	Penicillins	Inhibits cell wall synthesis
Streptomycin	Gram-negative bacteria	100 µg/ml	10 mg/ml	4 days	Aminoglycosides	Inhibits translation (30S subunit)
Kanamycin	Gram-negative bacteria	100 µg/ml	10 mg/ml		Aminoglycosides	Inhibits translation (30S subunit)
Tetracycline	Broad-spectrum bacteria	10–50 µg/ml	5 mg/ml		Aminoglycosides	Inhibits translation (30S subunit)
Gentamicin (Gentamycin)	Broad-spectrum bacteria, mycoplasma	50 µg/ml	5 mg/ml	15 days	Aminoglycosides	Inhibits translation (30S subunit?)
Lincomycin	Mycoplasma, Gram-positive bacteria	50 µg/ml	5 mgl/ml			Inhibits translation (50S subunit)
Tylosin	Mycoplasma Gram-positive bacteria	10 µg/ml	5 mg/ml		Macrolide	Inhibits translation (50S subunit)
Amphotericin B (Fungizone)	Fungi, yeast	2.5 µg/ml	250 µg/ml	4 days	Polyene	Alters membrane permeability
Nystatin (Mycostatin)	Fungi, yeast	20 units/ml	2000 units/ml		Polyene	Alters membrane permeability

(Reprinted, with permission, from Harlow and Lane 1988.)

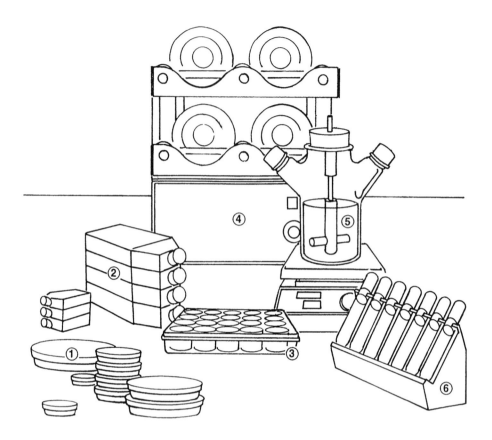

FIGURE 3.

Cell culture containers. **Key:** (1) *Dishes.* Generally used for adherent cells, most are treated to maximize attachment of cells. The 100-mm size, which holds 10 ml, should not be confused with bacterial dishes of the same size, as bacterial dishes are not treated for cell attachment. The 60-mm size holds 4–5 ml, and the 35-mm, 1–2 ml. (2) *Flasks.* Available with straight or canted necks: Straight necks minimize sloshing, which is good for suspension cultures, and canted necks permit easier access to the culture surface, which is useful when manipulating adherent cells. However, either neck type can be used for either adherent or suspension cultures. 25 cm^2 (50 ml), 75 cm^2 (250 ml), 175 cm^2 (750 ml) are common sizes. (3) *Multiple-well tissue culture plates.* A standard size of 86 × 128 mm is divided into 6-, 12-, 24-, 48-, or 96-well sizes, and is compatible with automatic diluters and plate readers. These are used for hybridoma and monoclonal antibody work, titrations, toxicity testing, and any experiment that requires a comparison of different cell treatments. They can be used for adherent and nonadherent cells. Plates are usually purchased treated, and some sizes are available with flat or round-bottomed wells: Most instruments require flat-bottomed wells. (4) *Roller bottles.* Usually used for maximum yield. Adherent or suspension cells can be grown in roller bottles. Can be used in an open or closed system. (5) *Spinner bottles.* Designed to spin gently, without subjecting cells to harsh mixing. Used for suspension and microcarrier cell cultures, as well as for insect cultures. Different gas mixtures can be added, and the bottles can be used in an open or closed system. (6) *Tubes.* For adherent cells. Round bottoms allow adherence on all parts of the tube. Leighton tubes have one side flattened, permitting microscopic observation.

Cell Medium

Most labs either buy the medium *already prepared and bottled,* or as a *powder that must be rehydrated and filter sterilized.* Of course, the latter choice is less expensive, and especially makes sense if the medium is being used in bulk.

> *Commercially prepared medium has an expiration date, which should be nonrigidly adhered to. Use expired medium for cell washes.*

Cell media look alike, since most contain phenol red or another dye as a pH indicator. But they are not alike, so don't just use what medium is available. Check the *formulation* you need, and order it from a company that guarantees its media to be mycoplasma-free.

Medium with a phenol red pH indicator will look

Lemon yellow below	pH 6.5
Yellow at	pH 6.5
Orange at	pH 7.0
Red at	pH 7.4
Pink at	pH 7.6
Purple at	pH 7.8

Most cells grow best when medium is around pH 7.4.

Yellowish medium is *acidic* and can indicate
   An overgrown culture
   Bacterial contamination
   Too much CO_2 in the incubator

Purplish medium is *alkaline* and can indicate
   A sparse and non-growing culture
   Mold contamination
   Too little CO_2 in the incubator

Some cells require the addition of other components to the prepared medium. L-Glutamine is a common addition, as some cells will fairly quickly exhaust the glutamine in the medium. Filter-sterilized and frozen aliquots can be thawed and added to the medium at the time of use.

Cell culture medium contains many heat-labile components, so you should store the media in the cold. However, medium should be warmed to 37°C before being added to cells: Never shock the cells by the addition of cold medium. But don't leave your bottle of medium in a 37°C water bath until you get around to feeding your

> *Be careful when adding anything directly to cells, especially compounds dissolved in DMSO, ethanol, or methanol. These compounds are toxic to cells at high concentrations, and you should shake or stir the container while adding the compound to dilute the compound as quickly as possible.*

cells, because many ingredients, such as some antibiotics, have a shorter half-life at 37°C. Warm medium 10 minutes before use. Better yet, remove and warm only what you will need.

> *Even on slow-growing cells, the medium must be changed regularly, because the cells still will metabolize and may exhaust some of the medium components.*

It is convenient to buy or make medium in 500-ml bottles. If you are using a 500-ml bottle a week, then add the serum and other labile components to this bottle. Don't forget to only have (or remove) enough medium in the bottle so you can add the other components for a final 500-ml volume.

> If you will be adding 10% serum and 5 ml of antibiotics, set up bottles of medium with 445 ml of medium. Add the serum and antibiotic aliquots only as you need fresh medium.

Serum

Serum supplies needed growth factors and nutrients. Some cells, particularly transformed cells, have a very low serum requirement of around 0.5%. Some cell lines have been "trained" to survive in medium with low serum. As the needed components for serum are defined, more and more cells can be cultured with supplements and individually added components. This is a fortunate situation for you if your cells can be cultured without serum.

> *Serum is very expensive. Always aliquot and freeze serum, and add it to medium just before use. Store unused portions of thawed aliquots in the refrigerator, where it will be fine for several weeks.*

These are the serum variables you must consider:

- **The percentage of serum.** Most cells require 5–20% in the medium for good growth.
- **The type of serum.** Some cells like horse serum. The standard for tissue culture cells is calf serum. Some cells require the more expensive fetal calf (also known as fetal bovine) serum, and some cells (usually human) require serum of their own species, the most expensive serum proposition of all.
- **Whether or not the serum is heat-inactivated.** Serum is subjected to heat to inactivate components such as complement.

> ### To heat-inactivate serum
> Thaw the frozen serum at room temperature. This may take 5 or 6 hours for a 500-ml bottle of serum. Incubate the thawed serum at 65°C for 30 minutes. Aliquot the serum. Aliquot for the percentage of serum and the amount of medium you usually use. Freeze and store. Thaw aliquots in a 37°C water bath as needed.

- **From where you should obtain the serum.** Ask someone in the lab, or who has worked on the cells, as particular cells only tolerate certain serum. There is great competition among companies selling serum, but this is not the place to save money!

Serum varies from lot to lot. Many labs assay lots of serum for their ability to support cell growth and function and buy bulk quantities of the best lot. There is also company-to-company variation, so always check with someone in the lab for the tried and tested best source of serum for your cells.

How to split cells

Each cell line grows at its own rate and will require splitting at an individual schedule. The density at which a cell grows profoundly affects its physiology, so you must take pains to maintain cells at a healthy density and to always use cells grown to the same density for experiments.

Cell cultures should be split so that they are seeded to a defined density. In theory, this means that the cells should be counted every time they are split. In practice, cells are often split at a particular ratio of old-to-new medium—say, at 1:4 (10 ml of cells are added to 30 ml of medium). Well, it is sloppy, but it does work for some cells. If you split your cells this way, check them before and after splitting sometime so you know what your cell numbers are. Always record the split ratio.

It is convenient to split cells twice a week. Most cell lines have a doubling time of approximately 24 hours, and so will grow to the original number in just a few days. You could split to a lower number of cells, but too sparse a culture won't grow. You could just wait and split once a week, but the cells will stop growing at high density and may not be as healthy a culture.

Common mistakes in culturing cells

- Letting stock cultures overgrow because you don't have time to split them on the proper day

- Using cultures that are obviously the wrong density for an experiment instead of waiting another day or splitting the cells again

- Using old media instead of making fresh media

Cells growing in a monolayer must be dislodged from the culture vessel and put into a single cell suspension. Since cells secrete extracellular matrix components to which they will bind tightly, and may be attached to each other by Ca^{++}-dependent receptor-ligand interactions, it can be difficult to do. Dislodging can be done physically, by scraping, but this does cause cell injury. Generally, cells are loosened by enzymatic degradation of the cell adhesion and extracellular matrix components with trypsin. Particularly strongly adherent cells are also treated with EDTA for chelation of Ca^{++} and with varied proteinases to digest the matrix.

Use the gentlest treatment that works on your cells.

TABLE 3. Cell Dissociation for Transfer or Counting; Procedures of Gradually Increasing Severity

1.	Shake-off	Mitotic or other loosely adherent cells
2.	Trypsin[a] in PBS (0.01–0.5% as required, usually 0.25%, 5–15 min)	Most continuous cell lines
3.	Prewash with PBS or CMF, the 0.25% trypsin[a] in PBS or saline-citrate	Some strongly adherent continuous cell lines and many cell lines at early passage stages
4.	Prewash with 1 mM EDTA in PBS or CMF, then 0.25% trypsin[a] in citrate	Some strongly adherent early passage cell lines
5.	Prewash with 1 mM EDTA, then EDTA 2nd rinse, and leave on, 1 ml/5 cm	Epithelial cells, although some may be sensitive to EDTA
6.	EDTA prewash, then 0.25% trypsin[a] with 1 mM EDTA	Strongly adherent cells, particularly epithelial and some tumor cells (*note:* EDTA can be toxic to some cells)
7.	1 mM EDTA prewash, 0.25% trypsin[a] and collagenase,[a] 200 units/ml PBS or saline-citrate or EDTA/PBS	Thick cultures, multilayers, particularly collagen-producing dense cultures
8.	Scraping	All cultures, but may cause mechanical damage and usually will not give a single cell suspension
9.	Add dispase (0.1–1.0 mg/ml) or pronase (0.1–1.0 mg/ml) to medium and incubate until cells detach	Will dislodge most cells, but requires centrifugation step to remove enzyme not activated by serum. May be harmful to some cells

(Reprinted, with permission, from Freshney 1994; copyright by Wiley-Liss, Inc.)
[a]Digestive enzymes are available (Difco, Worthington, Boehringer Mannheim, Sigma) in varying degress of purity. Crude preparations, e.g., Difco trypsin 1:250 or Worthington CLS grade collagenase, contain other proteases that may be helpful in dissociating some cells but may be toxic to others. Start with a crude preparation and progress to purer grades if necessary. Purer grades are often used at a lower concentration (mg/ml) as their specific activities (enzyme units/g) are higher.

PROTOCOL

Splitting Adherent Cells

1. Aspirate medium from the cell monolayer.

2. Gently add warm (37°C) PBS or culture medium without serum. Pipet the medium onto a wall of the culture vessel, not onto the cells, to avoid dislodging loosely adherent cells.

3. Aspirate the PBS or medium wash from the monolayer.

4. Add 0.25% trypsin/PBS, just enough to cover the cells when the culture vessel is tilted.

> *Cells are washed to remove traces of serum, which inhibits trypsin. You can use old medium without serum for washes.*

5. Aspirate the trypsin, almost immediately: Leave it on the cells only 10–30 seconds before removing it.

6. Incubate the cells at room temperature for 5–15 minutes, checking every couple of minutes to see whether the entire monolayer slides when you tilt the culture vessel. (You can see this macroscopically.) When it does, you can end the incubation. Alternatively, you could incubate the cells at 37°C for 5 minutes.

7. Add fresh medium (the same volume you removed) and pipet vigorously to break cell clumps. Check on the inverted scope to be sure you have a single cell suspension and pipet until you do.

8. Remove 1 ml of cells to a microfuge tube.

9. Count the cells.

10. Figure out the dilution you must make to get to the recommended seeding concentration.

11. Remove that quantity of cells to a fresh culture flask.

12. Add the calculated amount of fresh medium (which has been warmed to 37°C).

Example:

If you have counted the cells and they are at 1.0×10^6 cells/ml, the desired seeding concentration is 10^5 cells/ml. The final volume in the flask will be 10 ml. You want to dilute the cells at 1:10. Add 1 ml of cell suspension to 9 ml of medium.

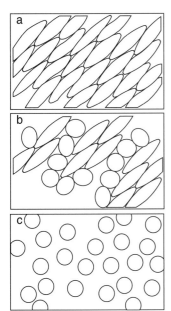

FIGURE 4.

Dissociation of adherent cells. The cells of the monolayer (*a*) appear flat and of low contrast. As cells are released from the substratum they will still be clumped together (*b*). Quite quickly after this, all cells are released from the surface, most are single cells (*c*), and fresh medium can be added.

13. Rotate the flask gently to be sure the cells are dispersed evenly over the surface.

14. Place the cells in the incubator. Be sure the cap is loose.

> *If you are using 100-cm plates for culturing your cells, be sure you are using tissue culture dishes, and not bacterial culture dishes. Tissue culture dishes are treated to promote cell adherence; cells will not stick to bacterial dishes.*

PROTOCOL

Splitting Suspension Cells

1. Gently shake the culture flask so you can get an even suspension of cells. Remove 1 ml of cells to a microfuge tube.
2. Count the cells. Don't forget to look at the cells while you are counting, to check for the general condition.
3. Figure out the dilution you must make to get to the recommended seeding concentration.
4. Remove that quantity of cells to a fresh culture flask.
5. Add the calculated amount of fresh medium (which has been warmed to 37°C).
6. Place the cells in the incubator. Be sure the cap is loose.

> *Look at the cells on the inverted microscope to check on your dilution. You should learn what different concentrations of cells look like.*

7. Also incubate the original flask, without adding medium. Whenever you split cells, retain one of the original flasks as a backup in case of contamination. Write "Backup" on the flask, and discard that flask when you next split cells.

Example:

If you have counted the cells and they are at 2.3×10^6 cells/ml,
The desired seeding concentration is 5×10^5 cells/ml.
The final volume in the flask will be 10 ml.
($2.3 \times 10^6 = 230 \times 10^5$ so you can ignore the 10^5.)

$23 : 5$ as $10 : x$ where x is the # ml of cells.

$x = 2.2$

Add 2.2 ml of cell suspension to 8.8 ml of medium.

Microscopic Count of Viable Cells

A sample of cells are mixed with *trypan blue*, a dye which is excluded by living cells, but stains dead cells a dark blue color. The cells are placed on a kind of gridded slide called a *hemocytometer*, and are counted manually under a microscope.

Materials

- Hemocytometer (improved Neubauer type), cleaned and dried each time. (Other hemocytometers can be used: the grid will look different.)

- Hemocytometer coverglass (reusable), cleaned and dried each time.

- 0.4% trypan blue (w/v) in PBS.

- Counter.

- Cells in suspension, either a suspension culture or a trypsinized adherent culture. Be sure adherent cells are trypsinized enough that they are single cells (see Fig. 4) and that you swirl the flask and take a representative sample.

- Pipettors, tips.

- Microfuge tubes.

- Phase contrast microscope, upright or inverted, with 10X objective.

- Sterile cell medium for dilutions.

Estimation of the number of cells is important in maintaining and freezing cell lines, and you should set yourself up so you can do it quickly and easily. Keep a hemocytometer and trypan blue stain ready.

A Coulter counter can also be used to count cells. Hemocytometer counting is more practical for single samples and has the added advantage of allowing you to actually look at the cells.

Procedure

1. Place the coverslip evenly on the middle of the hemocytometer.

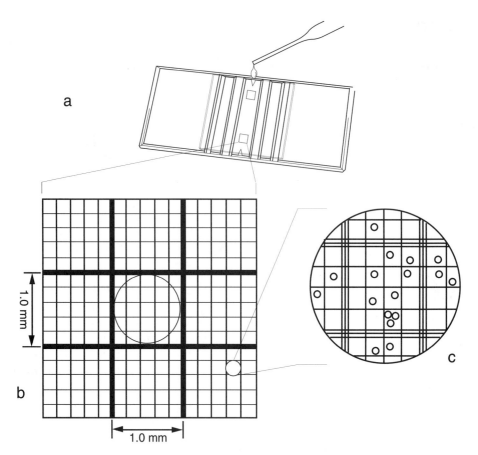

FIGURE 5.

Counting cells with a hemocytometer (Improved Neubauer). The hemocytometer is loaded with cells in both of the chambers on either side of the central trough (*a*). As you look at the slide with a 10X objective (100X total magnification), each 1-mm-square grid will take up the field of view. Each 1-mm square is divided into 25 smaller squares (*b*). Each of the 25 squares is divided into 20 smaller squares, to aid in counting small cells or sparse numbers of cells (*c*). It is the cell count for a 1-mm square that is used to calculate the cells/ml. (Modified, with permission, from Freshney 1994; copyright by Wiley-Liss, Inc.)

2. Remove 500 μl of cells and medium to a microfuge tube. If sample volume is low, take 100 μl.

3. Place 50 μl of the cells and 50 μl of the trypan blue solution in a microfuge tube. Tap the tube to mix.

> *Not having a well-suspended and well-mixed sample to add to the counting chamber is the major source of error in hemocytometer counting.*

4. Remove 50 μl from the cell/trypan blue mix with a pipettor. Add 20 μl to each side of the coverslip by allowing a drop held at the end of the tip to be taken under the slide by capillary action. (If you have two different samples,

you can carefully load them one on each side.) Fill both sides of the chamber even if you only have one sample, or the cell count won't be accurate.

> *If you have fewer cells than 30, you could concentrate the cells by spinning an aliquot and resuspending in a smaller volume, but it usually isn't worth it. Make three independent counts to be able to best estimate your cell numbers.*

5. Place the hemocytometer immediately on the stage of the microscope, and locate the grids in the hemocytometer at low power. You will only count cells in any one of the 1-mm-square areas, so move to a corner and up the magnification so that one entire grid takes up the field. You can count at low power, but it is more difficult to distinguish dead from living cells. If you are using an inverted microscope, drop the objective so you can get enough light—adjusting this will make a big difference.

6. Roughly count the cells in a 1.0-mm area, 25 boxes worth, to see if your cells need to be diluted or concentrated. Ideally, you should have between 30 and 300 cells/mm. If you have more, make a 1:5 or 1:10 dilution (For 1:10, mix 50 μl of cells from tube in step 2 with 450 μl of medium or buffer; mix and take 50 μl to add to 50 μl of trypan blue as in step 3.)

> *To avoid counting cells twice, count only cells that lie on the top and left-hand-side lines of each box, and don't count cells that lie on the bottom and right-hand-side lines of each box. **Uniformity of counting**—counting the cells the same way every time—is the only way to get reproducible numbers.*

7. Count the viable cells in a 1-mm square. Dead cells will stain blue all over the cell, whereas viable cells will not stain (although they may have a blue rim or appear to be granular). It helps to have a counter with two channels, so you can count both dead and living cells and get a percentage of viable cells.

> *If your counts are very different from each other, say, over 20% different, you may not have resuspended the cells well enough or there may be clumps.*

8. Count the cells in a total of three different 1-mm squares, and divide by three to get an average number of cells/1-mm square.

9. Calculate the number of cells per ml.

Example:
You have counts of 113, 99, and 118 (with an average of 110).
$110 \times 10,000 = 1.1 \times 10^6$ cells/ml
Since you mixed 50 μl of cells with 50 μl of trypan blue, your dilution factor is 2.
  $2 \times 1.1 = 2.2 \times 10^6$
  2.2×10^6 cells/ml is the number of cells in the original culture.

The average number of cells/1-mm square X 10,000 X dilution of sample = number of cells/ml in original sample.

10. Calculate the percentage of viable cells in the original culture. Divide the number of viable cells in three 1-mm areas by the total number of viable and nonviable cells in three 1-mm areas and multiply by 100.

> *A viability of less than 80–90% indicates an unhealthy cell population. The most likely explanation is that the cell culture is too dense, but it may also indicate contamination or a problem with the medium or serum.*

FREEZING AND STORAGE OF CELLS

As cells grow the phenotype may change, or drift. Since it is important that your cells be predictable, you should freeze every cell line as soon as possible.

 Before freezing cells

Check the requirements for freezing your particular cells.

> *Unfortunately, it is still not possible to freeze and thaw most primary cells.*

- Check the ATCC catalog for the formulations for freezing the particular cell type.

- Certainly, check with lab members for modifications of the recommended freezing medium and conditions, but be wary of this information because many lab members have never themselves consulted the ATCC catalog or any literature but have fallen back on general techniques that usually work, will probably work, but may not be maximum in effectiveness for these particular cells.

- If it is a new cell line, call the originator of the line (check the literature).

- If you can find no information for your cells, do use one of the basic recipes given below.

Be sure you have sterile freezing ampoules (cryotubes). These must be screw-cap plastic ampoules, made to resist severe cold. They may be flat or round bottomed, either of which is fine for freezing (but you may want the flat bottomed for centrifuging). Glass ampoules may also be used. *Don't use snap-cap microfuge tubes.*

Make sure you already have space for your cells in liquid nitrogen. Liquid nitrogen tanks are notoriously crowded, and you don't want to get there with your thawing cells, searching for a tower. Also, if you put your cells in the wrong place, someone may dump them.

PROTOCOL

Freezing Cells

1. Grow cells to log phase in the usual maintenance medium/serum.

2. Perform a viable count. Do not freeze down cells with greater than 20% dead cells.

> *Too few cells, and the culture may never start to grow upon refreezing: too many, and the culture will be unhealthy.*

3. Determine how many cells and ampoules you will need. Each ampoule will take 1×10^7 cells (or between 4×10^6 and 2×10^7 cells) in 1 ml of medium.

> **Freeze cells down at a concentration at which, when they are diluted 1:10 at thawing, they will be at 5x the normal seeding concentration.**
>
> Example:
> If the normal seeding concentration is 5.0×10^5 cells/ml, you want cells after thawing and resuspension in fresh medium at 2.5×10^6 cells/ml. Since the cells will be diluted 1:10, freeze cells down at 2.5×10^7/ml.

4. Prepare freezing medium, 1 ml/aliquot plus 10%. Freezing medium typically contains regular culture media, 10–20% serum, and 5–10% glycerol or DMSO. If you don't know what freezing medium to use, freeze the cells in 20% serum and 10% DMSO.

5. Resuspend the pellet in freezing medium by pipetting gently.

6. Dispense 1 ml per ampoule. Keep cells on ice.

7. Place the ampoules in a freezer box you have lined with paper towels. Put in your vials and place the box near the top of a freezer that is –60°C or less. Leave them there for 16 to 24 hours.

> *Label each ampoule, even if you are preparing a box of ampoules. Write the cell type, the passage number, number of cells, the date of freezing, your name. Do not use tape labels, which become brittle and break off in the cold. Write on the vial or ampoule with a permanent lab marker, one that doesn't wash off with ethanol.*

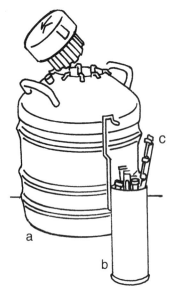

FIGURE 6.

Liquid nitrogen tank (*a*), canister (*b*), and canes (*c*). Remove the cap of the tank, and lay it aside. Grasp the hooked end of the canister and lift it up and out of the tank. Remove the appropriate cane from the canister, and snap out (or in) the tube. *Immediately* replace the cane, canister, and cap. Wear gloves and face protection, even to remove one tube.

8. Pour a bit of liquid nitrogen into an ice bucket, and place your tubes in here while you transport them to the liquid nitrogen freezer. If you can't get liquid nitrogen, place the vials on dry ice.

> *If you have a programmable freezer, cool the ampoules at $-3°C/min$ until $-60°C$ is reached.*

9. Put the tubes in the appropriate place and immediately record their location in your files, and in a liquid nitrogen book, if one is kept.

Using liquid nitrogen

- Cells are kept either in a liquid nitrogen tank, which is filled with liquid nitrogen, or in a liquid nitrogen freezer, which is hooked up to a large tank of nitrogen. Tanks must be refilled manually every few weeks with more liquid nitrogen.

- Automatic fill tanks should be checked periodically to be sure they are working properly and that the tank is not empty.

> *Don't open the tank or freezer if the liquid nitrogen is low. You want to keep the contents as cold as possible.*

- Wear heavy gloves when manipulating canes, racks, or boxes. Liquid nitrogen can cause bad burns.

- Wear, at least, latex gloves when removing a tube from a box or cane.

- Don't hang into liquid nitrogen tanks or freezers, or deeply breathe the vapor. Use your hand to "brush" away the vapor, and you will see the liquid nitrogen below.

- Protect your eyes with safety glasses when you do any manipulations with liquid nitrogen, because vials can suddenly break and shatter in the extreme cold.

- Never put loose vials in a tank or freezer. Each tube must be in the appropriate box or cane. Request space well in advance of the time you will need it from the person in charge.

- Don't disable the alarm. Check periodically to be sure no one else has disabled it.

- If you hear an alarm from a liquid nitrogen freezer or tank, immediately notify the lab. If it is the weekend or 3 A.M., first check the alarm panel to see if, indeed, the liquid nitrogen level or temperature is low. Then call the person in charge.

CONTAMINATION

Contamination happens, but it is usually a drag and can be a disaster. Good aseptic technique will prevent most problems, but remain vigilant always to detect contamination in its earliest stage. Look at every flask you take out of the incubator; in fact, get in the habit of running your eyes over all the flasks in the incubator, whenever you open the door.

> *If you see a contaminated flask belonging to someone else, notify that person immediately.*

Contamination can be caused by bacteria, yeast, fungi, mold, mycoplasma, and by other tissue culture cells.

How to Recognize Contamination

 Macroscopically. Look at the flask or dish of cells as you pick it up, and hold it to the light, checking for:

- **Cloudiness.** Even in a dense culture, the medium should be clear. Look for cloudiness in the medium or patches of cloudiness that move and shift with movement of the flask. Some molds may actually form colonies that float on the medium surface.

- **Medium color change.** The phenol red pH indicator in red medium will turn yellow in acidic conditions, magenta in alkaline conditions. A good bacterial infection will often turn the medium yellow, and fungal contamination may turn it hot pink.

- **Smell!** Obviously, don't open the flask and stick your nose in the flask. But many contaminants have a noticeable and characteristic odor that might even be detected as you open the incubator door.

> *Check the flask before throwing it away! A rapidly growing or overgrown cell culture might also turn the medium yellow, and a problem with the CO_2 level in the incubator could cause yellow (too much CO_2) or pink (not enough CO_2) medium.*

Microscopically. Look at the flask or plate on low power (10X objective) first and then, more thoroughly, at higher power (40X objective, 400 total magnification) on an inverted microscope, scanning up and down with the focus knob to examine different "depths" of the medium. Look for:

> *To determine if a shape is a microorganism, look for regularity. There are occasionally mineral precipitates from the medium, or cell granular extrusions and debris, but these will be irregular in appearance.*

- **Other organisms.** At low power, the mycelia of *fungi* will appear as long strands, often across the entire field. *Yeast* may also be visible at this magnification, and will appear to be smooth balls, sometimes with budding.

  At high power, bacteria may be seen. These may be rods, or cocci, singly or in chains or clumps. They may be associated with the cells, and be seen apparently within the cells. The cells may be lysed. There may be so many that the cells are obscured. There may be only one contaminant every two fields (which still counts as contamination!). They may be motile.

> *Don't confuse motility with Brownian motion, as all particles will gently vibrate back and forth. Cell granules may gently shake, and can resemble bacterial contamination.*

- **Damaged cells.** An infection can kill cells: It can even cause every cell to lyse and/or cause a monolayer to lift off the plastic completely. More likely, the cells become more irregular looking (and smaller or larger), with a dark granularity visible even at low power.

> *Unless they are extremely rare and almost impossible to obtain, do not try to rescue contaminated cells by pulsing them with antibiotics! Throw the cells away!*

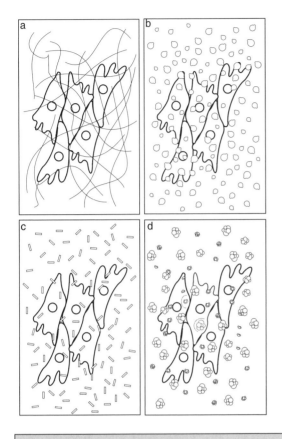

FIGURE 7.

Contaminants in an adherent cell culture under 400× power on the inverted microscope. (*a*) Mold; (*b*) yeast; (*c*) bacteria, small rods; (*d*) bacteria, clumps of cocci. Some of the cocci have been internalized by the adherent cells.

Suspension cultures are harder to observe microscopically than adherent cultures, especially at higher power.
- After you place the flask on the microscope stage, leave it for a minute to let the turbulence slow.
- Focus on the bottom of the flask, and look carefully for slightly adherent cells that may have attached microorganisms.
- Focus up through the flask, and whenever you have cells in focus, use your fine focus knob to examine the medium around the cells for contamination.

If you have a doubt about the presence of contamination

1. Make a wet mount or a stained slide (see Chapter 16). Centrifuge 1 ml of medium from the cells and resuspend in 50 μl of medium or buffer. Put on a slide and add a coverslip for a wet mount, or smear, fix, and stain with methylene blue or a Gram stain, and observe under high power.
2. Streak some of the cells/medium on a nutrient or blood agar plate, and incubate at 37°C for 3 days. Colonies? Contamination!
3. Remove 1 ml of cells/medium to a sterile microfuge tube and incubate for 3 days in the incubator. Observe for cloudiness, and make a wet mount.

Mycoplasma Contamination

 Recognizing mycoplasma contamination. A difficult and ubiquitous problem! Mycoplasmas are the smallest self-replicating organisms, as small as 0.3 μm, and can generally not be seen with an inverted microscope. These bacteria have no cell wall, and are not susceptible to commonly used antibiotics. Investigators usually don't know their cells are infected until the viability decreases or the cells don't function as they should.

Without the aid of special stains, or unless the cells have been visibly damaged by a particularly heavy infection, the only way mycoplasma infection is suspected is that experiments stop working. The only way to detect and treat mycoplasma contamination is to routinely screen cells for it, a very simple procedure.

 Preventing mycoplasma contamination. Use only media and serum that have been certified to be mycoplasma free. Most companies can make this guarantee. Only obtain cells that are guaranteed to be mycoplasma free. This is easy when ordering commercially, more difficult when you obtain cells from another investigator. Ask directly whether the cells have been checked for mycoplasma contamination.

> *The most common way in which mycoplasma are introduced to cells is through newly acquired, already infected cell lines. Test new cell lines for mycoplasma, and never freeze a culture until it has been checked.*

Routine screening is a commitment, and investigators and labs who only employ cells for short-term experiments don't want to bother. Fine. They might never know that the reason they couldn't raise antibodies against a cell surface protein, or express a protein effectively, was that they were using mycoplasma-infected cells.

 Screening for mycoplasma contamination. If the integrity of the cells is important to you, screen them routinely every 4–6 weeks. There are a number of ways to do this:

- **Fluorescent staining of mycoplasma** is the easiest, cheapest, and most common way to screen.

- **PCR detection using mycoplasma-specific primers** might be the easiest way if your lab is geared up for running gels and doing PCR. You can make your own primers, or order them (and the appropriate controls) from a company.

- **Send a sample away to one of the many companies that does mycoplasma testing.** The company may provide mailers, but this isn't as fast (although it is easier and more expensive) as doing it yourself.

 And if you find mycoplasma contamination... Good luck.

- The best bet is to throw the cells out and start with another thaw.

- You could ignore it.

- There are methods to "cure" a culture of mycoplasma, but they are difficult and should only be used for irreplaceable cells. The best bet is to contact a company that manufactures kits for removal of mycoplasma. ICN and Boehringer-Mannheim have effective kits: Call and ask them for suggestions.

> *Most non-cell biology labs do nothing, on the "why fix it if it ain't (obviously) broke" belief. But mycoplasma contamination can cause changes in cell function that aren't obvious. It can cause chromosomal abnormalities, loss of the characteristic of interest, reduced capacity to support viral growth.*

Cross Contamination

Cells can infect other cell cultures. This cross contamination is thought to be quite widespread, with many investigators inadvertently growing, using, and freezing contaminating cells instead of the intended one.

This is very preventable.

- **Obtain your cells from a reputable place,** or check the identity of the cells yourself. There are companies that can check this.

- **Don't ever work on more than one cell line at a time.** Don't even have flasks of different cells in the hood at the same time.

- **Never use the same pipet** for different cell lines.

- **Never use the same bottle** of medium or trypsin for the same cell line.

- **Never put a pipet back** into a bottle of medium after you have used it to pipet cells.

- **Use plugged pipets** for cell maintenance.

Check the cells for cross contamination if your cell line suddenly grows or functions differently than usual, and you have ruled out mycoplasma contamination. (Change can also be explained by mutation or drift.)

CO_2 INCUBATORS AND TANKS

CO_2 is used in an open culture system to regulate the pH of the cell medium. It is purchased as a cylinder of compressed gas and is dispensed into an incubator that can monitor and report the CO_2 content as well as maintain a set temperature.

CO_2 Incubators

- Never put any cells in an incubator unless you have checked with the other incubator users.

- Water in a stainless steel pan in the incubator prevents the cultures from drying out. Also, CO_2 detectors are accurate only in a humidified atmosphere. Keep the pan filled with sterile distilled water, and change the water once a week. Don't use bacterial growth inhibitors in this water, which may damage the stainless steel.

- Frequent cleaning of the trays that hold the cultures will help prevent contamination. Wipe down the trays with 70% alcohol at least weekly. Autoclave the trays monthly.

  > *Never use Clorox or another chlorine bleach to clean trays. It is toxic to the cells.*

- Minimize opening and closing the incubator door. Don't leave the door ajar while you carry your cells to the hood. Fluctuations of temperature and CO_2 levels aren't good for many cell lines.

- The incubator alarm will sound when the CO_2 runs low.

- Most CO_2 incubators are set at 37°C: Some may not be, so check. A buzzer or alarm will sound when the temperature rises above or falls below the setpoint. Reset the temperature. If the incubator needs to be repaired, a temporary incubator must be found.

  > *Never change any setting on an incubator without consultation with all lab members.*

- A thermometer is often kept on one of the trays in the incubator, to confirm the temperature readings of the incubator's temperature sensor. Be careful not to break the thermometer in the incubator! The most accurate thermometers are mercury filled, and an incubator contaminated with mercury might never be able to support cell growth again. To accurately check the temperature, place the thermometer in a beaker of water in the incubator.

- A buzzer, but possibly an alarm, will sound when the water jacket needs water. This water jacket is needed to maintain the temperature. Fill it with a hose attached to deionized water (not distilled). Do not add antibacterial agents to the water. If the incubator does not have an alarm, look for condensation on the roof on the chamber, which indicates that the water in the jacket is low.

> *If the alarm goes off for a CO$_2$ incubator (indicating that the gas has run out) and you don't have another tank, don't open the incubator door! The gas inside will last about a day if you don't open the door.*

- Most incubators are set on 5% CO$_2$, but the setting depends on the particular cells and the medium used.

- CO$_2$ readings on the incubator readout can be inaccurate. Occasionally, and whenever changes in medium color make you suspect a problem, you should determine the proper CO$_2$ percentage in the chamber with the use of a Fyrite gas analyzer. This instrument is the best way to get an independent CO$_2$ reading, but it must be done carefully to get accurate results.

 Measurement of CO$_2$ levels with a Fyrite gas analyzer. The Fyrite (Bacharach, Inc.) uses a volumetric gas analysis method involving selective absorption of CO$_2$ in a chemical solution. The aspirator bulb pumps the gas sample into the analyzer and purges the measuring chamber of the previously analyzed sample.

Always store the Fyrite in the hard plastic carrying case. Don't be put off by the long directions. Analysis of the CO$_2$ concentration in an incubator will take about 30 seconds.

1. Hold the Fyrite upright and away from your face. Press the plunger momentarily to vent the tester.

2. Invert the Fyrite to drain the liquid from the top.

3. Turn the Fyrite upright, and allow the fluid to drain to the bottom.

4. Hold the Fyrite at eye level. Loosen the locknut at the rear of the scale. Slide the scale until the top of the fluid column lines up with the zero on the scale. Tighten the locknut.

5. Attach the open end of the rubber gas sampler hose to the sample port on the incubator. Do not attach the tube to the Fyrite tester at this time. Pump the aspirator bulb a few times to clear the air from the sampler line.

6. Hold the Fyrite upright, and place the rubber connector tip for the sampler tube over the plunger valve, and pump the aspirator bulb at plunger valve during the final squeeze.

7. Invert the Fyrite, and allow all the liquid to drain from the top. Turn upright, and allow all the liquid to drain to the bottom. Repeat once.

8. Momentarily hold the Fyrite at a 45° angle to allow the fluid droplets to drain to the bottom.

9. Hold the Fyrite upright. Allow the fluid a few seconds to stabilize. Determine the percent CO_2 from the level of the fluid column. A delay of 5–10 seconds in taking the reading may result in a slight error; a longer delay may result in a substantial error.

10. Repeat steps 6–10 until two consecutive readings agree.

11. Remove the Fyrite hose from the sample port to allow the chamber to breathe.

The dark red fluid floating on the top of the Fyrite solution is normal. It has been added to the solution to prevent excess foaming at the meniscus and does not indicate defective fluid.

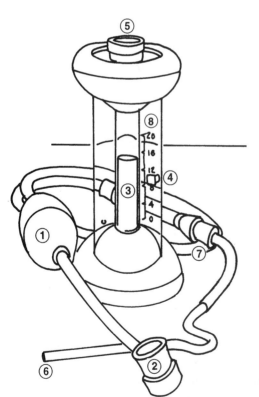

FIGURE 8.

Fyrite gas analyzer. **Key:** (1) *Aspirator bulb.* (2) *Connector tip.* (3) *Fluid.* (4) *Locknut.* (5) *Plunger.* (6) *Sampler hose.* (7) *Saturator filter.* (8) *Scale.*

Precautions for using the Fyrite

- The reagent used for the chemical absorption and measurement of gas in the Fyrite is potassium hydroxide that has been dyed red. Potassium hydroxide is corrosive and poisonous. If you get some on your skin, *flush with water.* Follow that washing with a rinse with vinegar: If your lab or your lunch doesn't happen to have vinegar, flush longer with water. If it gets in your eyes, flood with water and then wash with a 5% boric acid solution. Seek medical help.

- Do not invert the Fyrite when the plunger is depressed.

- Do not hold the Fyrite near your face when the top plunger is depressed.

- Always hold the Fyrite by the fins to prevent heat transfer from your hands.

- Always moisten the filter in the sampling tube before taking a sample. Failure to do so will result in inaccurate readings.

- For maximum accuracy, the Fyrite must be at ambient temperature. Do not store the Fyrite in a location subject to extreme temperatures, such as a windowsill.

- Check the strength of the Fyrite fluid whenever the instrument is used. After taking a reading with the Fyrite, do not vent the sample. Invert the Fyrite again, and take another reading. If there is an increase of 1/2% or more on the second reading, fluid replacement is necessary. Follow the manufacturer's directions. Fresh Fyrite fluid should be good for approximately 350 samples.

- With the Fyrite vented and in the vertical position, it should be possible to adjust the zero scale to the top of the fluid column. If this is not possible, fluid should be added or removed. To add fluid, hold the Fyrite upright and press the plunger. Add clean tap water a few drops at a time. To remove fluid, consult a manual or the manufacturer.

CO$_2$ Tanks

- A tank of compressed CO$_2$ is attached to the incubator and delivers CO$_2$ at a level determined by presetting the incubator.

- The tanks and attachments to the incubator look more complicated than they are. If you are careful, there is very little danger.

- CO$_2$ tanks are usually delivered to a central location at the institution, and are brought to the lab as needed. The tanks are rented, so return the empty tanks as

> *Be careful when using compressed gases. Carbon dioxide (and argon, helium, and nitrogen) are inert, colorless, odorless, and tasteless, but can cause asphyxiation and death in confined, poorly ventilated areas. They can cause severe frostbite to the eyes or skin. If treated carelessly, tanks of compressed gas can explode.*

soon as possible to reduce costs. Returns are usually handled at the same central location as deliveries.

- The cylinder cap protects the cylinder valve from mechanical or weather damage. It should be removed from the cylinder only when the cylinder is supported and ready to be attached to the incubator.

- Many incubators have an automatic CO_2 tank switch, a small box that usually sits on top of the incubator. This system monitors the regulated CO_2 supply into the incubator, and will switch from the empty tank to a full one. It also sounds an alarm if all tanks are empty, and turns off the CO_2 supply during a power failure to prevent toxic CO_2 accumulation in the incubator.

The regulator

The gas in cylinders is at very high pressure; in fact, dangerously high pressure. The regulator reduces the pressure of the gas so it can be used safely.

- There are two basic types of pressure regulators, single stage and two stage. They look the same. The two-stage regulator will deliver a more constant pressure

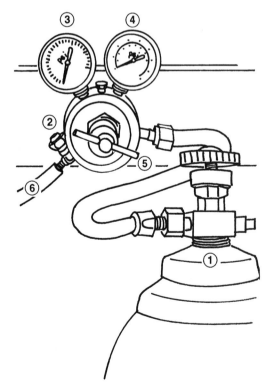

FIGURE 9.

A pressure regulator. **Key:** (1) *Cylinder valve of the gas tank.* (2) *Flow control valve.* (3) *Gauge for delivery pressure.* (4) *Gauge for tank pressure.* (5) *Pressure adjusting screw.* (6) *Tubing to incubator.*

under more stringent operating conditions than the single-stage regulator. You can't tell one from the other.

> *The gauge with the smaller numbers measures the flow, the one with the larger numbers measures the remaining pressure of the gas in the tank.*

- Most regulators (whether single or two stage) will have two gauges. One measures the tank pressure, and one measures the flow or delivery pressure.

- Some regulators don't fit some cylinders: This is done to prevent interchange of equipment for incompatible gases. If the regulator doesn't fit, don't force it.

Precautions to take when using cylinders of compressed gases, including CO$_2$

- When storing or moving a cylinder, have the cap securely in place.

- When moving large cylinders, have them capped and strapped to a properly designed wheeled cart.

- All cylinders must be restrained by straps, chains, or a suitable stand to prevent them from falling.

- Do not expose cylinders to temperatures over 50°C.

- Never use a cylinder that cannot be properly identified: Don't rely on color to identify the contents.

- Use the appropriate regulator on each cylinder. Don't use a cylinder that has been altered or tampered with.

- Never lubricate, modify, or force a cylinder valve. Don't loosen or remove the safety plug or rupture disc.

- Rapid release of a compressed gas will cause an unrestrained hose to whip dangerously and may also build up a static charge that could ignite a combustible gas.

- Never bleed a cylinder completely empty; leave a slight pressure to keep contaminants out.

- When not in use, cylinder and bench valves should be tightly closed.

- Don't order a surplus of cylinders. They are a safety hazard and, in most places, there is a daily rental fee.

- Remove the regulators from empty cylinders and replace the protective caps. Mark the cylinder "Empty" and return to Purchasing, or to whomever will send it back to the company.

- Don't use damaged or corroded cylinders, or cylinders with a test date more than 5 years old stamped on the shoulder. Return them to the vendor.

- Some gases are flammable (acetylene, butane, ethane, hydrogen, methyl bromide, propane), some highly reactive (oxygen), some toxic (sulfur dioxide, ammonia, chlorine), so check for the hazard of the particular gas before using it.

- Tanks are sometimes attached to a manifold, a series of pipes and metal tubing that permits connection of several cylinders to a common supply line and regulator for a larger continuous flow of gas. Effectively, multiple (usually, up to four) tanks are regulated as one, preventing wear and tear of cylinder mounting, and saving time. However, since several incubators in the lab may be supplied with CO_2 from the same set of tanks, this dependence on one source can leave the laboratory vulnerable.

 ## How to change CO_2 tanks on an incubator

1. Turn off the empty tank by screwing closed the cylinder valve.

2. Recap the empty tank and roll it or cart it out of the way.

3. Move the new tank into place, and strap it.

4. Attach the regulator to the cylinder valve outlet.

5. Turn the pressure-adjusting screw counterclockwise until it turns freely.

6. Open the cylinder valve slowly until the tank gauge on the regulator registers the cylinder pressure. Check that it is the expected value. If not, the valve may be leaking.

7. With the flow-control valve at the regulator outlet closed, turn the delivery-pressure adjusting screw clockwise until the required delivery pressure is reached (consult manual for incubator).

Control of flow can be regulated by means of a valve supplied in the regulator (the flow control valve) or by a supplementary valve installed in a pipeline downstream from the regulator. **The regulator itself should not be used as a flow control by adjusting the pressure to obtain different flow rates.** This defeats the purpose of the pressure regulator.

RESOURCES

Alberts B., Bray D., Lewis J., Raff M., Roberts K., and Watson J.D. 1994. *Molecular biology of the cell,* 3rd edition. Garland Publishing, New York.

American Society for Cell Biology (ASCB).
http://www.ascb.org/ascb
E-mail: ascbinfo@ascb.org
Phone: (301) 530-7153

Bacharach, Inc. 1980. FYRITE instruction manaul #11-9026. Bacharach, Inc., Pittsburgh.

Banker G. and Goslin K. 1991. *Culturing nerve cells.* MIT Press. Cambridge.

Bioconcepts 3 (2):6. 1997. *ICN Biomedical research products,* vol. 3, pl. 6. ICN Biochemicals, Costa Mesa, California.

Forma Scientific. 1990. Water-jacketed incubators. In *Instruction manual #7043158.* 1990. Forma Scientific, Inc., Marietta, Ohio. (This contains all information on the use of the Fyrite.)

Freshney R.I. 1994. *Culture of animal cells. A manual of basic technique,* 3rd edition. Wiley-Liss, New York.

Gershey E.L., Party E., and Wilkerson A. 1991. *Laboratory safety in practice: A comprehensive compliance program and safety manual.* Van Nostrand Reinhold, New York.

Harlow E. and Lane D. 1988. *Antibodies: A laboratory manual.* Cold Spring Harbor Laboratory, Cold Spring Harbor, New York.

Hay R., Caputo J., Chen T.R., Macy M., McClintock P., and Reid Y. 1994. *ATCC Catalog of cell lines and hybridomas,* 8th edition. American Type Culture Collection, Rockville, Maryland.
12301 Parklawn Drive, Rockville, MD 20852-1776.
Phone: 1-800-638-6597
Fax 1-301-2331-5826

Heidcamp W.H. 1995. *Cell biology laboratory manual.* Gustavus Adolphus College, St. Peter, Minnesota.
http://www.gac.edu/cgi-bin/user/~cellab/phpl?index-1.html

Kirsop B.E. and Doyle A., eds. 1991. *Maintenance of microorganisms and cultured cells. A manual of laboratory methods,* 2nd edition. Academic Press, New York.

Veile R. 1990. *Appendix: Operation and maintenance of Nuaire incubators.*
http://hdklab.wustl.edu/lab_manual/12/12/_10.html

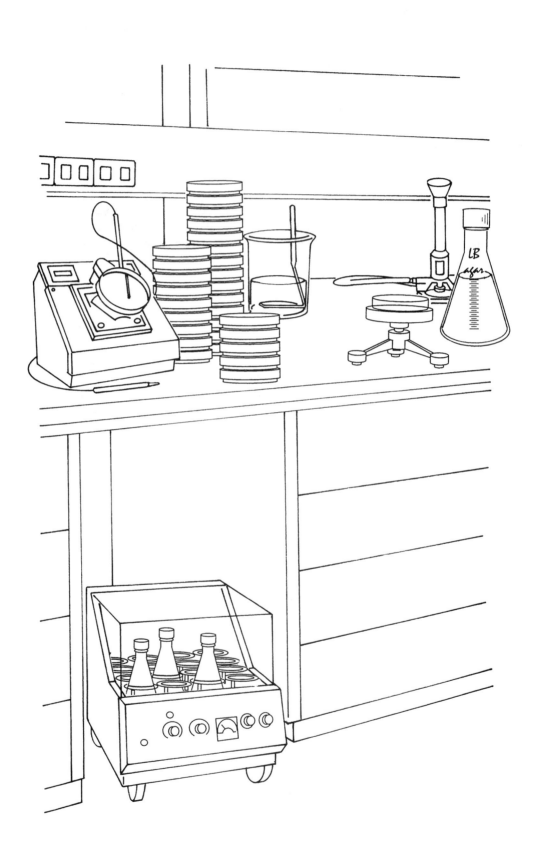

11

Bacteria

YOU MAY VIEW BACTERIA as a wondrous form of nature, and study how they grow, why they cause disease, what they need to prosper. Or you may see bacteria only as bags of enzymes, useful for gene manipulation and protein expression. If so, beware. Bacteria really are living entities, and must be cultivated and treated correctly to give you dependable and clean results.

SETTING UP

You will be able to do most of your work at your own laboratory bench.

Microorganisms are functionally classified by the extent of their ability to infect individuals and cause disease. The classification will affect the manner and the place you use to work with a particular organism.

The bacteria used routinely in molecular biology, such as nonpathogenic strains of *E. coli* and *Bacillus subtilis*, are Class 1 (no risk) and a few, such as *Salmonella* and *Shigella*, are Class 2 (low risk). Most listings do not distinguish between Class 1 and Class

SETTING UP	245
WORKING RULES	247
OBTAINING BACTERIA	248
GROWTH AND MAINTENANCE	249
Making tubes or flasks of liquid medium	251
Making plates of solid medium	252
REVIVING CULTURES	255
ANTIBIOTICS	257
OBTAINING ISOLATED COLONIES	259
Streaking with a wire loop over an agar plate: One strain	259
Streaking multiple samples on an agar plate	261
Picking colonies with a needle or toothpicks	262
COUNTING BACTERIA	263
Using a Petroff Hausser counting chamber	265
Viable plate counts	267
Changes in turbidity as a measurement of growth	270
STORAGE	273
FREEZING BACTERIA	274
Freezing bacteria for long-term storage	274
CONTAMINATION	276
RESOURCES	276

2 organisms. You can work at your bench for most manipulations (BL1), and in a biosafety cabinet for procedures that create aerosols (BL2 precautions).

See Chapter 9, Working without Contamination, for a description of biohazard classification and the containment facilities each requires.

Class 3 organisms, which present a high risk of causing disease by inhalation, must be used only in a BL3 containment lab. Examples of Class 3 organisms are *Mycobacterium tuberculosis, Mycobacterium bovis,* and *Francisella tularensis.* A containment lab is physically isolated from surrounding rooms, with no air exchange with other rooms via doors, ducts, or ventilation. The room is under negative pressure so if the security of the room is breached, air can only come in: Potentially contaminated air from the containment lab will remain in the room. All work is done in biosafety cabinets, protective clothing is worn, and access is controlled.

If you intend to work with a Class 3 organism, speak with EHS at least a month before you would like to start. Working in a containment lab requires instruction, as most lab routines are rigidly controlled. Not only is access to a containment room usually controlled with keys and key cards, but users must often be certified before they can use the room, and such processes don't always move swiftly. Do not try to evade this process by borrowing a key, or you and the lendee will likely be barred from the room.

All Class 3 organisms—even sealed, freeze-dried tubes—must be stored *within* a BL3 facility. There can be no temporary storage in "ordinary" freezers or liquid nitrogen tanks.

BL4 maximum containment labs, suitable for work with Class 4 organisms of high risk to individuals and the community, are found in very few facilities. Most Class 4 agents are arboviruses, arenaviruses, and filoviruses. A government license is usually required to work in such a facility.

Only Class 1 and Class 2 culture is considered in this manual.

 ## The lab bench

- The procedures you are likely to do include
      Selecting mutants
      Growing the organisms
      Determining the concentration of bacteria
      Centrifuging cultures
      Transformation
      Plasmid isolation
  These procedures can all be done at the bench.

- The setup of the lab bench should be as for the typical lab bench described in Chapter 3. You will be working aseptically, so your lab bench should be maintained to minimize motion and mess.

- A vortex, Bunsen burner, and aspirator are needed.

- All trash used with *E. coli* and other organisms is biohazard waste. You need a separate sharps, liquid waste, dry waste, and radioactive waste disposal for the waste you generate while culturing microorganisms.

In addition, you will need access to

- An incubator or warm room, set at 37°C. For some bacteria, a different temperature (and therefore, a different incubator) might be required.

- A shaking incubator, shaker, or wheel in a warm room, for the aerobic growth of *E. coli*.

- Centrifuges—microfuge and high-speed.

It is useful if you have access to

- A biosafety cabinet for making plates and filter-sterilizing medium components and antibiotics.

- An electroporator, for transformations.

- A spectrophotometer, for monitoring growth.

WORKING RULES

- **Follow the universal lab safety rules** (Chapter 1). No eating, drinking, mouth pipeting, open-toed shoes, or lab coats outside of the lab.

> *All material which has come in contact with microorganisms is referred to as infectious or biohazard material.*

- **Wash work surfaces at least once a day and after any spill of bacteria.** Start the morning by wiping down your bench with a disinfectant such as 70% ethanol. Immediately wipe any spills or drips and disinfect the area.

- **Decontaminate all infectious waste before disposal.**

- **Wash your hands after handling infectious material and before you leave the laboratory.** You should do this even if you wear gloves while working, since other people might leave bacterial traces on phones, doorknobs, computer keyboards, and pens.

Liquid waste

Add Clorox to approximately a final 10%. Let sit for 30 minutes. Pour down the sink, while running tap water.

Dry waste

Dispose of dry waste as biohazard disposal. Autoclave. This may be a lab or institutional responsibility, but you must at least store and label the waste appropriately (see Chapter 8).

- **Perform procedures in a way that minimizes aerosols.** Avoiding the generation of aerosols is the best way to reduce the chance of infection by a pulmonary route, and to minimize contamination. Aerosols are generated by obviously disruptive procedures such as detergent lysis or sonication, but they are also made by pipeting, pouring, and opening centrifuge tubes. Don't pop open tubes: Open them slowly and gently. Pour without splashing. Blow out the last bit of fluid and air from a pipet with the pipet tip held close to the surface of the fluid to minimize splashing.

- **Don't accumulate plates and tubes.** As soon as you have the bacteria you need, and have stored samples of them, throw away all the old cultures. Even in the refrigerator, old plates can become wonderful sources of contamination, serving as growth medium for mold and *Bacillus* species, among other little creatures.

"It's just E. coli..." Wrong! Don't let the ease of culture of E. coli cause you to loosen your vigilance. Safety issues may not seem to be much of a problem with E. coli, but the effect of usually benign microorganisms on immunocompromised hosts is real. And contamination—especially by other strains of E. coli, which might really mess up your experiments—could easily occur with sloppy technique. Treat all bacteria with care.

OBTAINING BACTERIA

Bacterial strains can be obtained from

- **Lab members.** Most strains will be obtained from fellow lab workers, since they are likely to be working on the same organism. Ask for a frozen culture (newly started cells are acceptable) and stand your ground if you are pooh-poohed. But don't ask just anyone. There may be a person in charge of maintaining lab stocks, and this is your first choice. Otherwise, try to ask someone who seems organized.

- **Other investigators.** If you come upon a description in the literature of a strain you need, E-mail or write to request it. If you don't hear back in 2 weeks, follow up with a phone call. But do not request strains that are available commercially: Go to the source probably mentioned in the Material and Methods section of the paper, or call to find out the source.

- **American Type Culture Collection (ATCC).** The ATCC is a nonprofit organization that preserves and distributes bacterial strains, as well as cultures of viruses, DNA probes, plant cells, and animal cells. This is a great source, since most strains used will be sent here by the investigators, and the integrity of the strains is checked: For a nominal fee, you can obtain almost anything.

- **Other collections and service organizations.** There are many organizations and collections for particular strains. Also, NIH grants are awarded to investigators to fund the maintenance and distribution of particular strains. The usual way to find out about these sources is through the literature or word of mouth: If you don't have time for this, try to call ATCC or the Centers for Disease Control (CDC) or do a search on the Internet.

- **Companies.** This will be your main source for bacteria used for gene manipulation—strains for propagating phages and bacteria, and for expressing protein. Before you buy, check with the technical division of the company to be sure that the strain you want is what you need.

> *Check every new bacterial strain to be sure it is what you think it is. This includes bacteria from companies, not just from possibly mistake-prone lab members. Just because the culture comes in a fancy box, with a fancy price, doesn't mean that human hands haven't been involved and a mistake made. Grow a culture from a single colony, and do an enzyme digestion or functional assay to confirm the identity of the strain.*

Bacteria change. Over time and with repeated culture, certain characteristics may be selected for, and the strain may be phenotypically and genetically different from the parent strain. Avoid obtaining strains that have been passaged continuously.

There is a prejudice that phenotypic drift is true only for exotic bacteria (to some labs, this is anything that isn't *E. coli* or *Salmonella*), but any store-boughten, protein-pushing *E. coli* can drift with repeated culture and become unable to do what you hired it for.

GROWTH AND MAINTENANCE

Bacteria are grown in a variety of ways, some dictated by the needs of the bacteria (aerobically or anaerobically, shaking versus stationary, etc.), and some by your convenience (liquid culture or culture on semi-solid medium).

> *Generally, don't grow bacteria unless you need them, to avoid selection of variants and contamination.*

The main advantages to liquid culture of bacteria are the sheer numbers that can be generated, and the ease of harvesting.

Semi-solid medium is liquid medium to which agar has been added as a hardening agent, giving the medium the consistency of a tough jello. It is aliquoted into convenient sized plates before hardening. Bacteria can be incorporated into the medium, or can grow on top of the medium. Since each colony that grows on the semi-solid medium is derived from one bacterium, plate culture is ideal for isolation and selection of particular colonies and strains.

You must have some knowledge of the physiology of your organism to grow it properly. For example, *E. coli* is a facultative anaerobe, able to grow either in the presence or absence of molecular oxygen: It will use O_2 as a terminal oxidizing agent when it is available, and when it is not, will obtain energy by fermentation. However, it grows better and faster under aerobic conditions. This is why you shake a flask of *E. coli* when you are growing it, and why you should leave a lot of room in the flask for vigorous aeration.

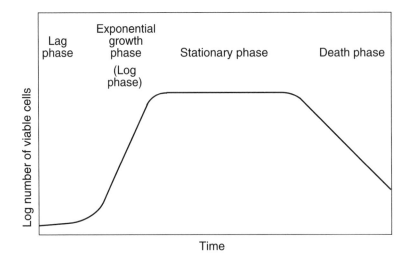

FIGURE 1.

Normal growth curve of bacteria in liquid culture. The phases of bacterial growth must be considered when setting up and harvesting cultures for experiments or storage.

Bacteria have a characteristic growth pattern in liquid culture, which can be separated into distinct phases (Fig. 1). When the bacteria are first inoculated into the medium, they do not grow: during this **lag phase,** cell mass increases as the bacteria adapt to the new environment and synthesize needed components.

The culture enters the **exponential growth phase,** also known as the logarithmic phase, so called because there is an exponential increase in cell numbers.

Changes in the chemical and physical environment will signal the start of **stationary phase.** Although there is no net increase in cell numbers, bacteria in this stage still require an energy source to remain viable. When the energy source has been depleted, the culture undergoes a **death phase.** Cell numbers may actually decrease during this time.

Different applications require bacteria to be in a particular growth phase: Usually this is late log or stationary phase. Ignoring the instructions on growth stage can have a seriously detrimental effect on the success of a procedure or experiment. Bacterial growth is best monitored by change in turbidity in the culture.

PROTOCOL

Making Tubes or Flasks of Liquid Medium

The media needed for *E. coli* and company will generally be extremely easy to make: For some formulations, you need only weigh out one to three ingredients, autoclave, and dispense.

Materials

- Ingredients for 500 ml of the appropriate medium

- Water bath set at 37ºC

- Pipets

- Pipettor

- Bunsen burner (only if you are using glass pipets and tubes)

Procedure

1. Make the medium, leaving out thermolabile substances such as antibiotics, growth factors, or vitamins. pH if required.

2. Autoclave the medium for 20 minutes.

3. After the medium has been removed from the autoclave, place it in the water bath for 30 minutes. You can also let it cool on the bench or in a warm room.

4. Filter-sterilize any heat-labile ingredients. Aseptically add the antibiotics and/or other heat-labile ingredients to the flask. Swirl to mix.

5. Work with the flask to the left of your working area. Use aseptic technique (see Chapter 9) to remove and dispense medium into tubes. Flame all glass pipets and tubes as you work.

> *If it is possible, prepare all media in a laminar flow hood.*

6. Label tubes with your name, the kind of medium they contain, and the full date. Be sure to include the identity of any antibiotics in the medium.

7. Store tubes at 4°C. Media without antibiotics or other heat-labile ingredients can be stored for several months. Media with antibiotics should be used within the week.

> *If you are worried that you might have contaminated the medium while dispensing it, incubate it overnight at 37°C, and see if anything grows.*

PROTOCOL

Making Plates of Solid Medium (Pour Plates)

Many departments have a media maker, a person who will pour and package plates for departmental members. Even if you are fortunate enough to have access to the services of such a person, there will be times when you need to quickly pour some plates for yourself.

> *Do not use 100-mm cell tissue culture plates instead of bacterial plates. It won't hurt anything, but specially treated tissue culture plates are much more expensive.*

Plates will be filled with 15–20 ml of medium that contains 1.5% agar. Too little medium results in plates that dry up very quickly in incubators. Plates of medium containing antibiotics should be used within a week or two.

Materials (for 25–30 90-mm plates)

- A 1000-ml flask.

- Material for 500 ml of the appropriate medium.

- 7.5 grams of agar. Bacto-agar (Difco) is excellent for most plates. Don't use agarose.

- Sterile plates/dishes. Disposable plastic plates. 90 mm is the typical size for culture.

- Water bath set at 45–50°C. Set it at 50°C for the first few times you pour plates. When you are swifter, you can set the water bath to 45°C without worry that the agar will solidify again before you are finished pouring.

- Bunsen burner.

Procedure

1. Make the medium, leaving out thermolabile substances such as antibiotics, growth factors, or vitamins.

2. Autoclave the medium for 20 minutes.

3. After the medium has been removed from the autoclave, place it in the water bath for 30 minutes.

4. While the medium is cooling to a workable temperature, prepare the plates. Remove them from the sleeves, and label them with the type of medium and the antibiotic it will contain, if any. Label the bottoms of the plates, since plates are incubated upside down. Set the plates up in stacks to the left of your working area.

   Many laboratories use a code and pattern of colors to indicate the kind of medium.

5. Filter-sterilize the heat-labile ingredients, if necessary. Have them ready to add. If there is a sizable volume of additives, be sure they are at room temperature so they won't change the temperature of the medium when added.

   Even if you can hold the flask with gloves at a temperature higher than 50°C, wait until the medium has cooled to 50°C. Pouring plates with too-hot medium results in excessive condensation.

6. Remove the flask from the water bath. At 50°C, you might require heat-protective gloves, whereas at 45°C, you can work bare-handed or with latex gloves.

7. Aseptically add the antibiotics and/or other heat-labile ingredients.

8. Remove the cap from the flask and place it on the bench. Immediately pick up the flask in your right hand and flame the open mouth. With your left hand, open the lid on the plate.

9. Pour approximately 15 ml of the medium into the plate, until the level reaches a few centimeters from the top. Flame the flask again, and maintain it at a 45° angle.

> *Don't allow medium to run down the outside of the flask. It may drip into the plates and contaminate them. Wipe drips away.*

10. Place the lid on the plate, and start a stack of poured plates, placing each newly poured plate on top of the others. Lift it carefully to avoid spilling over the sides.

11. Open the lid of another plate, flame the flask, and pour. Occasionally swirl the flask to be sure the suspension is even.

12. Carry on until all of the medium has been poured. By the end of the pouring, the medium will probably be starting to solidify. Once it has, do not pour any more plates.

> *The surface of the plate must be smooth. If bubbles form on the surface of the plate, quickly apply the flame of the Bunsen burner to the surface to pop the bubbles. Be careful not to melt plastic petri dishes.*

13. Place a flask or bottle of hot water on top of each stack of plates to reduce condensation. Let the plates sit for 20–60 minutes.

14. Dry the plates of remaining condensation by incubating them in a warm room or in a laminar flow hood for several hours. You may leave the lids slightly ajar in the hood.

15. Either wrap the plates in plastic wrap or bags, or place them in the sleeves from the empty plates. Fold the top over and close it with tape. Label the bag, and store it in the refrigerator.

> *If the antibiotic in the plates is light sensitive, wrap the plastic-wrapped plates in aluminum foil, or place them in a box. Tetracycline is light sensitive.*

 Making tubes of solid medium (slants). Slants are tube containers with solid medium: They are called slants because the medium with agar is allowed to solidify in the tube with the tube tilted, leaving a flat and angled surface for streaking. These tubes can also be used for stab cultures, in which an inoculating needle is used to pierce the medium and allow bacterial growth within the agar.

   The basic procedure is the same as for plates. Instead of pouring the warm medium/agar mixture, pipet it into sterile tubes so the tubes are 1/3–1/2 full. Place the tubes on an angle, either in a special rack or by resting them on a piece of styrofoam, and leave the caps on loosely to prevent condensation.

Any size tube can be used. Many investigators use the small glass vials usually used for scintillation counting, because these vials are inexpensive and the size is convenient for storage or mailing.

REVIVING CULTURES

Cultures of bacteria may come to you in any number of ways. If you get a culture from someone in the lab, you may receive a frozen vial, a streak on a plate, or a stab culture. The ATCC is likely to send you a lyophilized culture, and a commercial organization will send you frozen bacteria on dry ice.

DOUBLE-VIAL PREPARATIONS

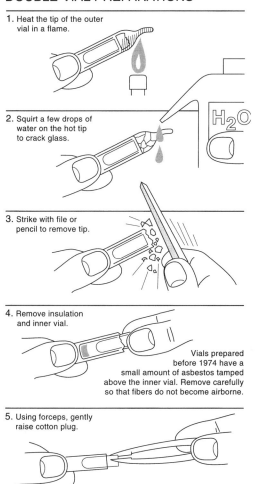

1. Heat the tip of the outer vial in a flame.

2. Squirt a few drops of water on the hot tip to crack glass.

3. Strike with file or pencil to remove tip.

4. Remove insulation and inner vial.

   Vials prepared before 1974 have a small amount of asbestos tamped above the inner vial. Remove carefully so that fibers do not become airborne.

5. Using forceps, gently raise cotton plug.

SINGLE-VIAL PREPARATIONS

1. These preparations may be enclosed in a thin skin of cellulose; this skin must be removed (either with a sharp blade or by soaking in water for a few minutes). Score the ampule once briskly about 1 inch from the tip.

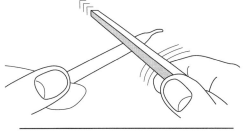

2. Disinfect the ampule with alcohol-dampened gauze.

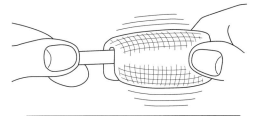

3. Wrap gauze around the ampule and break at the scored area. Care should be taken not to have the gauze too wet or alcohol could be sucked into the culture when the vacuum is broken. Rehydrate material at once.

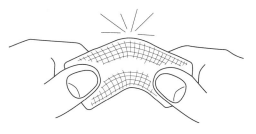

FIGURE 2.

How to open vials containing freeze-dried cultures. (Redrawn, with permission, from Pienta et al. 1996, *American Type Culture Collection Catalogue of Bacteria, Phages, and rDNA Vectors 1996.*)

Procedure: Reviving a Freeze-dried Culture

1. Wipe the outside of the vial with 70% ethanol.

2. Add 0.4 ml of the appropriate sterile medium (warmed) to the vial.

3. Pipet gently with a pipet or sterile pasteur pipet until the bacteria are in solution.

4. Add the bacterial suspension to a tube filled with 5 ml of the appropriate sterile medium (warmed). Retain about 10 µl.

5. Pipet the remaining 10 µl of bacterial suspension onto an agar slant or a plate. Streak for isolated colonies (see p. 259).

6. Incubate the tube and the plate or slant at the appropriate conditions.

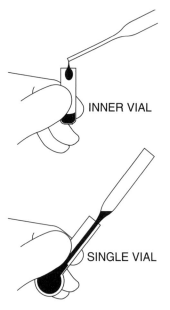

INNER VIAL

SINGLE VIAL

FIGURE 3.

Use a sterile pasteur pipet to rehydrate, resuspend, and transfer the bacterial culture to broth and plate. The pasteur pipet should be plugged with cotton. Discard the pasteur pipet in a biohazard sharps disposal box. (Redrawn, with permission from Pienta et al. 1996, *American Type Culture Collection Catalogue of Bacteria, Phages, and rDNA Vectors 1996.*)

Procedure: Reviving a Frozen Culture

Most frozen cultures of bacteria (for example, most strains of *E. coli*) do not have to be thawed completely in order to be recultured.

1. Remove the tube from dry ice or the freezer to a microfuge rack, and take it immediately to the bench or hood where you will be working.

2. Flame a loop (or use a sterile, disposable loop), let it cool for several seconds, and touch the top of the frozen culture.

> *Revived cultures may have a prolonged lag phase, so give the cultures twice as long to grow as would be expected.*

3. Put the culture on ice.

4. Streak a plate or a slant. Always streak for isolation.

5. Immediately put the frozen culture back in the freezer, at least at −70°C.

> *Do not repeatedly freeze and thaw bacterial cultures.*

6. Incubate the plate or slant in the appropriate conditions.

Procedure: Reviving a Frozen Culture of Fussy Bacteria

Slow-growing or otherwise fastidious bacteria may require a large inoculum to start growing again. Sometimes an old culture of *E. coli* must be revived in this way.

1. Remove the tube from dry ice or the freezer.

2. Incubate the tube in a water bath at 37°C until thawed.

3. Using a sterile pasteur pipet, transfer approximately half of the bacterial suspension to 4 ml of the appropriate culture medium. Put the remainder of the original culture on ice.

> *Usually, you should include antibiotics in the medium if your culture bears a plasmid for antibiotic resistance. However, strains carrying Tet^r, Amp^r, Kan^r, or Cam^r should be grown in medium without antibiotic to allow expression of the antibiotic resistance before antibiotic selection is applied (Miller 1992, p. 27).*

4. Incubate the newly inoculated culture as needed.

5. Store the original culture in the freezer at least at −70°C.

ANTIBIOTICS

- Genetically engineered plasmids usually contain genes for at least one antibiotic resistance gene. This enables the plasmid, with whatever other gene the investigator wants to have expressed, to be selected for: Only bacteria that are expressing the plasmid will survive in medium with that antibiotic.

- Almost all the plasmids routinely used contain one or more resistance genes for ampicillin, tetracycline, chloramphenicol, and kanamycin (neomycin).

- Antibiotics are heat-labile, and are added to the medium after it has been sterilized and cooled. Frozen aliquots are often used, but others make the antibiotics only as they are required.

- If a particular antibiotic is used infrequently, buy the size of antibiotic vial you can use without weighing the contents; for example, 100 mg. It will cost more than buying in bulk, but it is cheaper than eventually discarding an expired item.

- There is a range of antibiotic concentration that will be effective, and you will find different sources recommend different concentrations, all of which are probably okay. Use the concentration used by others who work on the same strain and are doing similar manipulations to yours.

TABLE 1. Antibiotics Commonly Used for Selection of Plasmid-carrying Strains

1. **Tetracycline (15 mg/ml stock solution)**
   Weigh out 15 mg of tetracycline and dissolve in 0.5 ml of sterile H_2O and 0.5 ml of ethanol (under fume hood). Wrap the test tube in foil. Add 1 ml of the stock solution directly to 1 liter of cooling agar. (Final concentration: 15 µg/ml)
2. **Streptomycin (100 mg/ml stock solution)**
   Make more stock solution than will be needed since some volume is lost in filter sterilization. Weigh out 200 mg of streptomycin and add 2 ml of H_2O. Filter sterilize. Add 1 ml of the stock solution directly to 1 liter of cooling agar. (Final concentration: 100 µg/ml)
3. **Kanamycin (30 mg/ml or 50 mg/ml stock solution)**
   Depending on the type of plates, prepare a 30 mg/ml or a 50 mg/ml stock solution. Make more stock solution than will be needed since some volume is lost in filter sterilization. Weigh out 60 or 100 mg of kanamycin and dissolve in 2 ml of H_2O. Filter sterilize. Add 1 ml of the stock solution directly to 1 liter of cooling agar. (Final concentration: 30 or 50 µg/ml depending on type of medium)
4. **Ampicillin (100 mg/ml stock solution)**
   Make more stock solution than will be needed since some volume is lost in filter sterilization. Weigh out 100 mg of ampicillin and add 1 ml of H_2O. Filter sterilize. Add 1 ml of the stock solution directly to 1 liter of cooling agar. (Final concentration: 100 µg/ml)
5. **Chloramphenicol (20 mg/ml stock solution)**
   Weigh out 20 mg of chloramphenicol and add 1 ml of ethanol (under fume hood). Add 1 ml of the stock solution directly to 1 liter of cooling agar. (Final concentration: 20 µg/ml)
6. **Rifampicin (50 mg/ml stock solution)**
   Weigh out 100 mg of rifampicin and dissolve in 2 ml of methanol (under fume hood). Vortex immediately to prevent rifampicin from sticking to the bottom of the tube. Add ~5 drops of 10 N NaOH to facilitate dissolving the rifampicin. Add 2 ml of the stock solution directly to 1 liter of cooling agar. (Final concentration: 100 µg/ml)
   Rifampicin is light-sensitive, so plates should be stored in the dark or wrapped in aluminum foil. The lifetime of plates can sometimes be increased by adding minimal A salts (100 ml of 10X minimal A salts per liter of medium).
7. **Nalidixic acid (100 mg/ml stock solution)**
   Weigh out 100 mg of nalidixic acid and dissolve in 1 N NaOH. Add 0.3 ml of the stock solution directly to 1 liter of cooling agar. (Final concentration: 30 µg/ml)
8. **Trimethoprim**
   When used in media, weigh out under sterile conditions 10 mg of trimethoprim and add the powder directly to 1 liter of cooling agar. (Final concentration: 10 µg/ml)

The concentrations given are standard concentrations, but a particular strain may have a different requirement. Use sterile distilled water in all recipes where H_2O is indicated. Store aliquots at –20°C. (Reprinted, with permission, from Miller 1992.)

OBTAINING ISOLATED COLONIES

It is absolutely vital that you learn to streak bacterial cultures for isolation of single colonies. A colony is an island on a plate of semisolid medium, **a clone derived from a single bacterium:** Unless you start a culture with a single colony, you may grow a mixed culture, or a contaminant, instead of the strain you thought you had. Generating and picking isolated colonies must become second nature to you, or you will never be sure that you have isolated and are working on the right bug.

PROTOCOL

Streaking with a Wire Loop over an Agar Plate: One Strain

Isolated colonies are obtained by diluting the bacteria until a single colony can be manually picked without touching another colony.

> *Streaking is indispensable for isolating one colony type out of a mixed culture, or checking to be sure that a colony really is only one colony.*

Materials

- A metal (usually platinum) loop. Disposable loops are available. They are expensive but handy, especially for BL3 organisms.

- A Bunsen burner or flameless loop heater

- Plate of semisolid media

- Bacterial sample from broth or semisolid media

> *Arrange your materials to minimize extra movements and reduce the chance of contamination.*
> - *If you are right-handed, have the Bunsen burner to your right.*
> - *Put plates to be streaked to the left.*
> - *Bacterial samples are set up in the middle.*
> - *Loosen the caps of tubes or flasks.*

Procedure

1. Label the plate, on the bottom, with your name, the date, and the bug. Lightly mark the bottom of the plate into quadrants, if you are worried about the streaking, and label 1, 2, 3, and 4 clockwise.

> *Incubate all plates upside down, so condensation doesn't drip onto the colonies.*

2. Flame the loop. If you are using a Bunsen burner, always start about 6 inches from the loop, and flame toward the loop. This avoids splattering of bacteria that may be left on the loop. If you are using a flameless loop heater, keep the loop all the way in for the recommended time.

> *Flaming not only kills surface bacteria, but convection from the heated surface prevents other bacteria from settling onto the surface or into an open tube.*

3. Take the tube in your left hand, swirl to resuspend, and remove the cap with the last two fingers of the right hand. Flame the open tube by passing it for 1 second through the flame.

4. Insert the loop (which will be cool enough) into the tube, without touching the sides of the tube. Insert it only as far as you have to go to touch the inoculum and remove.

5. Pass the tube through the flame again, replace the lid, and put the tube back in the rack. Move quickly but deliberately, and don't wave your loop around.

> *If your bacterial sample is on a plate, be sure to pick as isolated a single colony as you can see and touch it very gently with the top of the cooled loop. You do not need to touch the entire loop to the colony!*

6. Hold the plate in your left hand. Use the last three fingers as a platform, and your thumb and forefinger to hold and lift the lid 1–2 inches open at the end away from your hand.

7. In the first quadrant, touch the loop to the surface of the plate, near the rim. Don't dig the loop into the surface. Rhythmically move the loop on the surface back and forth, moving toward the center of the plate, but staying in the quadrant. Don't cross over a line you have already made.

8. Close the lid of the plate, and reflame the loop. Start flaming away from the loop and work toward the loop, for a total of 5–10 seconds.

> *To be sure the loop isn't too hot, touch it lightly on a not-streaked area of the plate before you touch the bacterial streak. Designate this the cooling area of the plate, and don't streak over this bumpy surface.*

9. Rotate the plate 90º, open the lid, and touch the loop to the 1st quadrant, near the center of the plate (the end of the streak). Cross over the last streak once, then streak your loop into the empty quadrant. Keep moving the loop over the empty quadrant, never crossing over a past streak or into any other quadrant, and fill the quadrant.

10. Repeat steps 7, 8, and 9 twice to streak in the remaining quadrants.

11. Reflame the loop and set it down.

12. Incubate the plates, upside down, at the appropriate temperature.

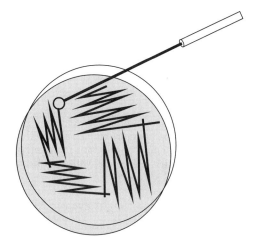

FIGURE 4.

The streak lines you have already made will be visible if you open the lid slightly and angle the plate toward the light.

PROTOCOL

Streaking Multiple Samples on an Agar Plate

For multiple samples, and only when you are starting with a one-colony inoculum, streak multiple samples on a plate to save time and materials. This is the type of streaking that will be done in most cloning experiments. Only do this kind of streaking when you are adept at one-plate streaking, for it is harder to obtain single colonies with a multiple sample plate.

Materials

- A metal (usually platinum) loop. Disposable loops are available. They are expensive but handy, especially for BL3 organisms.
- A Bunsen burner or flameless loop heater.
- Plate of semisolid medium.
- Bacterial sample from semisolid medium or broth.

Procedure

1. Label the plate on the bottom with your name, the date, and the bug.

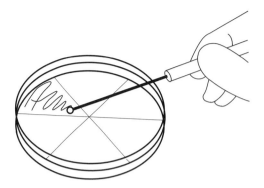

FIGURE 5.

When streaking multiple samples, start with as small an inoculum as possible to be sure you get isolated colonies. (Reprinted, with permission, from Miller 1992.)

2. Lightly mark the bottom of the plate, dividing it into six or eight even sections. Label each sector with the sample name or number.

3. With a flamed and cooled loop, lightly touch the single colony to be picked up. If your sample is a broth culture, do not immerse the entire loop in the culture, but touch the edge of the loop to the broth.

4. Starting at the edge of the plate, lightly touch the plate and rhythmically streak the loop lightly across the surface, moving toward the middle of the plate. Don't cross over the sector lines, or over any streaks.

5. Repeat for each sample, reflaming the loop each time.

6. Incubate the plate upside down at the appropriate temperature.

Slants and stabs

Use only a single colony as inoculum. To streak, start from the bottom of the tube and streak toward the top, rhythmically moving the needle or loop back and forth as you progress. To stab, use an inoculating needle to pierce the agar once, as deeply as you can go. Usually a slant is streaked and stabbed.

PROTOCOL

Picking Colonies with a Needle or Toothpicks

Use this method when you have many well-isolated colonies as your inoculum. You may also use a needle (reusable, as is the loop, but with a blunt end), but it will be much more tedious.

Materials

- Plate of semisolid medium.

- Template. Make a cardboard template representing a plate divided into 30–100 numbered sectors.

- Bacterial sample: colonies on semisolid medium. If you need to know what colonies you are picking, have the colonies to be picked numbered and organized before you start.

- Sterile toothpicks. Autoclave on the dry goods cycle. A small beaker, covered with aluminum foil, is a convenient receptacle.

- Biohazard sharps container for disposal of toothpicks.

Procedure

1. Label the plate on the top (there will be no room on the bottom) with your name, the date, and the bug. Lightly mark the bottom of the plate with orientation marks, so you can identify each colony by the template, and number each row.

2. Place the plate right side up on the template.

3. Touch a colony with a sterile toothpick, and then touch the toothpick lightly to the appropriate place on the plate.

4. Dispose of the toothpick and repeat for all the desired colonies.

COUNTING BACTERIA

There are two main ways to count bacteria: by *viable plate counts*, and microscopically, using a *counting chamber* such as the Petroff Hausser chamber. They can also be counted in a Coulter counter.

Most investigators use **viable plate counts** as the standard way to do growth curves, titer a culture, or examine the effect of various conditions on bacterial survival. Dilutions of the culture are streaked on plates and are allowed to grow: Only the bacteria that can grow will be counted. A clump of bacteria will only be counted as one viable unit.

Counting with the **counting chamber** is best suited to times when you need an immediate answer on the number of bacteria in a culture—for example, if you want

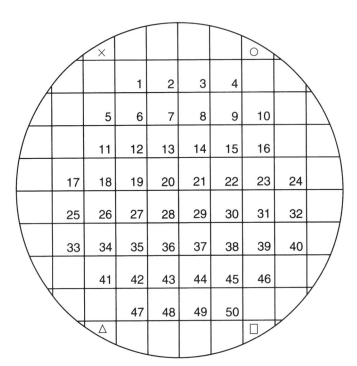

Template for 50 colonies

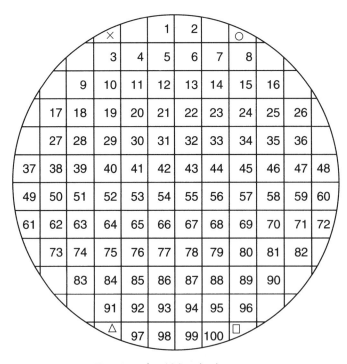

Template for 100 colonies

FIGURE 6.

Templates for 50 and 100 colonies, with orientation marks. Draw 3 or 4 orientation marks on the grid and the plate and keep those marks aligned as you work. (Reprinted, with permission, from Miller 1992.)

to know how many bacteria you have in a culture before you use them for an infection. You simply take a sample of the culture, put it on the Petroff Hausser slide, look at the slide on the microscope, and count the bacteria. Of course, you will be counting both dead and live bacteria.

Instead of counting cell numbers, the growth of cultures is often and easily monitored by the change in turbidity that occurs as the number of organisms increases. This is the simplest and the most rapid way to check for the growth of bacteria. Singular readings are only meaningful if you have already compared optical density readings with actual cell numbers and so can extrapolate the cell number from an O.D. reading.

> *Stains are available that can differentiate between dead and living bacteria.*

PROTOCOL

Using a Petroff Hausser Counting Chamber

Materials

- Petroff Hausser or other bacterial counting chamber such as a Helber. Do not use a hemocytometer.
- Special and reusable coverslip.
- Pipettors and pipet tips.
- Medium for dilutions.
- Microfuge tubes.
- Counter.
- Light microscope, upright or inverted.

Procedure

1. Aseptically remove 0.5 ml of culture with a 1- or 2-ml pipet to a microfuge tube. Be sure culture is well mixed before you take an aliquot. You could take less of the culture if it is scarce, but it is better to use a pipet than a pipettor.

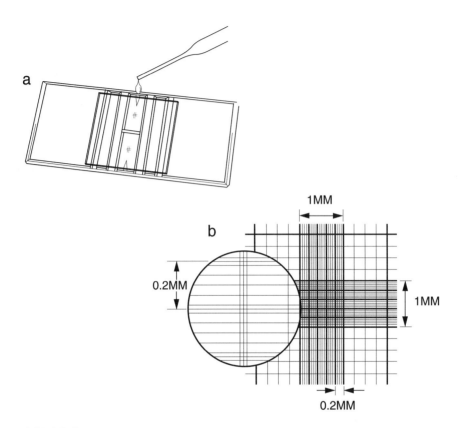

FIGURE 7.

Petroff Hauser counting chamber. (*a*) Load the chamber by allowing a drop of bacterial suspension to enter the chamber by capillary action. (*b*) View of the Petroff Hauser grid at high power. The ruled surface is 0.02 mm below the coverslip, so the volume over a square mm is 0.02 cubic mm.

2. Set up your counting chamber. Clean it with water and finish with 70% alcohol, dry with a Kimwipe. Place the coverslip over the slide, with the chamber in the center.

3. Add 50 μl of bacterial culture to the chamber. First, shake the tube to resuspend the bacteria before sampling. Remove 50 μl with a pipettor but do not dispense it immediately. Gently push the button as if you were dispensing, but stop when you have a drop hanging from the edge of the pipet tip. Touch the drop to the coverslip at one end, and by capillary action, the fluid will be drawn under the slide. Be careful not to overfill the chamber. If fluid runs into the troughs, wash and dry the chamber and try again.

4. Allow the chamber to sit for 5 minutes, so the bacteria can settle.

5. Place the chamber on the microscope and find the grid under 10X. Find the center grid, then go to 40X.

6. Do a rough count to determine whether you need to do a dilution. In 25 squares there should be 100–500 bacteria. If there are too many bacteria, your count will be inaccurate. If you do have too many bacteria, you will save a great deal of time by counting a 1:5 or 1:10 (or more) dilution.

7. Count your sample. Count the bacteria in at least 25 squares. Count each organism, count organisms touching the lines. Divide this by the number of squares counted. Repeat count twice and average your three numbers.

8. Calculate the number of cells/ml in the original culture. Multiply the number of bacteria/square times 2×10^7. If you have made a dilution, multiply your total by the dilution factor to give the number of bacteria/ml of the original culture.

Example

A sample is removed and added to the chamber. A rough count of 90/square is seen, so the original sample is diluted 1:10 by adding 100 µl of sample to 900 µl of medium in a microfuge tube.

This sample is counted. The counts are 200, 171, and 192 for each 25 squares. This is 563 bacteria, divided by 75, which equals 7.5 for a final bacteria/square.

7.5×10 (dilution factor) $\times 2 \times 10^7 = 1.5 \times 10^9$/ml in the original culture.

PROTOCOL

Viable Plate Counts

Materials

- Diluent. Use media or 0.1% peptone in water. Be sure diluent is sterile and at room temperature before use (cold shock may prevent reproduction). Only use saline or distilled water if you know it is okay for your organism.

- Pipets. Pipets or pipettors and tips are fine.

- Sterile tubes. Most tubes will do; glass or plastic, the cheaper the better, as long as it is clean and sterile, has enough room to allow vigorous mixing, and is big enough to allow a pipet or tip in.

- Solid culture medium in petri dishes. Medium should have the appropriate antibiotics, and be at room temperature for use. Inspect each dish for contamination.

- Vortex.

- Broth bacterial culture.

- Bunsen burner.

- Turntable (optional).

- Glass spread rods. You can make these yourself, from glass rods, or purchase them from one of the large distributers.

- 70% ethanol (100–200 ml) in a 500-ml beaker.

- Colony counter (optional).

> *In a pinch, you can make a glass spread rod with a long-tipped pasteur pipet. Heat the pasteur over a flame, and use a forceps to pull the heated glass into the shape you want.*

Procedure

Making the dilutions (see dilutions, Chapter 7)

1. Prepare the dilution tubes. 1:10 dilutions are typical. A volume of 900 µl will save medium yet allow accurate mixing and pipeting. Make 8–10 plates if you are unsure of the growth characteristics of the bacteria.

2. Remove 100 µl of bacterial culture, and add it to dilution tube 1 (10^{-1} dilution). Discard the pipet or tip. Touch the tube gently to the vortex to mix.

> *Flame glass dilution tubes when you remove or add a sample.*

3. Remove 100 µl from dilution tube 1 and transfer it to tube 2 (10^{-2} dilution). Discard the pipet. Vortex. Continue to transfer 100 through the series of dilution tubes.

Spreading the plates

1. Label the plates with the dilution, your name, date, and the sample. Duplicate plates are an excellent idea.

2. Remove 100 µl from the last dilution, and add to the appropriately labeled plate in a series of droplets. Discard the pipet.

3. Put the plate on the turntable or on the bench.

> *If you are fast, you can add all the dilutions to all the plates at once, using the same pipet and working from the most dilute to the most concentrated dilution. You should have multiple glass rods to do this, as one rod won't cool fast enough to be safely dipped into the ethanol.*

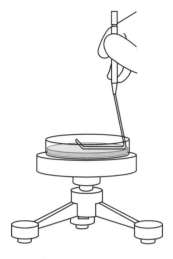

FIGURE 8.

The use of a turntable facilitates the spreading of the bacteria.

4. Dip a glass rod into the ethanol. The ethanol must only touch the bottom part of the rod, and the first inch of the stem.

5. Flame the rod. A flame should travel the length of the rod and quickly extinguish.

6. Cool the rod by touching it to the agar, away from the place you have added the bacteria.

7. Spread the rod back and forth across the plate, covering the entire plate and spreading the liquid as evenly as possible. If you have a turntable, hold the rod steady while you twirl the turntable.

8. Allow the plate to sit 5 minutes before inverting it for incubation. Check plates daily and remove as soon as colonies are clearly visible. Don't allow plates to overgrow.

Counting colonies and calculating the cell number

1. Examine all the plates. Look for a plate containing between 30 and 300 colonies, but take one as close to this as you have. You only need one plate to count, or two plates, if you did duplicates.

2. Count the colonies.

3. Multiply the number of colonies by the reciprocal of the plate dilution and the sample dilution plated to find the number of bacteria/ml in the original culture.

The low-tech method is to count by marking the plastic lid above the colony with a dot (use a sharpie) and keeping a mental note of the number. Make a notation on the plate for every 100 colonies. An electronic marker pen which beeps and records the number is available through a large distributer. An illuminated screen or a light box makes counting even easier.

Example

278 colonies were counted on the 10^{-4} dilution plate.
278 (# colonies) × 10,000 (plate dilution) × 100 (sample dilution plated) =
$2.78 × 10^7$ ml

PROTOCOL

Changes in Turbidity as a Measurement of Growth

As the numbers of bacteria in the medium increase, the amount of light that is transmitted through the medium will be reduced. This amount, called the absorbance or optical density, is usually measured in a spectrophotometer.

Absorbance can also be measured with other instruments, including a Klett-Summerson colorimeter. The Klett, and some spectrophotometers, can be used to measure O.D. without removing a sample, since a long sidearm of a special flask can be inserted directly into the machine.

Materials

• Bacterial culture, freshly inoculated. Use a large volume so removal of samples won't impact on the culture.

• Medium for spectrophotometer blank.

• Cuvettes. Disposable plastic or glass cuvettes. Do not use quartz cuvettes, which are only suitable for UV readings.

• Spectrophotometer.

• Pipets.

Procedure

1. Turn on the spectrophotometer. Set the wavelength at 420 or 660, and zero the machine.

2. Blank the machine against medium. If the spectrophotometer is old and will not allow this, blank it manu-

The best wavelength to use is the one at which the bacterial culture absorbs the most light, and this will depend on medium components, pigmentation, and other qualities. This can be determined by scanning the culture at all visible light wavelengths.

ally by reading the O.D. of the medium and subtracting it from the reading for the bacterial culture.

3. Take a bacterial sample. Swirl the flask before you remove the sample, so you can obtain as representative a sample as possible. Do all manipulations aseptically, especially if you are doing a growth curve.

4. Add the sample to the cuvette and quickly read it, before the bacteria settle.

5. Repeat readings at regular intervals. For quickly growing bacteria such as *E. coli*, with a doubling time of 20 minutes, a reading every 10 minutes might be necessary. At very high bacterial numbers, the O.D. readings may no longer have a linear dependence on cell numbers. If your culture gives O.D. readings over 1.2 or so, dilute it 1:5 and take another reading. Don't forget to multiply the O.D. by the dilution factor when plotting the growth curve.

6. As you go through the time course, plot the absorbance of each sample versus time. When the exponential growth ceases, it is time to stop the growth curve.

Calculation of generation time (*g*). It is invaluable to know the growth kinetics of generation time of the organisms you work on. Armed with that information, you can set up all your cultures to maximize yield and conserve time and materials.

Do a growth curve, taking samples of a growing culture and counting the number of bacteria in each sample. From the change in cell number over time is calculated μ, the growth rate constant, and from μ is calculated *g*.

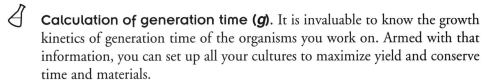

$U = (\log_{10}Z - \log_{10}Z_0)/(t-t_0)$
$U = \ln2/g = 0.693/g$
where
Z_0 is cell number/ml at zero time
Z is cell number/ml (or any cell component, such as weight) at a time point
t = time
t_0 = time at zero time, or the earlier time point
U = the rate of increase of cells, the growth rate constant
g = generation time, doubling time

- Start the growth curve as early in the morning as possible, and you might be able to avoid a very late night. Inoculate your inoculum the night before.

- Perform the growth curve under the same conditions in which you will use the organism.

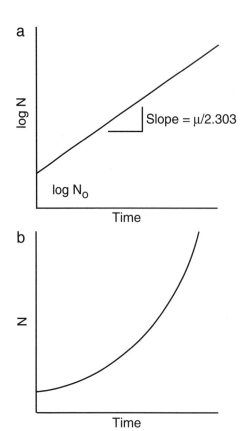

FIGURE 9.

Comparison of methods of plotting growth data. Plotting the logarithm of cell density (number of cells/ml, N) of a culture undergoing balanced growth as a function of time yields a straight line (*a*); the slope of the lines is the growth rate contant (μ) divided by 2.303, and the intercept is log N_0. Plotting the cell density directly as a function of time yields an exponential curve (*b*). (Reprinted, with permission, from Stanier et al. 1976.)

- Take time points at regular intervals. Base the intervals on an estimation of *g*. If the organism has an approximate *g* of 30 minutes, take a reading every 15 minutes. If the organism has an approximate *g* of 24 hours, take a time point every few hours.

- Use a volume large enough that the culture won't be affected by volume loss after sample taking. 100 ml is a good minimum.

- Cell numbers can be determined by direct counting or by viable plate counts. If you have previously correlated cell numbers with O.D. readings, you can use O.D. readings to find *g*. If you haven't done that correlation, do it now: It is much easier to monitor growth by O.D.

- The inoculum must be healthy, and should be in log or late log growth. A very small inoculum will give a long lag phase: A large inoculum might result in no apparent lag phase at all. A 1:100 dilution should do for most rapid growers.

- Continue the growth curve until you have reached, at least, stationary phase. Some organisms will not exhibit a death phase.

STORAGE

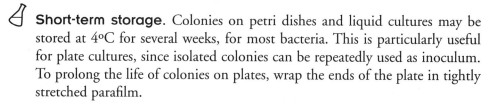 **Short-term storage.** Colonies on petri dishes and liquid cultures may be stored at 4°C for several weeks, for most bacteria. This is particularly useful for plate cultures, since isolated colonies can be repeatedly used as inoculum. To prolong the life of colonies on plates, wrap the ends of the plate in tightly stretched parafilm.

Long-term storage. The method of long-term storage will depend on the bacteria you are using. Some strains don't survive well under conditions in which other strains thrive. When you obtain bacteria, find out the recommended procedure for storage. Unless you have reliable information, or test your culture for its ability to survive particular storage protocols, you cannot be sure you will have viable bacteria when you want them. The dictates of your own facilities, how often you will use the culture, and the relative replaceability of the strain will also help determine how you store a particular strain of bacteria. There is no perfect storage method. Some options are considered below:

- **Subculture.** A culture is inoculated, grown up, and stored, and the process is repeated at intervals so there is always a fresh culture growing before the preceding one dies. This is not recommended.
  Advantages: Immediate access to a viable culture. Inexpensive.
  Disadvantages: Loss of viability, increased chance of contamination, loss of stability of phenotype.

- **Drying.** Water is removed, and rehydration is prevented. This method is most commonly done with fungi, although some bacteria survive well, for several years. There are several matrixes upon which the samples are dried (these include silica gel, paper, starch, and gelatin discs; see Snell, p. 26.), and the survival for each method is very species-specific.
  Advantages: Inexpensive, contamination unlikely.
  Disadvantages: Information about using this method for a particular strain may be hard to find.

- **Freeze-drying.** Water is removed by sublimation from the frozen sample of bacteria. After drying, the samples are stored under vacuum, in glass ampoules. Samples are good for over 10 years, some for over 50 years.
  Advantages: Long-term cultures can be easily maintained.
  Disadvantages: Not all labs have the equipment needed. Inconvenient for frequently used strains. Some strains lose a great deal of viability.

- **Freezing and storage in a low-temperature freezer.** Water is not available to the microorganisms, and the dehydrated cells are stored at low temperature. They may be stored in a low-temperature freezer that is below –70ºC, or in the vapor phase (–140ºC) or liquid phase (–196ºC) of a liquid nitrogen tank.
  Advantages: Most cells can be adequately preserved, making this the default, best choice of maintaining long-term bacterial cultures.
  Disadvantages: High cost for freezers, high maintenance. Damage to cells during the cooling to freezing and thawing of the frozen cultures.

FREEZING BACTERIA

Consider these things before you grow your bacteria for storage:

- **Minimize subculturing.** With repeated transfers, mutation, or selection of variants, contamination may occur. As soon as you have the strain you want, prepare for freezing.

- **Grow the cells under ideal conditions.** Use early passage cells, grown under ideal conditions, utilizing the recommended medium, atmosphere, and temperature. In general, minimal medium works best.

- **Find out what the freezing conditions are for your bugs.** Freezing conditions are different for many bacteria: Find out what your bugs need before you label your vials.

- **Prepare freshly made freezing medium,** which is usually different from growth medium. Be sure your glycerol is sterile.

- **Documentation is critical!** You must have a book in which you record the strain, growing conditions, date, your name, and storage place. This list is separate from the freezer list, which should also be scrupulously updated when you store or remove bacteria.

PROTOCOL

Freezing Bacteria for Long-term Storage

The following freezing protocol will work for most bacteria.

Materials

- 20% glycerol/water, autoclave to sterilize
- Cryotubes (special screw-top freezing vials) and rack
- Ice
- Pipets
- Pipet aid

How many vials should you freeze? This depends on what you need the bacteria for, whether you will be giving them away, or perhaps just need a backup. Don't forget, since you can take a sample from the top of the frozen sample without thawing the tube, you get many more samples than tubes. And also don't forget that you can always grow and freeze more. For plasmid strains, library samples, experiments, freeze *5–10*. For strains you will use for years, freeze *50–100*.

Procedure

1. Grow the cells to the early stationary phase of growth. A too sparse or too overgrown culture may not survive freezing. If you have no specifications for medium, use a minimal medium.

2. Pellet the cells and decant the supernatant. Spin the cells gently, at 2000–5000 rpm on most centrifuges, for 10 minutes. Decant the supernatant into a flask, to be disposed of as biohazard waste.

3. Loosen the caps and label the vials while the bacteria are spinning. On each vial record the strain, the date, and your name. Do not merely label the box containing the vials.

4. Resuspend the pellet in 1/20th the original volume of fresh freezing medium.

5. Add an equal volume of 20% glycerol, to bring the glycerol concentration to 10%.

6. Dispense 1 ml of the suspension into the labeled tubes. Although you can reduce the volume, don't add more, as the contents will expand when frozen. An easy way to do this is to use a 10-ml pipet to fill 10 vials, opening and filling each tube separately. Aseptic technique is extremely vital here.

7. Place in freezer boxes; don't add loose tubes to the freezer.

8. Store below –50°C, in a freezer or in the vapor phase of a liquid nitrogen tank.

*Extremely useful when freezing bacteria is a **rack**, available from several companies, which holds the tubes steady and in place while you remove the cap.*

CONTAMINATION

- **Plates.** Every time you look at a plate, be sure there is only one colony type. Older (larger) colonies may sometimes have a slightly different pigmentation, but not very different, and the shape and texture should be the same. If you doubt the veracity of a colony, pick the isolated colony, grow it up, and test its identity. Slower growing organisms tend to get contaminated more often than faster growing organisms.

- **Yeast.** Yeast, although they are eukaryotic cells, are grown and cultured similarly to bacteria. They can be grown both on plates and in liquid culture, like bacteria, using most of the same ingredients. Lab strains have doubling times closer to those of bacteria than to mammalian cells. Most yeast are usually grown at 30°C.

- **Yeast and bacteria** should never be grown in the same incubator, and most labs maintain separate working quarters (hoods, even rooms) for each. This is more for the sake of the yeast, which more easily can get contaminated by bacteria than the other way around: Still, any sharing of equipment can lead to contamination of bacterial cultures.

> *When in doubt, throw it out. Really.*

RESOURCES

Bionet.Microbiology FAQ. V.2.3. 1995.
  Among many other things, lists microbiology newsgroups and bulletin boards.
  http://www.qmw.ac.uk/~rhbm001/BMFaq.html
Chen T. 1997. *Glossary of Microbiology.*
  http://www.hardlink.com/~tsute/glossary/index.htl
Collins C.H., Lyne P.M., and Grange J.M. 1989. *Microbiological methods,* 6th edition. Butterworth-Heinemann, Oxford.
Gerhardt P., Murray R.G.E., Wood W.A., and Krieg N.R., eds. 1994. *Methods for general and molecular bacteriology.* American Society for Microbiology, Washington, D.C.
Heidcamp W.H. 1995. *Cell biology laboratory manual.* Gustavus Adolphus College, St. Peter, Minnesota.
  http://www.gac.edu/cgi-bin/user/~cellab/phpl?index-1.html
Horton R.M. 1996. Internet on-ramp. Using newsgroups: Virtual conferences on specialized topics. *BioTechniques* **20:** 62–64.
Microbiology at the WWW Virtual Library.
  http://golgi.harvard.edu/biopages/micro.html
Miller J.F. 1992. *A short course in bacterial genetics. A laboratory manual and handbook for Escherichia coli and related bacteria.* Cold Spring Harbor Laboratory Press, Cold Spring Harbor, New York.

Pienta P., Tang J., and Cote R., eds. 1996. *ATCC bacteria and bacteriophages,* 19th edition, pp. 465–466. American Type Culture Collection, Manassas, Virginia.

Snell J.J.J.S. 1991. General introduction to maintenance methods. In *Maintenance of microorganisms and cultured cells. A manual of laboratory methods* (ed. Kirsop B.E. and Doyle A.), pp. 21–30. Academic Press, New York.

Stanier R.Y., Adelberg E.A., and Ingraham J.L. 1976. *The microbial world,* 5th Edition. Prentice-Hall, Englewood Cliffs, New Jersey.

U.S. Department of Health and Human Services Publication. 1988. *Biosafety in microbiological and biomedical laboratories.* Public Health Service, Centers for Disease Control and National Institutes of Health. U.S. Government Printing Office, Washington, D.C.

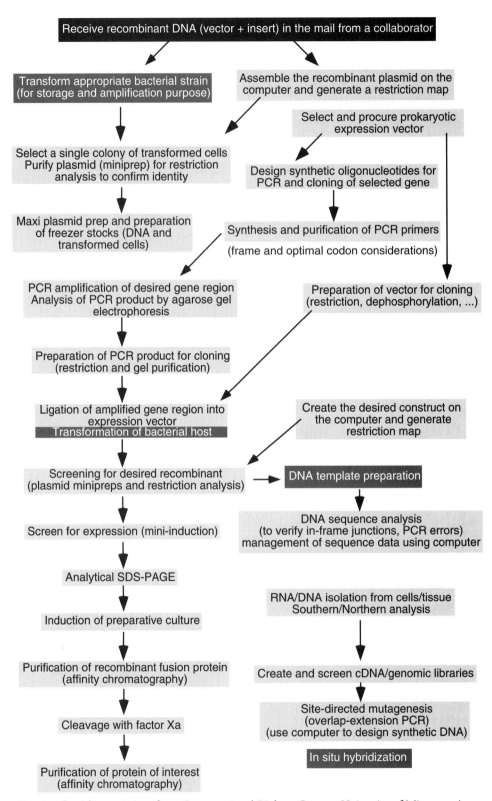

Receive recombinant DNA (vector + insert) in the mail from a collaborator

Transform appropriate bacterial strain (for storage and amplification purpose)

Assemble the recombinant plasmid on the computer and generate a restriction map

Select and procure prokaryotic expression vector

Select a single colony of transformed cells
Purify plasmid (miniprep) for restriction analysis to confirm identity

Design synthetic oligonucleotides for PCR and cloning of selected gene

Maxi plasmid prep and preparation of freezer stocks (DNA and transformed cells)

Synthesis and purification of PCR primers

(frame and optimal codon considerations)

PCR amplification of desired gene region
Analysis of PCR product by agarose gel electrophoresis

Preparation of vector for cloning (restriction, dephosphorylation, ...)

Preparation of PCR product for cloning (restriction and gel purification)

Ligation of amplified gene region into expression vector
Transformation of bacterial host

Create the desired construct on the computer and generate restriction map

Screening for desired recombinant (plasmid minipreps and restriction analysis)

DNA template preparation

DNA sequence analysis
(to verify in-frame junctions, PCR errors)
management of sequence data using computer

Screen for expression (mini-induction)

Analytical SDS-PAGE

Induction of preparative culture

RNA/DNA isolation from cells/tissue
Southern/Northern analysis

Purification of recombinant fusion protein (affinity chromatography)

Create and screen cDNA/genomic libraries

Cleavage with factor Xa

Site-directed mutagenesis
(overlap-extension PCR)
(use computer to design synthetic DNA)

In situ hybridization

Purification of protein of interest (affinity chromatography)

(Reprinted, with permission, from Computational Biology Centers, University of Minnesota.)

12

DNA, RNA, and Protein

RNA, DNA, AND PROTEIN are the bread and butter of the molecular biology laboratory. Until a few years ago, investigators worked in a "DNA lab," or an "RNA lab" or a "protein lab," and had great expertise only in that area. Increasingly now, investigators need to be familiar with techniques involving all three macromolecules, and laboratories are set up to accommodate this range. Even a small project can easily involve a bit of cloning, mRNA isolation, and Western blotting.

The problems associated with either DNA or RNA or protein are not the same, as the molecules have completely different properties. But thinking and working aseptically will help you avoid some of the major pitfalls of macromolecule work.

MOLECULAR BIOLOGY TIPS

- **Know the theory behind everything you do.** With kits and protocols readily available, it is particularly easy to do experiments in mol-

MOLECULAR BIOLOGY TIPS	279
DNA	280
DNA isolation	281
Alkaline-SDS plasmid minipreps	282
Phenol extraction of DNA samples	284
Ethanol precipitation of DNA	286
Using a vacuum concentrator	287
Determining nucleic acid concentration and purity by UV spectroscopy	288
Restriction enzymes	290
PCR	290
Oligonucleotides	293
Ethanol precipitation of oligonucleotides	294
INTRODUCING DNA INTO CELLS AND MICROORGANISMS	294
Prokaryotic cells	294
Eukaryotic cells	295
RNA	296
RNA isolation	296
Ethanol precipitation of RNA	297
Selective RNA precipitation	297
mRNA isolation	298
Determining RNA concentration	298
PROTEIN	298
Isolation	299
Chromatography	299
Dialysis	300
Preparing the tubing	300
Setting up dialysis	301
Cell lysis	302
Determining protein concentration	304
Antibodies	308
RESOURCES	310

ecular biology without a thought in your head. Know the components of a kit, and know what they do. Know why you use high salt versus low salt, ionic versus nonionic detergents. If you don't, you will end up changing protocols instead of ever troubleshooting.

- **Don't endlessly protocol-shop.** In no field of science will you be able to get more help than in molecular biology. The manuals are plentiful and excellent, there are numerous on-line sources for advice, and many of the techniques are taught in college and grad-school labs. It is easy to become infatuated with a nifty new technique. But if you have a protocol that works, stick with it.

- **Purchase kits judiciously.** They are completely invaluable. But if they are not purchased wisely, they can be an enormous waste of time. Check out the lab's resources before you order one. If, for example, the lab already has 90% of the reagents needed, it doesn't make sense to purchase the kit. Or if a "kit" only consists of an easily made buffer, control DNA, and enzyme, buy the enzyme, make or buy a control, and make the buffer.

- **Consult with other scientists about results.** Because of the enormous amount of written material around, you may feel that you "shouldn't" ask questions. But here as in all fields, a bit of advice could save you weeks of effort and money.

- **Be vigilant about the effectiveness of your reagents.** The reagents you purchase are still made by human beings, and could be ineffective, labeled incorrectly, or have any number of things wrong. There is a tendency to assume that a prettily packaged, labeled, and boxed reagent *must* work, and that the failed experiment must be your own fault. (In most cases, of course, it is your fault.) Include controls, where feasible, for all reactions. Don't hesitate to call the manufacturer or supplier if you have a doubt about a reagent: The technical services will suggest ways to determine whether the reagent is functional and will arrange for an immediate replacement if it is not.

- **Label everything.** Each sample may pass through several tubes on its way to its final treatment, and the contents of even the intermediary tubes must always be clear.

- **Discard old tubes as you go.** Racks of microfuge tubes will pile up quickly in the refrigerator and freezer, and they can become confusing and depressing. Keep a tube only until you have the next step completed satisfactorily.

DNA

DNA is pretty tough, as the material that holds and transfers most genetic information would have to be. But don't get too casual. The main worry is that of contamination of samples or reagents with other DNAs.

DNA Isolation

- The DNA isolated will either be genomic or extrachromosomal.

- Investigate DNA isolation kits. These have been fine-tuned to isolate genomic and extrachromosomal DNA, as well as DNA from agarose gels and PCR products from multiple amplification reactions. They utilize a DNA-binding resin or membrane, and are often little microfuge columns. They are worth the expense. Their use usually eliminates the need for phenol extractions and CsCl centrifugation.

  > *Read and follow carefully the instructions included with DNA isolation kits. Details that may seem minor—such as the O.D. of a bacterial culture—can be very important.*

- Extrachromosomal DNA is isolated as phage or plasmid DNA.

- Large pieces of DNA, for example, genomic DNA, must be handled carefully to avoid breakage. It is isolated and stored differently from small DNAs.

- Preps may be referred to as mini, midi, and maxi (small, medium, and large). Mini preps are sufficient for a surprising number of uses.

- Find out what quality of DNA prep is required. Certain procedures such as DNA sequencing or transfection of mammalian cells may require a high quality of DNA to work well, whereas others, such as screening clones by restriction mapping, may be more forgiving.

Units of Measurement

1 kb of DNA = 6.5×10^5 Daltons of double-stranded DNA (sodium salt)
1 kb of DNA = 3.3×10^5 Daltons of single-stranded DNA (sodium salt)
1 kb of DNA = 3.4×10^5 Daltons of single-stranded RNA (sodium salt)
1 kb of DNA = 37,000 Daltons = 333 amino acids of coding capacity
Average MW of a deoxynucleotide base = 324.5 Daltons
Average MW of a deoxynucleotide base pair = 649 Daltons
1 μg/ml of 1 kb of DNA = 3.08 nM 5′ ends

TABLE 1. Genomic DNA Sizes

Organism	Base pairs/ Haploid genome	Copy number of single-copy genes
Escherichia coli	4.7×10^6 bp	1.8×10^8
Drosophila melanogaster	1.4×10^8 bp	6.6×10^5
Mus musculus (mouse)	2.7×10^9 bp	3.4×10^5
Homo sapiens	3.3×10^9 bp	2.8×10^5

PROTOCOL

Alkaline-SDS Plasmid Minipreps

Minipreps allow you to isolate and analyze plasmid DNA from a bacterial culture. 12 or 16—as many as can fit in your microfuge rotor—can easily be run at once.

Materials

- 5 ml overnight culture. Use LB plus the appropriate antibiotic, and inoculate with a single colony. Incubate at 37°C, shaking or rolling.

- Sterile microfuge tubes.

- Ice.

- Solution I (Lysis buffer: 25 mM Tris-HCl, pH 8.0, 50 mM glucose, 10 mM EDTA), hold on ice to chill.

- Solution II (Denaturing solution: 0.2 N NaOH, 1.0% SDS), made fresh for each preparation. Hold at room temperature.

- Solution III (Renaturation solution: 5 M potassium acetate. To make: Prepare 120 ml of potassium acetate. Add 23 ml of glacial acetic acid and 57 ml of H_2O for a total volume of 200 ml.) Hold on ice.

- TE.

- 70% and 100% ethanol.

- RNase A (DNase-free). Make up a 2 mg/ml solution, aliquot it, and store at –20°C. You can use and refreeze this. There are protocols to make Rnase A free of DNase, but you can (and should) just buy DNase-free RNase A.

Procedure

1. Add 1.5 ml of the culture to a microfuge tube.

2. Centrifuge 2 minutes at 10,000*g*, preferably in the cold. Aspirate the supernatant.

3. Resuspend the pellet in 100 µl of cold Solution I. Vortex for 2 minutes.

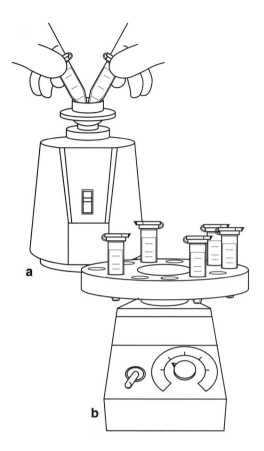

FIGURE 1.

Two tubes can be vigorously vortexed together by holding them bottom to bottom (*a*). If you have more than two tubes, use either a multi-tube vortexer or a standard vortexer with an adapter that holds multiple tubes (*b*).

4. Incubate the tube at room temperature for 5 minutes. The bacteria will be lysed and the DNA released.

> Some protocols call for the inclusion of lysozyme (Final 4 mg/ml) in Solution I to digest the bacterial cell wall, but this usually isn't necessary.

5. Add 200 μl of Solution II and mix the tube by inversion for 5 seconds. Vortexing would damage the DNA.

6. Incubate the tube on ice for 5 minutes.

7. Add 150 μl of Solution III and mix the tube by inversion for 20 seconds.

8. Incubate the tube on ice for 5 minutes. Plasmid DNA is selectively renatured.

9. Centrifuge at 12,000*g* for 5 minutes.

10. Remove the supernatant (which contains the DNA) with a pipettor into a new tube.

11. Add 5 μl of 2 mg/ml RNase A (DNase-free) to the supernatant and incubate at 37ºC for 5 minutes.

12. Add 450 µl of phenol-chloroform and extract (see protocol below) to remove the RNase A and proteins.

13. Extract with chloroform (see protocol below).

14. Add 1 ml of cold 100% ethanol and precipitate for 20 minutes at –80°C.

15. Aspirate the supernatant.

16. Wash pellet with 70% ethanol and dry under vacuum for 5 minutes. If you aren't in a hurry, invert the tubes onto a paper towel and let drain and dry for 30 minutes.

17. Resuspend the pellet in 25 µl of TE. Use 2–4 µl to run on a gel and store the rest at –20°C.

PROTOCOL

Phenol Extraction of DNA Samples

Phenol extraction is often done on samples of DNA (and RNA) to remove contaminating proteins. Phenol and water are not miscible, and will form separate phases when mixed. When the aqueous sample containing the DNA is mixed with phenol, the proteins partition into the phenol phase, the aqueous DNA is removed, and the sample is reextracted and concentrated by ethanol precipitation.

Materials

- Solvent-resistant plastic tubes. Try to work in as small volumes as possible. Most extractions can be done in microfuge tubes.

- TE-saturated phenol:chloroform:isoamyl alcohol 25:24:1 (see Chapter 7)

- Chloroform:isoamyl alcohol 24:1.

- Pipettor and tips.

Procedure

1. Add an equal volume of TE-saturated phenol-chloroform to the DNA sample. The total volume should not exceed 500 µl for a 1.5-ml microfuge tube.

2. Vortex the sample vigorously for 20 seconds.

3. Centrifuge the sample for 5 minutes at room temperature to separate the phases. This does not have to be a high spin, but it is often convenient to use the highest speed on the microfuge. Remove the samples carefully so you don't disturb the separated phases.

4. With the pipettor, remove as much aqueous layer as you can without disturbing the protein layer. Add it to a new tube.

> *If you have added hydroxy-quinoline to the phenol, the phenol will have a yellowish color.*

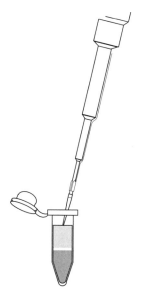

FIGURE 2.

After centrifugation, you should see two phases in the tube. The top phase is the aqueous phase, which contains the DNA. The bottom phase is the organic phase, containing the protein. There is usually an interphase of extracted protein, a thick or barely visible whitish band between the aqueous and organic phases. Don't touch the white junk when removing the aqueous layer!

To improve yield: If you think you have not gotten enough of the aqueous layer, you can reextract the phenol layer by adding a volume of TE, pH 7.5, approximately equal to the phenol layer. Vortex and centrifuge.

If the combined volume of the aqueous phases is under 500 µl, you may combine them in one tube. Usually, however, you will need another tube, and will end up with almost no DNA in that tube. It is not worth the time to routinely reextract the phenol layer.

To improve purity: If you think you might have picked up some of the protein layer, you can phenol extract the aqueous phase by adding a volume of phenol:chloroform approximately equal to the aqueous layer. Vortex, centrifuge, and carry on as in step 4. If you find that your enzymatic reactions with DNA aren't working, you probably need to do two extractions.

5. Add an equal volume of chloroform to the aqueous layer. Repeat steps 2, 3, and 4.

6. Label the tube. It is now ready for use or for concentration by ethanol precipitation.

> *Phenol-chloroform must be disposed of as hazardous waste. Do not discard it down the sink.*

PROTOCOL

Ethanol Precipitation of DNA

Precipitating the DNA sample enables you to resuspend it in a smaller volume, and so, to concentrate it. Precipitation also removes residual chloroform, which will inhibit many enzymatic reactions.

Procedure

1. To a maximum volume of 450 µl of DNA in water, add 1/10 volume of 3 M Na-acetate, pH 4.8. Invert briefly to mix.

2. Add two volumes of 95% or 100% ethanol. Invert well to mix.

3. Precipitate the DNA by placing the sample in the cold. Precipitations can be done at –20ºC overnight, –70ºC for 30 minutes, or on dry ice for 5 minutes.

> **Using dry ice for ethanol precipitations**
> Use a mallet to pound the dry ice into a powder, and insert your tubes into the powder, or break the dry ice into pieces, and add to a freezing-resistant dish. Add 95% ethanol to make a slurry, and insert your tubes. The ethanol will wipe out all markings except those done with a permanent sharpie.

4. Centrifuge the sample at high speed (at least 12,000 rpm) for 15–30 minutes, at 4ºC. If you don't have a refrigerated microfuge, place the microfuge at 4ºC.

5. Decant or aspirate the supernatant. The supernatants can be discarded down the sink.

6. Drain the tubes by inverting the tubes and leaving them upside down on a paper towel on the bench.

7. Wash the pellet with cold 70% ethanol.

8. Dry as described in step 6, or use a vacuum concentrator.

9. Resuspend the DNA in TE, pH 8.0 (10 mM Tris-HCl, 0.1 mM EDTA). If the DNA does not seem to go into solution, add more TE. Store at 4°C.

> *Caution is needed when handling large-molecular-weight DNA (over 30 kb). The DNA should never be vortexed, but should be mixed by inversion or on a wheel. Instead of precipitating the DNA with ethanol, traces of chloroform should be removed by dialyzing the DNA solution against large volumes of cold TNE or by extraction with water-saturated ether.*

PROTOCOL

Using a Vacuum Concentrator (Speed Vac)

If traces of ethanol remain in nucleic acids after ethanol precipitation, it is difficult to resuspend the pellets in water or buffer. If you are in a hurry, or have a large volume of volatile liquid to remove, a vacuum concentrator can be used.

A vacuum concentrator consists of a centrifuge, a pump used to create a vacuum, a heater, and a cooling trap. Models vary, and laboratory rules on usage vary even more.

Procedure

1. **Turn the cooling trap on at least 30 minutes before you are ready to use the concentrator.** In some models, you may have to add dry ice.

2. Turn on the vacuum pump.

3. Open the vent to release the vacuum inside the centrifuge.

4. Place your tubes in the centrifuge. They must be balanced, with the tops open. Cover the tubes with a piece of parafilm, and use a pin to poke a couple of holes in the parafilm. Theoretically, the tops can be left off, and the contents should be fine, as centrifugal force should keep the contents in the tubes. But if someone lifts the lid before the vacuum has been fully released and causes a bit of turbulence inside, the parafilm may help save your material.

> *If someone's samples are already spinning, slowly release the vacuum until the centrifuge is at atmosphere. Wait at least 10 seconds, a few seconds after you no longer hear the hissing of the air into the centrifuge. Then, and only then, can you turn off the centrifuge and load your own tubes.*

5. Close the lid, and turn the centrifuge on.

6. Once the centrifuge has achieved full speed, open the vacuum vent to the centrifuge.

7. Turn the heater on only if you have a lot of volume to dry, or can't wait the 10 minutes it takes to dry DNA precipitation pellets. Oligos will require several hours of spinning with heat.

8. To stop the run, release the vacuum in the centrifuge. Only then should you turn the centrifuge off!

9. Open the centrifuge when the rotor has come to a complete stop.

10. Remove the tubes, checking by eye to be sure they are dry. Cap immediately, to prevent losing the dry pellets.

11. Turn off the vacuum pump.

12. Follow lab procedure on cleaning the trap. Some require that you clean after every use, others that it be done once a day. If you evaporated a lot of liquid, you should clean it right way.

PROTOCOL

Determining Nucleic Acid Concentration and Purity by UV Spectroscopy

1. Turn the spectrophotometer on.

2. Turn on the UV lamp 20 minutes before you will take your readings. The visible light lamps can be used immediately, but the UV lamp takes a while to become steady. The amount of warm-up time needed depends on the lamp and the spectrophotometer.

3. Your sample will be DNA or RNA in water or buffer, with a blank of water or the same buffer. The amount of nucleic acid you add will depend on the source, so ask someone in the lab for a recommendation on the amount of material and the dilution you need.

4. Put the sample and the blank in a matched set of quartz cuvettes.

> *Only quartz cuvettes, not glass or plastic, will allow you to take accurate readings in the UV range.*

5. Set the wavelength to 260 nm.

6. Blank the machine against the water (or blank manually, if only one cuvette at a time can be measured).

7. Read the O.D. at 260.

8. Set the wavelength to 280. Reblank and read the O.D. at 280.

9. Calculate the concentration of the nucleic acid, using the following information:

    1 A_{260} unit of double-stranded DNA = 50 µg (50 µg/ml has an O.D. of 1 at 260 nm)

    1 A_{260} unit of single-stranded DNA = 37 µg

    1 A_{260} unit of single-stranded RNA = 40 µg

DNA concentration (µg/ml) = (OD_{260}) x (dilution factor) x $\dfrac{(50 \text{ µg DNA/ml})}{1 \text{ } OD_{260} \text{ unit}}$

Example: 10 µl of DNA is added to 390 µl of water, and the O.D. is 0.205.
0.205 x 40 x 50 = 410 µg/ml
The DNA concentration is 410 µg/ml.

---

10. Calculate the total yield of your preparation.

Yield = (DNA concentration in µg/ml) x (total volume in ml)
Example: If the 10-µl sample were taken from a 100-µl sample,
410 µg/ml x 0.1 ml = 41 µg or 0.41 mg
Note: If you removed 10 µl from the sample for assay, you would only have 36.9 µg left
(41 – 4.1 = 36.9).

---

11. Estimate the purity of the prep by figuring the 260/280 ratio. The ratio between the readings at 260 nm and 280 nm gives an estimate of the purity of the nucleic acid. Pure preparations of DNA should have a 260/280 ratio of 1.8, RNA a ratio of 2.0. A higher ratio would suggest extraction with phenol-chloroform to remove protein impurities.

Example: If OD_{260} of the DNA prep was .205, and OD_{280} was .114, the 260/280 ratio would be 1.8. Right on the nose!

Restriction Enzymes

Restriction enzymes are usually pooled for a laboratory or one or more departments. Some enzymes are expensive and infrequently used, and single investigators can't afford to keep a large selection. There will be one person in charge, and most of the dialogue will take place via sign-up and comment sheets.

- Always bring an ice bucket, labeled tubes, a pipettor, a box of sterile tips, and a sharps discard box (if there isn't one near the freezer) with you when you go to the –20°C freezer where the enzymes are kept. Don't bring tubes with DNA to the enzyme freezer.

- Remove one enzyme only, and place it in your ice bucket. Keep the freezer door shut: Don't stand with your body in the door, pipeting away.

- Take what you need. Use aseptic technique.

- Replace the stock enzyme tube in the freezer.

- Sign the sign-up sheet, or make a note of what you used and the amount you took.

- Take another enzyme, if you need one.

- Report all empty or almost empty tubes to the person in charge. Don't merely leave a note.

> *Use tips luxuriously. Use a tip once, and discard it immediately, so there is no chance of inadvertently using it again. Contamination of one enzyme with another is the major worry when working with restriction enzymes.*

> *If you need an amount of an enzyme that will deplete the stock, organize yourself to let the charge person know at least a few days before.*

Buffers for restriction enzymes

The buffer needs of most of the restriction enzymes can be met with five buffers, differing in the kind and concentration of salt used. Companies often supply the appropriate buffer with the enzyme, but you may not be the one who gets one of those tubes. If there are common buffer sources for restriction enzymes in your lab, don't use them: You must have your own buffers, because this is another source of possible cross-contamination. Either get hold of the manufacturer's tubes (you can make a set from different manufacturers) or make your own. It is easy enough.

PCR (Polymerase Chain Reaction)

PCR, an invention made by Kary Mulis at Cetus Corporation in 1985, is an in vitro method of DNA synthesis that allows a particular segment of DNA to be copied and amplified.

TABLE 2. Restriction Enzyme Buffers

Buffer	Label	10x Stock
Low salt buffer	x10 L	100 mM Tris-HCl, pH 7.5 100 mM $MgCl_2$ 10 mM dithiothreitol
Medium salt buffer	x10 M	10 mM Tris-HCl, pH 7.5 100 mM $MgCl_2$ 10 nM dithiothreitol 500 mM NaCl
High salt buffer	x10 H	500 mM Tris-HCl, pH. 7.5 100 mM $MgCl_2$ 10 mM dithiothreitol 1000 mM NaCl
Potassium buffer (KCl)	x10 K	200 mM Tris-HCl, pH 8.5 100 nM $MgCl_2$ 10 mM dithiothreitol 1000 mM KCl
Tris acetate buffer BSA-free	x10 T	330 mM Tris-acetate, pH. 7.9 100 mM Mg-acetate 5 mM dithiothreitol 660 mM K-acetate

(Reprinted, with permission, from Amersham Pharmacia Biotech, UK Limited.) Make 10x stocks of restriction buffers, and freeze in 1-ml aliquots. With 1-ml stocks of 0.1% BSA and 0.1% Triton X-100, the buffer needs of most restriction enzymes can be met.

The DNA template is first denatured by high temperature. The temperature is lowered, and two oligonucleotide primers that flank the DNA fragment to be amplified are annealed to their complementary sequences on opposite ends of the target sequence. With a DNA polymerase in the solution, the temperature is increased slightly: The primers are extended and the region between the primers is synthesized. The strands are again denatured, new primers are annealed, and DNA synthesis is allowed to take place again ... and again and again, 20 to 50 times.

A temperature cycler, a programmable water bath, is used to achieve the rapid changes of temperature the process requires. The DNA polymerase used is *Taq* DNA polymerase, which is derived from the thermophilic bacterium *Thermus aquaticus* and can thus function at high temperature. The process is brilliantly simple, but the problem is that any contaminating DNA can be amplified, sometimes in preference to the desired template.

Contamination of one DNA with another is the bane of the PCR user. With amplification possible with such minute pieces of DNA, it is horrendously easy to find spurious bands resulting from DNAs accidentally introduced during sample preparation.

The major source of contamination seen in PCR laboratories is the DNA obtained as a product from previous PCR procedures, which arises from the aerosols generated during the pipetting and manipulation of the PCR samples. Because of this, many labs have a separate sample preparation area, physically distant from the

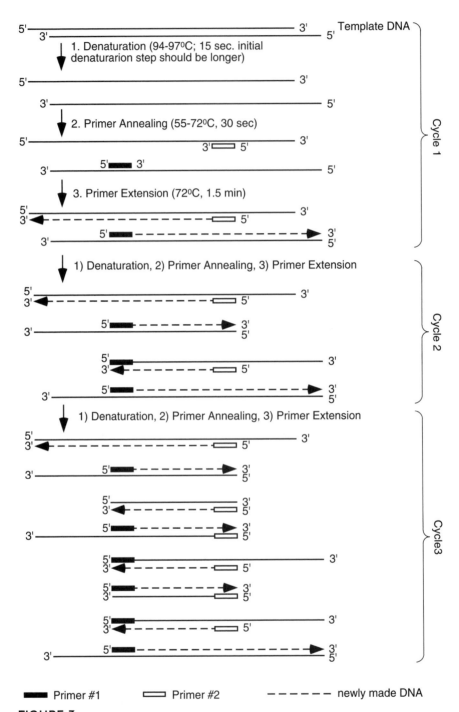

FIGURE 3.
Amplification of a specific sequence of DNA with PCR. After the first two or three cycles, the single-strand overhangs are ignored and the vast majority of the product is double-stranded target sequence. (Redrawn, with permission, from Zyskind and Bernstein 1992.)

PCR machine and from any area in which the post-PCR tubes will be opened. Another source of contamination of mammalian DNA is DNA from skin cells. Wear gloves.

🧪 Basic PCR Rules

- Prepare samples away from the PCR machine. Most labs have a separate sample preparation area, physically distant from the PCR machine and from the area where tubes will be opened after PCR. Whether or not there is an area dedicated to sample preparation, never prepare your samples near the PCR machine or where further manipulation of the sample will be done. Try to get a consensus to establish strict rules about sample preparation.

> *Briefly centrifuging the tube prior to opening will reduce aerosols.*

- Keep separate pipets and other supplies for setting up PCR reactions. A positive displacement pipettor will prevent aerosols and reduce the chance of sample carryover. Pipettor tips with filters will also prevent carryover from sample to sample.

- Wear gloves and change them frequently. This will help prevent contamination of the sample with epithelial cells from the hands.

> *Contamination can be removed physically and enzymatically (Dieffenbach and Dveksler 1995), but it is best to prevent it.*

- Add the DNA last to all reaction tubes.

Oligonucleotides

Oligonucleotide primers are synthesized in the lab, at a departmental facility, or by a company. It may be obtained as a crude, dried-down product, column- or HPLC-purified. You will be given instructions on how to further purify the product, if necessary, and how to store it. The more pure the product, the more expensive it will be.

There are software packages available to help in designing oligos. You can sit down with a pen and paper and do it, but a computer program can really help in designing the best primers and giving the optimum annealing temperature. Companies that supply oligos can help you with analysis. You could go on line, and use one of the programs available on the WWW (see Resources), or ask for a program recommendation from a newsgroup or another investigator.

PROTOCOL

Ethanol Precipitation of Oligonucleotides

1. Add 1/10 volume of 3 M NaOAc, pH 6.5, and three volumes of cold 95% ethanol.

2. Place at –70°C for at least 1 hour.

INTRODUCING DNA INTO CELLS AND MICROORGANISMS

After isolation, DNA is not only isolated and analyzed, but is often introduced into cells and microorganisms with the intention of altering the genotype of the recipient or harvesting quantities of the donated DNA or its translated protein.

Prokaryotic Cells

Transformation is the genetic change in a bacterium after exposure to and recombination with an isolated DNA. This is routinely done in order to amplify cloned DNA. Another common reason is to obtain quantities of a particular protein: The bacteria are transformed with DNA contained in an expression vector, and will pump out large amounts of the protein coded for by the DNA.

There are two main methods of bacterial transformation:

- *Incubation* with high concentrations of Ca^{++} ions, which causes the bacterial plasma membrane to admit foreign DNA. This is simple and takes a few minutes at the bench.

- *Electroporation.* Higher efficiencies of transformation are possible with electroporation. The conditions for maximum electroporation are different for different species and even different strains.

With either method, the bacteria must first be rendered competent; that is, able to take up DNA. The bacteria must be grown to a particular density, harvested, and washed with salts: Competent cells can then be aliquoted and frozen. There are slight variations between the methods for producing chemically competent versus electroporation-competent bacteria. Competent cells are available commercially.

Eukaryotic Cells

There are several methods of gene transfer for eukaryotic cells, and the success of a particular method is very species- and strain-specific. The process is termed transfection, a hybrid of transformation and infection: Virally mediated gene transfer is also called infection.

In a stable transfection the cells which have taken up the DNA are selected by expression of a reporter gene. (Traditionally, this is antibiotic resistance to hygromycin or neomycin: There are many alternatives, such as FACS selection of cells expressing Green Fluorescent Protein [GFP].) Cell lines can be made from individual clones of expressing cells. Transient transfections are more likely to be done to gather immediate information about the effect of the DNA on the cell. In general, transient transfections are of limited use since variable numbers of cells contain the gene of interest (the precise number is governed by the transfection efficiency), and the cells that do contain the appropriate DNA have variable copy numbers. In addition, results can be difficult to interpret since the recent transfection is extremely traumatic, and this damage is hard to control for. Analysis of transient transfectants can be of use in defining an early, preliminary sense of the phenotype that can be expected in the stable transfectants.

Transfection of eukaryotic cells is done in many ways, including:

- Calcium phosphate coprecipitation.

- DEAE-dextran-mediated transfection.

- Lipid-mediated transfection.

- Electroporation.

- Microinjection.

- Virally mediated transfer. Adenovirus, retrovirus, and SV-40 can be used to introduce DNA into cells.

Reporter genes are genes used to locate, identify, or analyze another gene. They may be coupled to the upstream sequence of another gene and transfected into cells to study the regulation potential of the potential upstream sequence: This is the more stringent definition of a reporter gene. The CAT gene, coding for chloramphenicol acetyltransferase, is the classic gene used to evaluate gene regulation in eukaryotic cells. More loosely, reporter genes may be transferred into cells or bacteria just to monitor whether or not the foreign DNA is being expressed: antibiotic resistance genes are an example.

Other reporter genes are β-galactosidase, β-glucuronidase, and alkaline phosphatase (if the enzyme is present and interacts with the substrate, a colored or fluorescent product results). GFP, an autofluorescent protein from the jellyfish Aequorea victoria, is becoming the reporter gene of choice, since it requires no activation or enzymatic activity to be visualized.

Since the efficiency of DNA transfer is so dependent on the cell type, you must investigate the transfection protocols used for your cells before you waste a lot of time. Check the literature, go on line, and make phone calls to ask about protocols.

Recommendation: Make sure you have access to an electroporator. You will be able to transform bacteria, yeast, mammalian cells, and many exotic cell types. Some older models lack the capacity to electroporate mammalian cells, but an attachment that allows this can be purchased.

The vector is of critical importance in determining the outcome of the transformation or transfection. In choice of vector, you will have a great deal of help. Companies such as Invitrogen or Promega offer vectors with inducible promoters, reporter genes, the ability to be propagated both in eukaryotes and in bacteria, and technical help.

RNA

RNA degradation was such a serious problem that, for years, people would avoid all RNA work like the plague. But a few rules, similar to those of aseptic technique, keep everything running smoothly.

 Basic rules

- Autoclave all plasticware and glassware that will touch anything that will touch the RNA.

- DEPC (diethylepyrocarbonate)-treat all water that will be used to make DNA buffers. Add DEPC to final 0.1%, leave overnight at room temperature, and autoclave for 15 minutes. Don't use DEPC for Tris buffers, as the DEPC will decompose into ethanol and carbon dioxide.

- Avoid alkaline buffers, as the hydroxy group in RNA makes the molecule very sensitive to alkali.

- Keep RNA buffers separate from other buffers, so they won't be accidentally used and contaminated with RNases.

RNA Isolation

Reagents such as guanidine hydrochloride or guanidinium isothiocyanate act as chaotropic agents and maintain the integrity of RNA. For RNA isolation, it makes sense to use a kit or prepared reagent. Many companies now offer an RNA-isolation reagent that allows the simultaneous isolation of DNA, RNA, and protein from cells or tissue samples. Even if you only need the RNA, these reagents are a worry-free way to work with RNA.

PROTOCOL

Ethanol Precipitation of RNA

Usually, RNA can be precipitated as can DNA.

Procedure

1. Add 1/10 volume of 1 M NaOAc, pH 4.8, and 2.5 volumes of cold 95% ethanol.

2. Precipitate overnight at –20ºC.

3. Wash the pellet with 70% ethanol.

Note: When you are working with small amounts of RNA (under 5 µg), add a carrier or coprecipitant to the RNA before precipitation. This material will precipitate with the RNA and give you a visible pellet that is much easier to work with. Two common carriers are molecular-biology-quality glycogen and yeast RNA.

PROTOCOL

Selective RNA Precipitation

This protocol has been adapted, with permission, from Epicentre Forum 1996, p. 10, Epicentre Technologies, Madison,Wisconsin. If you have a DNA–RNA mix (for example, after in vitro transcription reactions), you can precipitate just the RNA with ammonium acetate as the salt.

Procedure

1. Add 5 M ammonium acetate to the RNA to a final concentration of 2.5 M.

2. Chill the mixture on ice for 15 minutes.

3. Centrifuge in a microfuge at high speed for 15 minutes at 4ºC.

4. Remove the supernatant and wash the pellet with 70% ethanol.

5. Resuspend the RNA pellet in the desired volume of RNase-free water or buffer.

Note: Since ammonium acetate decomposes by loss of ammonia (and base is harmful to RNA), solutions should be prepared only from the pure salt which has been kept cool in a closed container. Sterilize the solution by filtration and store it at 4°C.

mRNA Isolation

mRNA is a small (generally 5–10%) proportion of the total RNA in a cell, the bulk of which is ribosomal RNA. Eukaryotic mRNA isolation methods take advantage of the polyadenylated tail present only on most of the mRNAs (there are a few mRNAs without poly(A) tails). Poly(A) RNA will bind to a resin made of oligo(dT)—cellulose will bind the mRNA under high salt conditions, and will be eluted with a low salt wash. This can be done in batch or in small columns. Some mRNA isolation kits allow the direct isolation of mRNA from cells.

Determining RNA Concentration

RNA concentration and purity can be determined by UV spectroscopy, as described for DNA. There are two differences:

* One A_{260} unit of RNA is 40 µg. The RNA concentration (µg/ml) =

    $(OD_{260}) \times (\text{dilution factor}) \times \dfrac{(40 \text{ µg of RNA/ml})}{1 \text{ OD}_{260} \text{ unit}}$

* Sample volume is usually kept as low as possible, to limit the use of the RNA to measure O.D. You can buy and use mini UV cuvettes, or determine the minimum volume your UV cuvettes can hold and give accurate readings.

PROTEIN

Degradation is the fear permutating protein work.

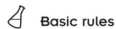 **Basic rules**

* *Ice, ice, ice.* Always have a bucket of ice handy when you are doing any protein work, and put tubes on ice immediately when removing them from freezers, centrifuges, etc.

- *Spin cold,* unless otherwise noted. Centrifuges can get quite warm.

- *Know your protein.* The properties of individual proteins vary greatly. Is it denatured by heat? Does it have disulfide bonds? Can it be repeatedly frozen and thawed? If you don't know, assume that it cannot be frozen and thawed, and that it can be heat-denatured.

- During and after cell lysis, include the appropriate *protease inhibitors* in all buffers.

Isolation

The ease of producing large amounts of protein with a bacterial or baculoviral expression system is not always accompanied by ease in isolating your protein. Despite the tricks for binding expressed fusion proteins, the characteristics of the particular purified protein can alter the way the system should work. Before you scale-up production, be sure you can isolate the protein effectively.

There are a lot of tricks to protein isolation. Although DNA, and even RNA, work can pretty much be done by following a manual, protein work is more complicated: Each protein has its own profile and personality. Seek help from someone in a protein lab.

Chromatography

Proteins, as well as DNA and RNA, are routinely separated and isolated by chromatography. This need not conjure up images of huge columns in the cold room or HPLC machines, as chromatography can as well be performed in a microfuge tube. The main kinds of chromatography done are gel filtration, ion exchange, and affinity chromatography.

- **Gel filtration:** The separation of compounds on the basis of molecular size.

  How it works: The stationary phase contains pores, which trap only smaller molecules.

  Example of materials: Sephadex (cross-linked dextran), Sephacryl (cross-linked copolymer of allyl dextran and *N,N'*-methylenebis(acrylamide), Sepharose (beaded agarose).

  Example of use: Removal of unincorporated nucleotides from a nick translation reaction on a G-50 (a kind of Sephadex) column.

- **Ion exchange:** The separation of compounds on the basis of charge.

   How it works: Association of the protein or other material with the charged groups of a solid support, followed by elution with an aqueous buffer of higher ionic strength. Column material can be anionic, cationic, or mixed bed (both).

   Example of materials: DEAE (Diethylaminoethyl) cellulose, amberlite, Dowex, CM-Sepharose.

   Example of use: Isolation of DNA from a gel by electophoresis onto DEAE paper.

- **Affinity chromatography:** The separation of compounds on the basis of natural binding site.

   How it works: The molecule to be purified is specifically and reversibly adsorbed by a ligand immobilized on an insoluble support.

   Example of materials: Oligo(dT) cellulose, biotin, heparin.

   Example of use: The binding of antibodies to Protein A.

> *Many chromatography materials need to be soaked and swollen before use, or they won't work effectively. Some materials require an overnight incubation in buffer.*

Dialysis

Dialysis is done to remove salts or other impurities from a sample. The sample is placed in a porous tubing: The size of the pores in the tubes will permit only molecules of sizes smaller than the pores to exit. The material in the dialysis bag is placed in a large volume of water or buffer, allowing the outward passage of contaminants and the eventual replacement of the buffer contents of the tubing by the dialysis buffer.

PROTOCOL

Preparing the Tubing

The tubing must be cleaned and prepared before use. Wear gloves for all manipulations.

> *Prepared dialysis tubing is a good item to share, as few single investigators can use it up before it should be discarded. Make an arrangement with other lab members to do this.*

1. Choose tubing of the appropriate MW cutoff.

2. Prepare the dialysis tubing. This can be done to a package, and the prepared tubing can be stored at 4ºC.

3. Place the tubing in a large volume (a liter for a full package) of 5 mM EDTA, 200 mM sodium bicarbonate in a flask.

Sodium bicarbonate	FW 84.01	use 16.85 g/l
EDTA	FW 372.24	1.86 g/l

4. Boil for 5 minutes.

5. Pour off the bicarb/EDTA, rinse the tubing briefly with deionized water, add another large volume of bicarb/EDTA, and boil again for 5 minutes.

6. Discard the second wash. Rinse the tubing well with deionized water.

7. Add a large volume of deionized water, and cover the flask with aluminum foil.

8. Autoclave for 10 minutes on the liquid cycle (slow exhaust).

9. Store at 4ºC in a sterile container with an opening large enough to permit easy removal and replacement of the tubing. If the tubing will be stored for longer than a few days, add sodium azide to a final 0.02% to the water and tubing.

Sodium azide will inhibit bacterial growth. Weigh it out very carefully, as it blocks the cytochrome electron transport system. Be aware that it can also inhibit some enzymatic reactions. Keep a small volume in the refrigerator of filter-sterilized 2% azide in water, and add 1 μl for every 100 μl of solution.

PROTOCOL
Setting up Dialysis

1. Cut a piece of tubing large enough to contain the material you want to dialyze. Allow approximately 2 inches at each end (4 inches in total) for tying off the tubing. (Special chambers can be purchased for "micro" dialysis.)

2. Either knot one end of the tubing, or use a dialysis clamp to close one end.

3. Open the other end with a gloved finger, and keep one finger in the tubing. Pipet or pour the material into the tubing carefully.

4. Tie off or clamp the other end. Remove air bubbles by pushing them before you clamp. Check for leaks, especially at the ends.

5. Place the filled tubing in as large a beaker or Erlenmeyer as you can find: 2–4 liters is a good size.

6. Add a stir bar and place on a magnetic stirrer, usually in a cold room. If the tubing sinks to the bottom of the container, and that worries you, tie the tubing on one end with string, hang it from the container, and attach it to a weight. You could also allow an excess of dialysis tubing at one end, which can be taped to the outside top edge of the beaker, with the filled tubing left suspended in the beaker. But unless the dialysis tubing is very turgid and immobilized on the bottom of the container, a gently turning stir bar will not break it.

7. Usually, dialysis is performed overnight. Change the buffer once if you have a 2–4 liter container, more often for smaller containers.

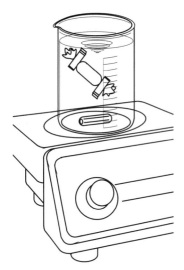

FIGURE 4.

Dialyze your material against as large a volume as is practical.

Cell Lysis

When isolating a protein, the cell or bacteria containing the protein must first be lysed.

 Physical lysis. This can be done physically, with machines of various disruptive potentials. For example:

- *Nitrogen cavitation bomb.* Nitrogen decompression is one of the gentler ways to open up eukaryotic cells. Nitrogen under pressure is allowed to equilibrate within cells. When the pressure is released, the nitrogen comes out of solution and the popping bubbles break the individual cell's membrane. No further disruption of the cell occurs, and organelles can be preserved intact. In addition, the reducing atmosphere and cool temperature provided by the nitrogen protect the proteins from degradation.

- *Homogenizer.* Basically a blender, subjecting the cells to shearing forces. Not suitable for bacteria, unless glass beads are added.

- *Ultrasonic processer (sonicator).* Sonic pressure waves create microbubbles, which can not only break open cells, but can shear DNA. Glass beads can be added to disrupt bacteria.

- *Freeze press.* In the freeze press, frozen cells are forced through a narrow orifice, causing shear stress and explosive decompression powerful enough to break open tough cell walls.

- *Bead mill homogenizer.* Bacteria, spores, or yeast, usually, are vigorously vortexed in a tube containing glass or zirconium beads. The movement against, and bombardment of, the cells by the beads breaks even tough cells open within minutes.

> *Cell lysis is relatively easy for eukaryotic cells, compared with yeast, bacteria, spores, and plant cells, with tough cell walls, and is usually accomplished by detergent lysis, nitrogen decompression, or homogenization.*

 Detergent. Detergents are sufficient to lyse many eukaryotic cells. The detergent used is dependent on the application for the lysed cells. Check the source of the detergent carefully, because the quality and purity of the detergent have a big effect on the success of protein isolation.

- Examples of anionic detergents are the salts of cholic acid, caprylic acid, sodium dodecyl sulfate (SDS), and deoxycholic acid.

- Examples of cationic detergents are cetylpyridinium and benzalkonium chloride.

- Examples of zwitterionic detergents are CHAPS and phosphatidylcholine.

- Examples of nonionic detergents are digitonin, Tween-20 (polyoxyethyl-enesorbitan, monolaurate), and Triton X-100.

Nonionic detergents are much milder, and don't perturb the nuclear membrane: They are often used to lyse cells prior to immunoprecipitations. A 0.1% Triton X-100 solution in water works to lyse most mammalian cells, and up to 0.5% will not harm most enzymes being isolated. Many enzymes, such as Proteinase K, remain active in the presence of Triton X-100.

 Protease inhibitors. When a cell is lysed and the contents released, proteases and other degradative enzymes are released as well. Unless proteases are included in the lysis buffer, the cell's own proteases will break down the cellular proteins.

Other inhibitors, specific to the protein you are studying, may also be used. For example, sodium vanadate, an inhibitor of protein phosphatases, is added to lysis buffers when a phosphorylated protein is being isolated.

TABLE 3. Protease Inhibitors

Inhibitor	Protease target	Effective concentrations	Stock solution	Comments
Aprotinin	Serine proteases	0.1–2 µg/ml	10 mg/ml in PBS	Avoid repeated freezing
EDTA	Metalloproteases	0.5–2 mM	500 mM in H_2O, pH 8.0	
Leupeptin	Serine and thiolproteases	0.5–2 µg/ml	10 mg/ml in H_2O	
α-Macroglobulin	Broad spectrum	1 unit/ml	100 units/ml in PBS	Avoid reducing agents
Pepstatin	Acid proteases	1 µg/ml	1 mg/ml in methanol	
PMSF	Serine proteases	20–100 µg/ml	10 mg/ml in isopropanol	Add fresh at each step
TLCK	Trypsin	50 µg/ml	1 mg/ml in 50 mM acetate, pH 5.0	Chymotrypsin unaffected
TPCK	Chymotrypsin	100 µg/ml	3 mg/ml in ethanol	Trypsin unaffected

Derived from Boehringer Mannheim Biochemicals (1987). (Reprinted, with permission, from Harlow and Lane 1988.)

Determining Protein Concentration

Which to choose

The most common methods of protein determination are the Bradford, BCA, and absorbance at 280 nm. Labs tend to be dedicated to a particular assay: **Try the lab assay first,** before you order new reagents. The Bradford is the best all-purpose assay to use.

- You cannot directly compare the results of one assay method with another. You must get used to working with the relative concentrations determined by one method. For example, BSA gives a value about twofold higher than its weight for the Bradford assay.

- The nature of your protein sample will also suggest which assay to use. If you know you have a purified protein without tryptophan, you shouldn't rely on absorption at 280 nm. And if you must have detergent in the protein sample, you must choose a method that is not particularly detergent sensitive, or you must remove the detergent (see below).

- For all methods you must run your unknown samples against a standard curve, every time you perform the assay. Any purified protein can be chosen as a reference standard, if only relative protein concentrations are desired. Bovine serum albumin (BSA) and IgG are commonly used: Use BSA unless you are measuring antibodies.

BCA

How it works. Copper sulfate, added to an alkaline solution of BCA (bicinchonic acid), gives an apple-green colored complex. When this solution is added to a protein solution, the Cu^{++} ions are converted to Cu^+ by interaction with the peptide bonds of the protein, changing the color of the complex to purple with an absorbance maximum of 562 nm. Pierce makes a BCA assay reagent.

Advantages. Fast, sensitive, accurate.

Disadvantages. Subject to interference by agents such as detergents and organic solvents. Time dependent, color develops for 24 hours.

Bradford

How it works. Utilizes the dye Coomassie blue G-250, which is red-brown at a pH below 1 but turns blue when binding to protein causes a shift in the pKa of the bound dye. Blue color is measured at 595 nm. The Bradford reagent is available from Bio-Rad.

Advantages. Fast, sensitive, accurate. Not time dependent.

Disadvantages. Detergent concentrations over 0.2% interfere with the assay.

Absorption at 280 nm

How it works. The aromatic amino acids, especially tryptophan, absorb strongly around 280 nm. All proteins that contain aromatic residues (or UV absorbing cofactors) have a unique extinction coefficient at 280 nm.

Advantages. Speed. Sample is not destroyed.

Disadvantages. Not as accurate as other methods.

Biuret

How it works. Measures the peptide bonds. O.D. read at 540 nm.

Advantages. Rapid. Good for monitoring protein separation, since salt interferes less than with the Bradford.

Disadvantages. Not very accurate for low protein concentrations.

Lowry (Folin-Ciocalteu)

How it works. Similar to BCA. O.D. read at 750 nm.

Advantages. Need very little material. Bio-Rad's detergent-compatible assay is based on the Lowry.

Disadvantages. Depends on the presence of tyrosine in the protein.

Detergent in the samples?

Detergents are a part of life with proteins, since they are used to lyse cells and to denature proteins. But they can interfere with determination of protein levels and with protein function.

To determine the protein level in a sample containing detergents, you have two options:

- Include the same percentage detergent in the standard curve. This is a necessity, and you may be lucky—you may get an accurate determination. More likely, however, the addition of detergent severely reduces the linear readings of your standards: You may be able to dilute samples (and hence, the detergent level) to be in the linear range, but this is not possible for low protein levels.

- Use a protein assay that is compatible with detergents. Several companies have reagents that can be used for samples with or without detergents. For example, the usual Bio-Rad protein assay is based on the Bradford, but does not accommodate detergent in the samples. However, the Bio-Rad DC Protein assay, based on the old Lowry, is compatible with both ionic and nonionic detergents.

If you are isolating a protein, you probably will have to remove the detergent. The method of detergent removal will depend on the detergent, the protein, and the buffer. Generally, detergents with a high critical micelle concentration (CMC) are easy to remove by dilution, and those with low CMC can be removed on the basis of molecular weights. You will need to seek advice for your particular situation: Especially if you have a hard-to-get protein, this is not the time to experiment. The wrong temperature or salt concentration can very quickly turn your precious solution into crystals or mud.

 Possibilities for detergent removal (adapted from Harlow and Lane 1988, p. 688)

1. Ionic detergents

   • Use gel filtration on a G25 column. For some proteins, equilibrate column in another detergent below its CMC.

   • Add urea to 8 M, then bind detergent to an ion-exchange column. Protein flows in 8 M urea: Dialyze to remove urea.

   • For ionic detergents with a relatively low micelle size and high CMC: Dilute as much as possible and dialyze. Add mixed bed resin to dialysate to increase the exchange rate.

2. Nonionic detergents

   • Use gel filtration on a G200 column. For some proteins, equilibrate column in another detergent below the CMC.

   • Dilute if possible, dialyze extensively against DOC, then slowly remove DOC by dialysis.

   • Use velocity sedimentation into sucrose without detergent.

   • Bind protein to affinity matrix or ion-exchange column, wash extensively to remove detergent, then elute protein. For some proteins, equilibrate column in another detergent below the CMC.

3. Amphoteric (Zwitterionic) detergents.

   • Dilute if possible, dialyze.

Antibodies

Antibodies are proteins secreted by lymphocytes and directed against foreign molecules. They are an important component of the immune system, and a vital tool of the lab.

Polyclonal antibodies are raised against an antigen in vivo by injection of an animal with the antigen. Polyclonal antibodies are a heterogeneous mixture of immunoglobulins of various affinities directed against different epitopes of the same protein.

Monoclonal antibodies are made in vitro, the product of a cell fusion between an immortalized myeloma cell and an antibody-secreting plasma cell. The entire culture will produce just one antibody, of one class (usually IgG), directed against one epitope.

 Obtaining antibodies

- Antibodies can be obtained commercially or from other investigators, or you can make them yourself. See Chapter 9 for suggestions on sources of antibodies which can be obtained from many of the same places as cells. The WWW site, The Antibody Resource Page, contains links to many antibody sources.

- Polyclonal antibodies are relatively straightforward to make. If you will require a regular supply of a polyclonal antibody, you should make (or have made) antibody. Don't attempt to make monoclonal antibodies unless you are in a lab or department in which this is done routinely.

- Be considerate when you ask other investigators for polyclonal antibodies. Unlike monoclonals, they are in limited supply. If your experiment is successful and you will need more antibody, you must make or buy your own.

 Uses. Antibodies can be labeled with a radioactive or enzymatic tag, allowing the protein they are recognizing to be visualized and quantitated.

- *Cell staining.* Labeled antibody can be used to localize cell proteins.

- *Immunoassays.* The antibody is a reagent used to test the function or presence of an antigen.

- *Immunoblots.* Also known as Western blots. The presence and amount of a protein can be detected on a sample immobilized on a filter.

- *Immunoaffinity.* The protein against which the antibody is directed can be isolated and purified.

TABLE 4. Immunochemical Techniques, Polyclonal versus Monoclonal Antibodies

Technique	Polyclonal antibodies	Monoclonal antibodies	Pooled monoclonal antibodies
Cell staining	Usually good	Antibody dependent	Excellent
Immunoprecipitation	Usually good	Antibody dependent	Excellent
Immunoblots	Usually good	Antibody dependent	Excellent
Immunoaffinity purification	Poor	Antibody dependent	Poor
Immunoassays			
labeled antibody	Difficult	Good	Excellent
labeled antigen	Usually good	Antibody dependent	Excellent

(Reprinted, with permission, from Harlow and Lane 1988.)

Storage

- Antibodies are best stored at –20°C, in aliquots: freeze-thawing is not good for most antibodies.

- A working aliquot can be stored at 4°C for at least 6 months.

- Sodium azide can be added to a final volume of 0.02% to inhibit bacterial growth.

Tips

- Know the animal from which your antibody has been derived, as this will determine the secondary antibody used in some assays. Polyclonals are usually from rabbit or donkey: Monoclonals are usually from mouse, rat, or hamster.

- Quickly spin your antibody in a microfuge before use to remove any precipitated material. This can prevent high background in a variety of assays.

- Protein A, a 42-kD polypeptide isolated from the cell wall of *S. aureus,* and Protein G, a 30–35-kD polypeptide isolated from some β-hemolytic streptococci, bind strongly to antibodies, and are useful tools to immunoprecipitate or localize antibodies. Protein A and G can be bound to beads, or labeled, and are good for most (not all) subclasses of antibodies.

RESOURCES

Antibody Resource Page.
    http://www.antibodyresource.com
Ausubel F.M., Brent R., Kingston R.E., Moore D.D., Seidman J.G., Smith J.A., and Struhl
    K., eds. 1991. *Current protocols in molecular biology.* John Wiley and Sons, New York.
    Updated protocols are sent regularly.
BioGuide-PCR
    J. Weizmann Institute of Science, Genome and Bioinformatics
    http://bioinformatics.weizmann.ac.il/mb/bioguide/pcr/contents.html
    Lists of programs for designing PCR primers.
Cell and Molecular Biology Online.
    http://www.tiac.net/users/pmgannon/faq.html#technique
    Recommended for its many links to protocol and reagent sources.
Clark D.P. and Russell L.D. 1997. *Molecular biology made simple and fun.* Cache River Press,
    Vienna, Illinois.
Comprehensive Protocol Collection. 1997.
    Ambros Lab, Dartmouth College .
    http://www.dartmouth.edu/artsci/bio/ambros/protocols.html
Dieffenbach C.W. and Dveksler G.S., eds. 1995. *PCR primer: A laboratory manual.* Cold
    Spring Harbor Laboratory Press, Cold Spring Harbor, New York.
Epicentre Technologies, Inc. Madison, Wisconsin.
    http://www.epicentre.com/f3_3/f3_3rna.htm
Harlow E. and Lane D. 1988. *Antibodies: A laboratory manual.* Cold Spring Harbor
    Laboratory, Cold Spring Harbor, New York.
Hengen P.N. 1997. Methods and Reagents FAQ list.
    http://www-1mmb.ncifcrf.gov/~pnh?FAQlist.html#section39
Hopkins T.R. 1991. Physical and chemical cell disruption for the recovery of intracellular
    proteins. In *Purification and analysis of recombinant proteins,* chap. 3 (ed. Seeetharam R.
    and Sharma S.K.). Marcel Dekker, New York.
Molecular Biology Methods and Reagents NewsGroup
    http://www.bio.net and go to bionet.molbio.methds.reagents
Molecular Biology Protocols.
    http://www.nwfsc.noaa.gov/protocols/oligoTMcalc.html
    Determine the T_m, MW of oligos.
Molecular Biology Protocols on the World Wide Web. 1996–1997.
    http://www.horizonpress.com/gateway/protocols.html
    A collection of protocols from different investigators and laboratories.
Pedro's BioMolecular Research Tools
    http://www.public.iastate.edu/~pedro/research_tools.html
    Links to Journals, GenBank, other databases.
Protocols, Melbourne Signal Transduction Group. 1995.
    http://biotech.bio.tcd.ie/paulb/protocol/index.html
Ramachandra S. 1990. Using the HETO Vacuum Concentrator.
    http://hdklab.wustl.edu/lab_manual/12/12_13.html

Recombinant DNA Technology Course, Computational Biology Centers, University of Minnesota, copyright 1994–1997.
    http://lenti.med.umn.edu/recombinant_dna/recombinant_flowchart.html
Technical Tips Online. Elsevier Trends Journals.
    http://tto.trends.com/
Zyskind J.W. and Bernstein S.I. 1992. *Recombinant DNA laboratory manual,* revised edition. Academic Press, San Diego.

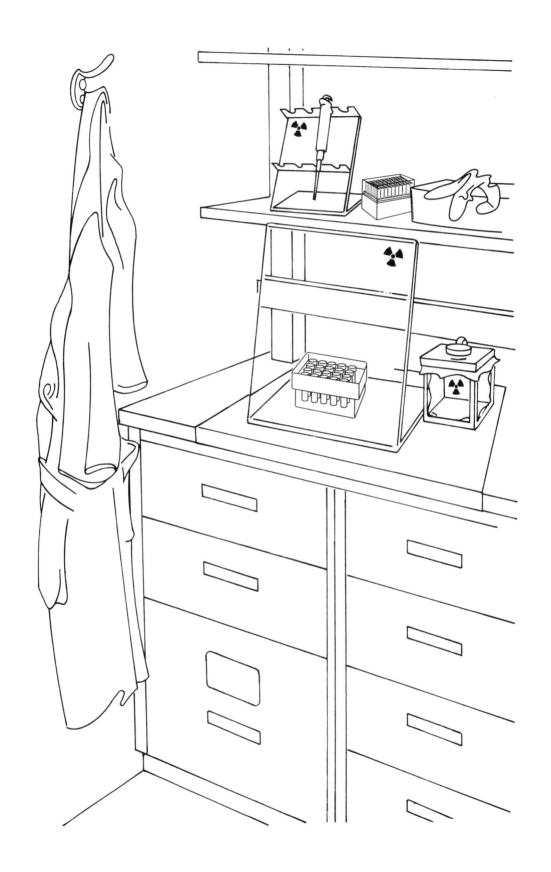

13

Radioactivity

RADIOACTIVITY IS CAUSED by the spontaneous release of particulate and/or electromagnetic energy from the nucleus of an atom. Practically, this means that a "normal" molecule can be labeled by the addition of a radioactive molecule, and that this radioactive molecule can be differentiated from normal molecules. The discoveries that a material could be metabolically labeled, and the fate of that label followed in in vitro and in vivo systems, helped to create the field of molecular biology. The use of radioactivity is still absolutely vital for most fields of experimentation.

There is an aura of danger surrounding radioactivity, but most of the radioactivity used in labs—when used with proper care—is no more of a threat than common solvents or infectious agents. However, there are alternatives to most uses of radioactivity, and these are quite worth investigating.

PROPERTIES OF RADIOACTIVE ELEMENTS	314
HOW TO OBTAIN RADIOISOTOPES	315
Certification	315
Deciding what you need	316
Ordering	320
DOING RADIOACTIVE EXPERIMENTS	320
Rad rules	320
Safety issues	321
Working routines	326
EXPERIMENTAL DETECTION OF RADIATION	329
Autoradiography	329
Exposing a membrane to film	332
Using an X-ray film processor	334
How to expose a sample	336
Liquid scintillation counting	337
^{32}P Cerenkov counting	338
STORAGE	338
DISPOSAL	339
ALTERNATIVES TO RADIOACTIVITY	342
RESOURCES	343

PROPERTIES OF RADIOACTIVE ELEMENTS

Radioactivity is measured in several ways, depending on the characteristics of the type of radiation of interest.

TABLE 1. Some Units of Measurement of Radioactivity

Measurement	Units	Description
Specific activity (1 g of ^{226}Ra e.g., Ci/g, mCi/ml, or µCi/ul)	Curie (Ci)[a] Millicurie (mCi) Microcurie (µCi) 1 Ci = 2.22 x 10^{12} dpm	How many nuclei decay each second
Exposure (photon irradiation in air)	Roentgen[b]	The number of ionizations to form one electrostatic unit in 1 cc of dry air
Absorbed dose (radiation exposure in tissue)	rad[b] (radiation absorbed dose)	100 ergs absorbed in one gram of matter
Dose and damage potential	Rem (rad equivalent, man)	Dose in rad x modifying factors

[a]The Becquerel (Bq;1 Bq = 1 disintegration per second) is the international standard unit of radioactivity, but the Curie is still in common use in the U.S.A. To convert:
$$1 \text{ Ci} = 3.7 \times 10^{10} \text{ Bq} \quad 1 \text{ Bq} = 2.7 \times 10^{-11} \text{ Ci}$$
[b]The rad is the amount of radiation exposure in tissue, the roentgen is the amount of radiation exposure in air: For most biological tissues, 1 roentgen produces 0.96 rad.

- The specific activity is the measurement that concerns the molecular and cell biologist, for that is a measurement of how "hot" a particular molecule is.

- Linked to the specific activity is the half-life of a radioactive element. Since the specific energy effectively says how many emissions or disintegrations occur per second, the amount of time it will take for half of the disintegrations to occur can be calculated.

- The emissions occur in several forms and include:

  α particles (2 protons plus 2 neutrons): ^{241}Au, ^{210}Po
  β particles (electrons): ^{3}H, ^{14}C, ^{35}S, ^{33}P, ^{32}P
  γ X-rays (electromagnetic energy): ^{125}I, ^{51}Cr
  Neutrons: ^{252}Cf

- When α or β particles pass through matter, they form ions by knocking electrons from the orbits of the molecules they pass through. These particles are often referred to as ionizing radiation. Ionizing radiation can be monitored by allowing the radiation to pass through dry air and measuring the numbers of ions formed. This is done, for example, in a Geiger counter.

HOW TO OBTAIN RADIOISOTOPES

Certification

The sale, transportation, use, and disposal of radioactivity are regulated by the federal government, or delegated to the state, and the first step in working with radioactivity is to be sure that you are legal.

 Institutional approval or certification. At most institutions you must be "certified" before you can use and/or order radioactive materials. The definition of certified varies with the institution, and you should check with EHS to find out the requirements. You may have to watch a movie, take a written test, or give a demonstration of your lab prowess.

In most cases you will be certified to work with particular isotopes, and must list what they will be. Consult with the head of the lab or with another lab member and find out what isotopes you are likely to use: These will probably be ^{32}P, ^{33}P, ^{3}H, ^{14}C, ^{125}I, or ^{35}S.

Most institutions have a broad license that includes commonly and uncommonly used isotopes. However, if you are contemplating the use of an uncommonly used isotope, check whether it is listed on the license before you make your plans. If it isn't, it can take months to amend the institution's license.

If you will work with ^{125}Iodine, you will have to have a background thyroid scan. Iodine can become concentrated in the thyroid, and personnel working with radioactive iodine are monitored by regular thyroid scans.

Other background biological monitoring might be done, depending on the isotope you will be working with.

 Laboratory approval. Radioisotope use is assumed in most labs. But you should still check with the P.I. or other lab members.

Most departments have a safety officer, a liaison between the laboratory or department and EHS, who can let you know what you must do and give you advice on ordering, storing, using, and disposing of radioactive material in that particular laboratory. You should inform the safety officer first if you intend to work on an isotope not yet used in the laboratory: It is important that storage and disposal of the material be arranged before the material is ordered. Radioisotope ordering may be centralized and certain radioisotopes shared in the department or lab, and the safety officer will know how this is handled.

> *Don't borrow radioisotopes to do experiments before you are certified.*

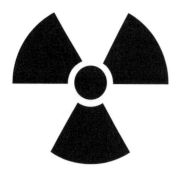

FIGURE 1.

The universal radioactive sign should be posted wherever radioactivity is used, stored, or discarded.

Deciding What You Need

The experiment you plan to do is based on, and is limited by, the nature of the radioactivity. To order the appropriate isotope, you must consider:

- The **molecule** you need to label
- Which **isotope** to use as the label
- The **specific activity**
- The **half-life**
- The **quantity**
- The **concentration**
- The **efficiency** of labeling and the **detection method** you will use

 The molecule you need to label. The application will, of course, determine which molecule should be labeled, but there are still choices to be made.

Metabolic labeling. To label a cell or organism metabolically, a precursor is given that will be incorporated into the molecule or structure you wish to study. Specifically labeling a particular molecule can be fairly tricky, as you need information about the pathway to know which precursor to utilize. The DNA synthesis pathway has been well studied and delineated, and the precursor thymidine is used to label the newly made DNA. Cells are labeled with 5-methyl [^{3}H]thymidine, which is incorporated into replicating DNA. The amount of incorporated label is quantitated by precipitating the DNA with trichloroacetic acid (TCA), collecting the precipitate, and counting the sample in a scintillation counter: In vivo incorporation is detected by autoradiography of the labeled cells.

Glucose

D-[6-³H]Glucose
D-[2-³H]Glucose
D-[5-³H]Glucose
D-[U-¹⁴c]Glucose
D-[6-¹⁴C]Glucose
D-[1-¹⁴C]Glucose
D-[3-³H]Glucose
L-[1-¹⁴C]Glucose

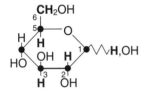

FIGURE 2.

Some molecules, such as this glucose molecule, can be labeled at different positions. Be sure the position of the label is suitable for your needs. (Redrawn, with permission, from Amersham Pharmacia Biotech.)

Alternatively, one could metabolically label many structures of the cell or organism by the addition of a nonspecific precursor such as ^{32}P. A great many molecules will be labeled, but a specific antibody or another binding protein can be used to isolate the desired molecule from the labeled mass. You must know what tools are available.

The position of the label in the molecule may or may not be very important. You must be sure that the label will not be enzymatically removed. Unless you are studying a very esoteric molecule, the catalogs and the technical division of companies that sell radioisotopes can help you.

Choice of probe for in situ hybridization. RNA, DNA, or oligonucleotide probes can be used to localize either DNA or RNA sequences. Generally, RNA probes can be labeled to very high specific activity with efficient incorporation of labeled nucleotide: Furthermore, single-stranded RNA probes are more sensitive than DNA probes, since the probes do not self-reanneal and the full-length probe is available for hybridization. But oligonucleotide probes, although less effectively labeled, are better used to distinguish between closely related sequences.

 Which isotope to use as the label. The chemical identity of an element is determined by the number of protons in the nucleus of the atom: Elements sharing the same number of protons but having different numbers of neutrons are known as isotopes. Radioisotopes are the radioactive forms of an element. For example, carbon (C) has 12 protons, but the radioactive isotope ^{14}C is used for metabolic labeling.

Each isotope has its own kind of emission and half-life. Of course, the molecule itself will dictate which isotope is used for a particular element, as it must have an element susceptible to being labeled. Some radioactive elements must be incorporated into the molecule; others can be nonspecifically bound.

The kind of emission will influence the detection method, and the nature and the amount of shielding required to work safely (see Safety Issues, this chapter).

Isotope	Emission	Half-life	Decays to	Energy (MeV max)
^{3}H	Low energy β	12.4 years	^{3}He	0.019
^{14}C	Low energy β	5730 years	^{14}N	0.156
^{35}S	Low energy β	87.4 days	^{35}C	0.167
^{33}P	Medium energy β	25.4 days	^{33}S	0.249
^{32}P	High energy β	14.3 days	^{32}S	1.709
^{125}I	γ rays	60 days	^{125}Te	0.035
	X-rays			0.027
	Auger electrons			0.030

Sensitivity versus resolution is the main issue you must decide before you choose the isotope you need.

DNA sequencing. One must achieve a balance between sensitivity (more sequence, strong signal, fuzzy bands) and resolution (more readable sequence, less fuzzy bands) for your particular need.

For sensitivity: ^{32}P>^{33}P>^{35}S
For resolution: ^{35}S>^{33}P>^{32}P

The best bet in a new situation is to go for the combination of sensitivity and resolution offered by the use of ^{33}P.

In vitro hybridization. **High energy isotopes** will give the highest sensitivity, but the high energy particles produced on decay of the isotope will travel further through the autoradiographic emulsion and produce a wide scatter of silver grains. Hence, less resolution. **Low energy isotopes** allow high resolution, but very long exposure times (weeks to months) are needed.

 Specific activity. The specific activity is the amount of radioactivity per amount of material. If the molecule that you want to label is rare, it is usually helpful to start with radioactivity of high specific activity. However, always ordering the highest specific activity material possible is not a good thing. It may be overkill for your detection system, and it makes the experiment more

TABLE 2. Features of Isotopes for Probe Labeling

Isotope	^{32}P	^{33}P	^{35}S	^{125}I	^{3}H
Energy of emission (MeV)	1.71	0.249	0.167	0.035	0.018
Resolution (µm)	20–30	15–20	10–15	1–10	0.5–1.0
Application	Macroscale in situ optimization of parameters	Localization at the cellular level	Localization at the cellular level	Subcellular localization	Subcellular localization
Advantage of label	Detection using X-ray film	Short exposure	Short exposure, medium resolution	High sensitivity, short exposure	High resolution
	Short exposure			Good resolution	
Disadvantage of label	Low resolution			γ-emitter	Long exposure times

(Adapted, with permission, from Amersham Pharmacia Biotech.)

dangerous. The specific activity does not change with time, but the total amount of radioactivity changes and your experiment may need to be adjusted for decay. For example, after 14.3 days, half of the ^{32}P will have decayed to ^{32}S.

> *The shorter the half-life, the greater the potential specific activity (number of nuclear disintegrations per minute per mole) achievable.*

Half-life. The half-life ($T_{1/2}$) of a radioactive isotope is the time needed for the initial number of radioactive atoms to decrease by half. The half-life determines both the remaining activity after storage or use, and the time that the isotope must be stored before disposal. This is only an issue for short-lived radioisotopes. However, there is a disposal issue for long-lived radioisotopes: Many institutions now charge for their disposal, an inducement to not order ^{14}C or ^{3}H unless you really need it.

> For example, using ^{33}P instead of ^{32}P or ^{35}S shortens the decay period of the waste, and reduces storage time before disposal. It has an energy 1/7th that of ^{32}P, and so reduces the potential exposure of workers to potentially harmful radiation, while providing better resolution and sensitivity than ^{32}P. ^{33}P nucleotides and deoxynucleotides are more expensive.

Time of use. Plan your purchases of labeled compounds to *avoid prolonged storage*. Take into account the half-life of your intended purchase: If your compound has a half-life of 14 days, it doesn't make any sense to order it immediately for an experiment in 3 weeks.

Quantity. Don't buy it *unless you need it!!* 1 mCi may cost $50.00, and 2 mCi may be $60.00, and it is very tempting to purchase the higher quantity, just in case. *It costs money to dispose of long-lived isotopes.* And you may be inspired to use it up with nonsensical and wasteful experiments.

> *Be aware that companies make particular compounds only on certain days or weeks, so it is not always possible to obtain your isotope just when you are ready for it. Check the catalog for the production and shipping schedule of the compound.*

Ordering

The ordering and delivery of radioisotopes is usually centrally controlled. In most cases, the institution itself is licensed to purchase radioactive material, and a department—usually EHS—will oversee the distribution of the purchased radioisotopes. You must check on the ordering procedure, which may be different from the procedure to purchase other supplies.

> *Save the data sheet when your product comes in. This contains vital information about the amount of radioactivity and use and storage conditions.*

When you receive your order, check it carefully. All vendors can make mistakes. Be sure the material and amount are what you ordered, and that the volume appears to be correct.

DOING RADIOACTIVE EXPERIMENTS

Rad Rules

- **Obtain necessary laboratory and institutional certification before you start any experiments.** The use of radioactivity in the lab is federally controlled. Unauthorized use is dangerous and can lead to a laboratory shut-down.

- **Work only in a place designated for radioactive work.** This may be your lab bench. Check which isotopes can be used on your bench: Many labs permit low-energy β emitters or small quantities of high-energy emitters on the bench but require that large labeling experiments be done in another area (the "hot" room).

- **Cover all work surfaces with spill paper or a tray.** Remove the paper or tray after the experiment.

- **Aerosol-generating procedures such as iodination, sonication, and homogenization should be done in a fume hood.** The fume hood used for iodinations must be approved for this use by EHS. If possible, open rotors and bottles behind a shield.

- **Wear lab coat and gloves when working with any radioactivity.** Use two pairs of powder-free latex gloves when working with ^{125}I and large amounts of ^{32}P. Change gloves frequently.

- **Monitor the working area frequently.** Do this **before** you work, **during** the experiment, and **after** the experiment. Pipettors commonly become contaminated. Don't forget to check the monitor itself.

- **Monitor yourself.** Wear the appropriate dosimeters when working with γ and high-energy β emitters. Pass a survey meter over yourself frequently while working. In particular, monitor your gloves frequently. Monitor yourself after working.

- **Minimize accumulation of waste and dispose of it only by appropriate routes.** Before you begin an experiment, know where you will dispose of radioactive glassware, trash, solvents, and biohazards.

- **Inform other lab members** when you will do an experiment involving over 10 μCi. Put a sign on any piece of equipment you will be using, such as centrifuges and incubators, so other lab workers can stay out of your way and minimize their own exposure.

- **Record all acquisition, use, and disposal of all radioactive material.** This information is required by EHS.

Safety Issues

Is it safe? No issue has such a cloud of fear around it as radiation does. Pregnant women sometimes won't go near it, lab workers might refuse to do a turn at radiation disposal. Yet the levels at which most lab workers use radioactivity make it much less dangerous than many other commonly used materials in the lab.

Not that working with radioactivity should be taken lightly. If you are working with radioactivity, you must plan every step of the way. Everything from procurement of the starting radioactive material to disposal of the remains of the experiment must be done with deliberateness. No guesswork is allowed, and you must follow the rules *every single time.* This is what is worrisome to many. But this deliberateness, this establishment of multiple safety nets, protects you in case there are mistakes.

Yes, by following the rules, it generally is safe to work with radiation. But there are some caveats:

- **Some isotopes pose more risk than others.** High-energy β isotopes (^{32}P) can potentially cause more damage than low-energy isotopes (^{35}S, ^{3}H, ^{14}C). All γ-emitting isotopes, even relatively low energy ones (^{125}I) can penetrate the body.

> *The complacency that comes from working with low-energy isotopes can also be a risk.*

- **Large amounts of isotopes pose more risk than small amounts.** Minimize the size of the experiments and the number of samples.

- **Certain procedures with isotopes pose more risk than do others.** Labeling a piece of nucleic acid will be much safer than labeling whole cells and isolating labeled cellular components, a procedure that involves a lot of label, cell lysis, and multiple centrifugation and pipeting steps. The simpler the experiment, the safer. Radioiodinating a protein is more dangerous than most routine lab labeling experiments because iodine itself is volatile.

- **You can control yourself, but you can't always guard against other people.** The **macho phenomenon** is the most alive in the field of radioactivity. Although some labs have all the safety devices needed, others take great pleasure in ignoring the rules, showing great bravery in handling radioactivity without appropriate protection.

- **Irrational fear is dangerous.** There is no place for fear and paranoia when working with radiation. You must be knowledgeable and you must remain vigilant, but if you are too fearful, you become the safety hazard.

Pregnancy. If you become pregnant, you should talk to EHS. There are federal guidelines for the amount of exposure considered safe for an unborn child. Most radiochemicals, used at standard lab dosages, are safe to use. Many solvents and biological reagents present much more of a hazard than routinely used radioisotopes. High-energy emitters, especially in mCi amounts, potentially present more of a problem, and you may choose to delay certain experiments. 8–15 weeks after gestation is the period in which the fetus is the most susceptible to the teratogenic effects of radiation. Another option is to ask a lab member to do any particularly hot experimental manipulations for you.

Before you use radioactivity in a lab, ensure that the work can be done safely there. If it can't, either buy what you need, or find another lab in which to do the experiment. Look after safety issues for yourself. If you think something is unsafe and needs to be changed, initiate the change yourself. Do not compromise with anyone on safety issues.

Reducing external exposure

Minimizing exposure to radiation is the key to cutting down on risk. This is done by:

- Shielding
- Protective clothing

- Controlling the duration of exposure
- Controlling distance from the source
- Proper monitoring

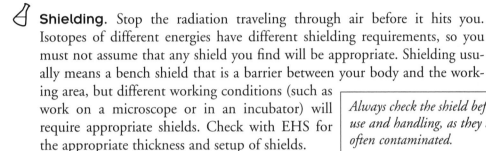 **Shielding.** Stop the radiation traveling through air before it hits you. Isotopes of different energies have different shielding requirements, so you must not assume that any shield you find will be appropriate. Shielding usually means a bench shield that is a barrier between your body and the working area, but different working conditions (such as work on a microscope or in an incubator) will require appropriate shields. Check with EHS for the appropriate thickness and setup of shields.

> *Always check the shield before use and handling, as they are often contaminated.*

The energy and kind of decay particle will determine the penetration of the radiation and therefore determine the degree of shielding necessary to protect the user.

- **Low-energy β** emitters such as tritium **do not require shielding, as the low-energy β** rays emitted do not penetrate the outer dead layer of skin. However, working behind a shield can reduce the risk of spilling radioactivity on your clothes, and cordons off the radioactive working area.

- **High-energy β** emitters (up to 20 millicuries) require an acrylic shield. **1 cm of acrylic will stop all βs**, and is appropriate for up to 10 or 20 millicuries of radioactive material.

- **High-energy β** emitters (greater than tens of millicuries) require at least 1 cm of acrylic, as well as some lead shielding.** This is because the absorption of the beta particles by the shield material gives rise to relatively high-energy *bremsstrahlung* radiation, against which lead is an effective shield. Leaded but see-through acrylic shields are available, or a secondary shield of lead could be placed between the acrylic and the worker.

- **X-ray and γ** emitters require a suitable thickness of lead or lead acrylic for shielding.

You must shield not only yourself, but other people in the lab, as well. If you use radioactivity on your bench, be sure the person on the other side of the bench is not being exposed. A simple slab shield will not protect anyone working to the side or back of the shield: You may need side panels, a workstation, or other shields placed in strategic locations.

All radioactivity must be in a shielded container during storage and transportation.

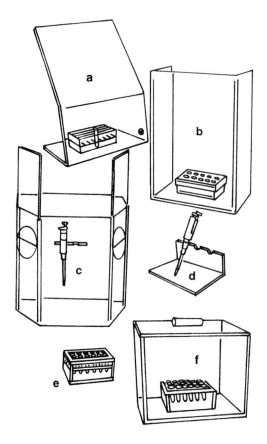

FIGURE 3.

Radioactive material must be shielded during storage and transportation, as well as during experiments. *a*, *b*, and *c* show shields and workstations of increasing protection, to be used while working. The hand and fingers can suffer the most exposure, and can be protected by a hand shield (*d*). Even if you are just crossing the hall, your radioactive samples should be carried in a shielded carrier, as shown in e. During storage in the refrigerator or freezer, all radioactivity should be restricted to a protective container (*f*).

Protective clothing. You should handle no radioactive material without wearing protective clothing. Many compounds, including some labeled with tritium (which is difficult to monitor), can be absorbed through the skin.

Gloves must always be worn. The gloves should be appropriate for the chemical nature of the material, not only for the radioactivity. You need protection, but you also must be able to manuever safely: Ask EHS for advice if you are using an organic-solvent-based isotope. Standard latex gloves are fine for most radioactive work. Whenever possible, wear a double set of gloves: This way, if the outer set becomes contaminated, it can be quickly shed. Gloves should be discarded as radioactive dry waste.

The lab coat you wear for hot experiments should not be used for non-radioactive work. One option is the use of disposable lab coats for radioactive work.

Use the Geiger counter or γ monitor to check your lab coat before you put it in the laundry. If it has been contaminated, ask EHS how to deal with it.

Duration of exposure. Reduce the time you are working with an isotope. The more smoothly the experiment goes, the less likely it is that you have excess exposure. Design the experiment so the label is added as late as possible. Do a dry run of the experiment without isotope. Make sure you have everything you need— pipets, disposal containers, tube holders, the most trivial component—so you don't have to search or plan for anything during the experiment.

Distance from the source. Keep your body as far from the work area as you safely and comfortably can. Doubling the distance from the source quarters the radiation dose. The radiation intensity decreases with the square of the distance.

Monitoring. By assessing and reassessing the amount of radiation you are exposed to, you can alter your behavior accordingly before and during experiments.

The Geiger-Muller survey meter (commonly known as a Geiger counter), is a type of gas-filled detector. Most counters in the lab have both a digital or analog meter and an auditory signal, as readouts. Be aware that

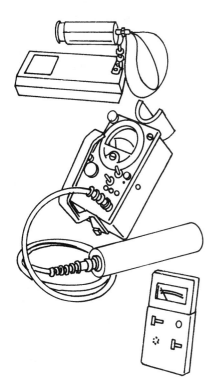

FIGURE 4.

There are many detector models in the lab, but you can't determine the capability by model appearance alone. There are β and γ meters, and within each group there are models with different efficiencies for different isotopes. Be sure to use one that can detect the kind of radiation you are using. Hold the detector about an inch from the surface to be tested and move it very slowly to survey for radiation.

there are different kinds of Geiger-Muller detectors, with the capability of measuring different kinds of ionizing radiation. Most cannot detect γ radiation. You must use the appropriate detector. Geiger-Muller detectors must be checked and calibrated routinely, usually by EHS.

NaI(Ti) (γ) survey meters can detect γ radiation, as well as *bremsstrahlung* radiation from high-energy β emitters such as ^{32}P.

Personal dosimeters (often known as badges) are worn on the body, and record the amount of radiation the body is exposed to. There are different kinds of dosimeters (for example, film badges, or thermoluminescent dosimeters [TLD] for work with high-energy β emitters) and the institutional lab or radiation safety department will determine

> *The probe on γ and Geiger counters can easily get contaminated. Keep a piece of thin plastic (Saran Wrap) on the probe, held on with a rubber band.*

which dosimeter should be worn and how often it should be checked. They may be shaped like a pen, or like a badge. Dosimeters are also made for hands or fingers, and these should be used if you will be doing a lot of manipulation with high-energy βs.

Working areas should be wiped or swabbed and counted regularly: Q-tips are handy for this, but dampen the tip slightly to increase efficiency. This may be done by the laboratory itself, or by EHS. This is particularly important for tritium, which, because of its low β-energy, cannot be monitored directly.

> *Turn your badge in, and pick up your new badge, at the required interval. Don't pile badges up in your drawer. Don't leave them where they can be accidentally exposed, and be sure to wear the badge when you are working.*

Working Routines

Establish for yourself a set of rules and routines that will ease worry about your next step. Unless you do radioactivity very rarely, you should use an area dedicated to radioactive work only. It may be a common area of the laboratory or a small area of your bench, but it is important that you work in an area in which everything—the pipettors, the aspirator, sharps disposal—can be used during the experiment.

 Before you start an experiment, check

- *The protocol.* Your protocol should be detailed, so you don't have to make any procedural decisions during the experiment. Hang it near the bench, where you will be able to consult it without fumbling through a notebook.

- *The correct supplies and equipment.* You don't want to break your concentration during the experiment to search for a coverslip. Think through the

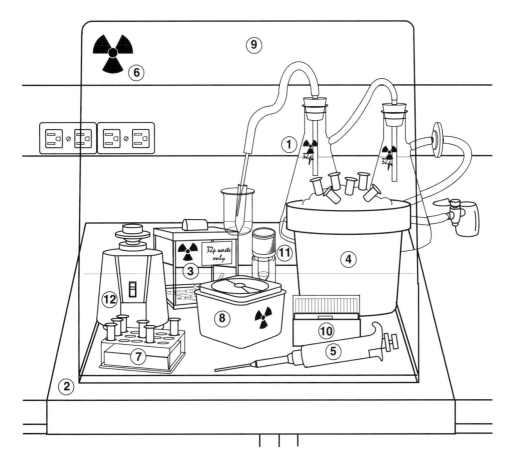

FIGURE 5.

Radioactive work area. As for work with an infectious agent, the bench used for radioactivity should be set up to minimize hand movements (and thus, accidents and spills). **Key:** (1) *Aspirator.* (2) *Bench paper.* (3) *Dry waste container.* (4) *Ice bucket.* (5) *Pipettor.* (6) *Radioactive symbol.* (7) *Samples in a β rack.* (8) *Sharps and tips container.* (9) *Shield.* (10) *Tips.* (11) *Vial of radioactivity.* (12) *Vortex.*

experiment and list your needs as you compose the protocol. Minimize reusable glassware if your samples are very hot, minimize disposables if the samples aren't very hot.

- *Disposal of waste.* You must have a designated place to put every piece of radioactive material while you are working. Paper towels, sharps, supernatants, used gloves, and tubes must be put safely out of the way.

  Most radioactive work areas require a dedicated aspirator (see Chapter 3). Each class of isotopes (long-lived isotopes together: short-lived isotopes together) requires its own flask setup. Infectious waste will require a separate setup than for other isotopes of the same class, as will hot organic waste. For details, check with EHS.

- *Safety.* Always have bench paper or a tray beneath the working area. This will contain spills, and make all cleanup afterward much easier. Be sure you have the appropriate shields and sample containers.

During the experiment

- Think aseptically! Much of aseptic technique is designed to save the material from contamination. In working with radiation, the main goal is to protect yourself. But thinking aseptically will help to minimize your exposure to radiation.

- Don't answer the telephone, or write a few notes in your notebook on your desk, or touch anything once you have put on your gloves for radioactive work. It is unsafe, makes it worthless to wear them, and scares people. Use a dedicated "hot" pencil to jot notes during the experiment, and transfer those notes immediately afterward to your lab book.

- *Concentrate.* Ask people not to talk to you during hot labelings.

Exposure to radioactivity can occur at times other than when you are directly performing the experiment. Conditions to be especially wary of:

Opening vials of radioisotopes. Aerosols may be generated when you open vials. Open all containers slowly and deliberately, behind a shield.

Frozen stock vials. Make sure the contents of the vial are completely thawed before you try to remove an aliquot. If the tip of a pipettor hits a frozen piece as you probe for fluid, it may easily knock the frozen (and radioactive) piece out of the vial and onto the bench or floor.

Centrifuging radioactive samples. Microfuges and centrifuges are inevitably contaminated by radioisotopes, even when all caps are tightly sealed. Most labs have certain centrifuges designated for radioactive work: If so, no other centrifuge can be used. Open all bottles behind a shield to protect yourself against aerosols: If possible, remove the rotor to a shielded area to remove the tubes.

Transporting radioisotopes. Even if you are going just down the hall, your samples should be carried in an acrylic or lead container.

Incubating labeled cells. Incubators look solid, but do not necessarily protect you from emitted radiation. ^{35}S, for example, will volatilize during incubation, and the shelf or roof above the sample can get quite hot. All flasks or dishes should be placed within an acrylic container or behind a shield. In addition, lab personnel should be informed of the radioactivity within the incubator the day before, so they can plan around your experiment.

After the experiment:

- Clean up. Absolutely nothing should be left behind. Remove the bench paper and dispose of it in the appropriate radioactive disposal. If you had a tray, wipe it clean with a paper towel or wash it (if permitted), and wash all reusable glassware. Empty the aspirator fluid into radioactive liquid waste and remove the sharps box (unless it is shielded). Everything you use for cleaning must also be discarded in radioactive waste.

> *A common cleaning agent is CountOff™, from New England Nuclear, which should be diluted before use. Keep a spray bottle of dilute CountOff near the sink.*

- Monitor. Use a survey meter to check your working area and all the tools you used. Check pipettors, pens, test tube racks, and the centrifuge. The incubator should be checked for contamination after the experiment, especially if you used a volatile substance such as ^{35}S. Check the floor, your body and lab coat, the shield: Check the monitor itself, if you used it during the experiment.

- Clean again. Wipe off any counts with a radioactive cleaning agent. Depending on the material, this agent will be a detergent or a mild acid: Check with EHS. Be particularly careful about what you use to clean the inside of centrifuges.

- Record. It is not always possible to completely document your experiment while it is under way, so do it now. Also record your radioactive usage for the experiment, and the amount of radioactivity you disposed of.

EXPERIMENTAL DETECTION OF RADIATION

The availability of varied and excellent detection methods is what makes the hassle of working with radioactivity worthwhile.

Autoradiography

Autoradiography is the localization and recording of a radiolabel within a solid specimen. The radiolabeled sample may be a *gel*, or a *filter*, or even *cell* or *tissue* samples.

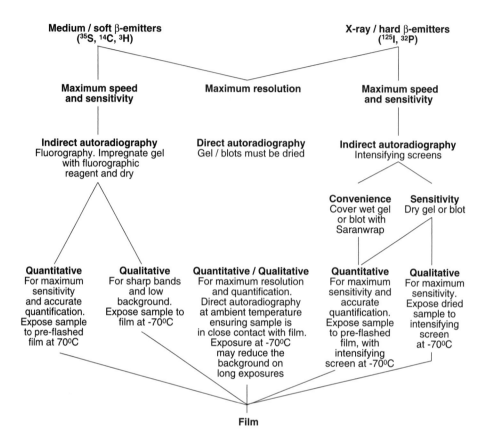

FIGURE 6.

Choose your isotope for autoradiography according to your needs. (Adapted, with permission, from Amersham Pharmacia Biotech.)

Applications for autoradiography

Band shift assays	In vitro transcription	RNase protection
Carbohydrate analysis	Kinase assays	RT-PCR
CAT assays	Library screening	S1 mapping
Cell proliferation	Microsatellite mapping	Slot Blots
Colony hybridization	Northern blotting	Southern blotting
DNA fingerprinting	Plaque lifts	SSCP
DNA quantitation	Primer extension	Short tandem repeat
DNA sequencing	Protein gels	TLC
DNA typing	RAPD	Western blotting
Dot Blots	RFLP	VNTR
Enzyme assays	RNA quantitation	

Detection and recording of the radioactivity may be done by film or phosphor-imager autoradiography. The sample must be properly prepared before detection of the radiation. The main preparation needed is the minimalization of the matrix of the sample so that the radioactive signal is not dampened or deflected, and so the distance traveled by the particles is as short as possible. This is done by drying the gel, filter, or cell or tissue sample to reduce water content.

Film autoradiography

Principle. The image is created by the interaction of a β particle or γ ray with the silver halide crystals in photographic emulsion, usually in X-ray film, but also in photographic emulsion.

Advantages and disadvantages. Most labs are set up for or have access to film autoradiography, with a darkroom, an X-Omat film processor, and boxes of film. No special cassettes are needed to hold the sample and film: Cardboard wrapped in aluminum foil to make it impenetrable to light works, as long as clips are used to ensure that the sample and film are in firm and uniform contact. The same film and film processor can be used for nonradioactive detection methods. Exposure times are longer than for the phosphorimager. A densitometer can be used to quantitate the data, but those data must usually be manually entered into a computer for analysis.

Use of an intensifying screen. Intensifying screens reduce the exposure time or increase the sensitivity in the detection of radiolabeled samples. They also decrease resolution. Conventional intensifying screens are effective with ^{32}P and ^{125}I, but not with ^{3}H, ^{14}C, ^{35}S, and ^{33}P. The screens work by generating photons through the interaction of the radiolabeled particles' energy and the phosphor in the intensifying screen. To make use of the screen, the isotope's particles must get through the film to the intensifying screen: Radioisotopes such as ^{3}H, ^{14}C, ^{35}S, and ^{33}P lack the energy to penetrate the screen.

Intensifying screens work best in the cold, between −60 and −80°C, since the cold is needed to lower the activation energy of the chemical reaction that makes the image on the film. If you use the screen at room temperature, more energy is needed to make an image, and you lose all the advantage the screen should provide. There are available intensifying screens that can work for weak to medium energy radioisotopes as well as for ^{32}P and ^{125}I. These screens don't depend on the energy of the isotope to penetrate the film to the screen.

Using two screens may increase the sensitivity, but it will also decrease the resolution. If you use two screens, orient them in the following way in the cassette:

Screen/specimen/film/screen.

Enhancing weak β *emissions: Fluorography.* Weak β emissions from isotopes such as ^{3}H, ^{35}S, or ^{14}C tend to be absorbed by the sample, and never reach the film to be recorded. By impregnating the gel or membrane with a scintillant, weak β particles are given the chance to transfer their energy to scintillator molecules, which then emit photons and are recorded on film.

After treatment with a scintillant such as Amplify (Amersham), the gel is dried and exposed at −70°C to film with an intensifying screen.

Film. Use a blue-colored base autoradiography film. The blue color is easier on the eye, and makes it easier to distinguish among gray bands. Buy films, cassettes, and screens of the same size gel format you usually use.

> *Preflashing—exposing film to a brief flash of light—is done to increase the linearity of the signal. It is not usually necessary.*

PROTOCOL

Exposing a Membrane to Film

Materials

- Film (There are several kinds. Most work fine.)

- Cassette. This can be a sturdy metal cassette, or a stiff cardboard folder.

- Intensifying screen for ^{125}I or ^{32}P.

- Whatman 3M paper. Other paper is fine, as long as it is a bit stiff and absorbent.

- Plastic wrap.

- Tape.

- Marker pen.

Procedure

1. As soon as the membrane has been through its final wash, touch the edge of it to drain the fluid off. Let sit at room temperature on the bench to dry briefly.

   > *A dried gel is treated in the same way as a membrane.*

2. Lay the membrane on a piece of Whatman's. Record your name, date, and all other pertinent information on the Whatman paper.

3. Put small pieces of tape, just barely attaching the corners of the membrane to the Whatman's.

4. Cover the membrane and Whatman's with the plastic wrap, taking care that the plastic wrap doesn't wrinkle or fold but is flat and flush with the surface of the paper and membrane. Fold it neatly in the back of the Whatman's.

5. Place the membrane in the cassette, and go to the darkroom.

6. With the safelight on, open the cassette on the bench. Always open it the same way, so you are always oriented. Place on the bottom of the open cassette, in order: the Whatman's with the membrane facing up, the film, and the intensifying screen.

   > *The film is inside an envelope, inside a cardboard box. The envelope should either be inverted in the box (so inadvertent opening of the box in light won't expose all the film) or should be carefully folded over. There are pieces of paper between each piece of film. Remove and discard the paper every time you take out a film—a box of paper can fool people into thinking you still have plenty of film.*

7. Close the cassette. Put away the film.

8. If you are using an intensifying screen, put the cassette in a –60 to –80°C freezer. Most labs have a specific place to put them—don't forget that the cassette isn't shielded. Be careful not to put a cassette with a strong signal on top of any other cassette, or you may ruin its film. Use plastic or lead sheets between cassettes. If you are not using a screen, expose at room temperature. This can be in a drawer, on a bench, in a closet, as long as it is shielded if it needs to be.

   > *Some films, rarely used, have emulsion on only one side. The emulsion side should face the membrane.*

9. Check with lab members for an estimated exposure time. Overexposure isn't a big worry, as you can always put the membrane down with another film for a shorter exposure. What you don't want to do is expose a low-energy emitter too soon. Times range from minutes for a strong ^{32}P signal to days or weeks for a weak ^{3}H signal.

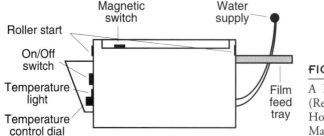

FIGURE 7.

A Kodak X-OMAT film processor. (Redrawn, with permission, from Holt 1990 in Donis-Keller Lab Manual 1995.)

PROTOCOL

Using an X-ray Film Processor, e.g., Kodak M35 X-OMAT (Adapted, with permission, from Holt M.S. 1990)

1. Films must be near room temperature before entering the processor. Remove film cassettes from the –80ºC freezer and allow them to warm to room temperature (usually 1–2 hours).

2. Turn on the water supply. This will probably be near the wall.

3. Turn the processor on by flipping the black toggle located at the left of the processor. Allow 15 minutes for the machine to warm up in the beginning of the day. Don't change the setting of the developer temperature.

4. Turn off the visible light and turn on the safelight.

5. Remove the first film from the film cassette and carry it to the feed tray. The film must be dry and at room temperature. Don't excessively shake the film to remove moisture, as the static buildup that may occur could leave marks on the developed film.

6. Push the roller-start button located near the top of both sides of the processor. The processor will buzz momentarily. Insert the film when the buzzer stops. The processor will draw the film in and buzz again, indicating that you may either insert another film or turn on the visible light.

7. Developed films drop into the tray at the left of the processor.

8. Shut off the power and the water supply at the end of the day.

Processor notes

- Film processors are usually shared equipment. There may be a sign-up list for use, and a list of particular rules to follow when using the processor.

- Some labs require that the first user in the morning wash the roller assembly before turning on the machine. To do this, remove the lid and the roller assembly cover. Carefully remove the roller assembly, taking care not to contaminate any of the inner tanks with liquid from the dripping rollers. Rinse the rollers under warm tap water, then rinse in distilled water. Gunk tends to accumulate at the ends of the rollers. Shake the excess water off, and/or wipe with a paper towel, and return the rollers to the processor. Don't forget to replace the roller assembly cover before putting on the lid.

- A common morning ritual is running a test film (any old film) through the processor before processing new films. Debris that has accumulated on the rollers while the processor was idle overnight should come off on the test film and not on the new film.

- The processor will cycle at regular intervals to keep the rollers wet. If the processor buzzes repeatedly, check the lid to be sure the magnetic switch is seated properly.

- A rapid thumping noise means one of the roller assemblies is dirty and is jamming. Wash the roller assembly, as described above.

- A gel may inadvertently be inserted into the processor, either because it was stuck to a film, or because the filter paper it is on was mistaken for a film. It may make it through, but it is more likely to get stuck in the rollers or contaminate one of the tanks. It must be removed immediately. Try not to do this.

Phosphorimager autoradiography

Principle. A phosphorimager employs a reusable screen instead of film for radioisotopic gel and blot analysis. Exposure of a storage phosphor screen to ionizing radiation induces latent image formation on the screen. This image is scanned by a laser, causing BaFBr:Eu+2 crystals in the screen to release blue light (phosphorescence) and return to the ground state. Blue light is collected by a fiber optic bundle, is channeled to a photomultiplier tube, and is digitized and measured to form a quantitative representation of the sample.

Advantages and disadvantages. Everything is done on the lab bench under normal lighting conditions, exposure times are a fraction of the times necessary for film autoradiography, and the exposure range is several magnitudes wider than for film. Images can be quantitated and manipulated with the software that is part of the phosphorimager computer. But the equipment is expensive, and is appearing slowly in labs and departments.

How to Expose a Sample

1. Prepare sample as you would for film autoradiography. Do not use enhancers or fluors.

2. Erase the storage phosphor screen by exposing it to visible light on a lightbox, or following the manufacturer's instructions for erasing.

3. Place your sample in the cassette and lay the screen on top to begin the exposure. For a first exposure, use 1/10 the exposure time you would expect from film use.

4. Slide the screen face down into the phosphorimager.

5. Scan and analyze.

Liquid Scintillation Counting

Low- and high-energy β radionucleotides can be detected in liquid scintillant, in a scintillation counter.

Principle. When β-particles are absorbed by special fluorescent chemicals called scintillants, they result in the emission of light. The light pulse may be seen by a pair of photomultiplier tubes. A scintillation counter records the faint light pulses and registers each one as a radioactive event or count. Usually the unit is given as counts per minute (cpm).

- If the percentage of actual radioactive decays that result in a collision with a scintillant (that is, the efficiency of counting by that particular machine) is known, then disintegrations per minute (dpm) can be calculated. This can be done by counting a standard of known activity and dividing the obtained values by the actual value to obtain the efficiency:

$$\text{Efficiency of counting} = \frac{\text{net cpm of standard}}{\text{dpm of standard}}$$

- Standards for ^{3}H tritium and ^{14}C are often purchased by the lab and are stored near or in the counter, or they can be obtained from EHS. Standards for shorter-lived isotopes can be made by counting an amount of isotope and calculating the dpm with the formula 1 Ci = 2.22 x 10^{12} dpm. To be accurate, you must use a half-life table for the isotope (found in the supplier's catolog) to know the remaining specific activity.

- γ counters are modified scintillation counters. The scintillant is a crystal placed outside the sample chamber: γ emissions can exit the sample vial and enter the fluorescent crystal. ^{125}I must be counted in a γ counter, without scintillant: In a pinch, it can be counted on the ^{3}H channel of a liquid scintillation counter.

- Different channels allow different wavelengths of light to be recorded, and these must be set for each isotope. In this way, both isotopes can be counted in dual-labeled samples.

> **Scintillation cocktails (fluors)**, a mixture of organic ingredients, have always presented toxic (fumes from the organic solvents used in fluors) and waste disposal problems. However, there are now available biodegradable cocktails with a low flash point and toxicity, capable of handling dry and aqueous samples, and these should always be used preferentially. Examples of these fluors are Ready Safe™ by Beckman, Ultima Gold™ by Packard, and Cytoscint™ by ICN. Samples with high salt, protein, organic content, or acid, may require another scintillant.

- Mix the sample and the scintillant well by inversion or with a vortex.

- Use glass mini-vials (7 ml) with hard caps. 20-ml vials should only be used in extraordinary circumstances.

- Limit the amount of counts you put in your vials. Most counters cannot count above 10^7 cpm, and counts between 1,000 and 10,000 are the best range in which to work.

- Count longer when the number of counts is small. With high counts, one minute of counting is sufficient. With low counts, count each sample 10 minutes.

- Substances that absorb the UV photon emitted by the scintillant (color quenching) or energy from the sample or scintillator (chemical quenching) reduce the efficiency of counting. With quenching, there is a shift of the counts toward a lower energy range, a shift in the windows. Use an internal standard (known cpm added to a sample vial) to find out if there is quenching and to determine the true efficiency of counting if quantitation is important.

- Remove your vials from the counter as soon as they have been counted.

- Scintillation counters can also be used to measure light generated by chemical reactions. The light is transmitted directly so no scintillant need be used.

> *Disposal of scintillation vials is separate from all other radioactive waste!*

^{32}P Cerenkov Counting

Cerenkov counting is a less efficient way than liquid scintillation counting to quantitate high-energy β emission, but it is faster to set up and reduces the danger and waste disposal problems associated with liquid scintillation counting.

Principle. High-energy β particles traveling through water cause the polarization of molecules along their trajectory, which then emit photons of light (350–600 nm) as their energy returns to the ground state (the Cerenkov effect). This can be measured by using the ^{3}H channel (open wide, so all possible counts will register) on the scintillation counter. No scintillant is used.

- Good for relative counts (incorporated vs unincorporated label).

- Efficiency.

<blockquote>
Percent of ^{32}P energy spectrum above 0.5 MeV   = 80%
(the threshold for Cerenkov counting)

Counting efficiency: glass vials   = ~50%
                plastic vials   = ~60%

The efficiency of counting will be approximately 40%.
</blockquote>

- Quenching. Cerenkov emissions are subject to sample quenching, from optical differences. Take care that all sample volumes are the same to avoid irregular counts, and check for quenching by the addition of an internal standard.

STORAGE

Check the data sheet that accompanies your radiolabel to find the recommended storage conditions. Store only in areas approved for radioactive use.

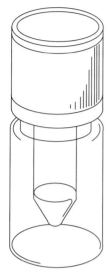

FIGURE 8.

It is sometimes difficult to see small volumes inside the manufacturer's vials. Tap the tube gently before opening to bring small drops from the lid to the bottom of the vial. (Redrawn, with permission, from Amersham Pharmacia Biotech.)

Temperature. Store your labeled compounds at $4°C$: Do not freeze unless this is recommended on the data sheet or by the company. The crystallization of the solvent during freezing can cause the formation of radiochemical aggregates that concentrate the sample and accelerate decomposition.

Aliquot. Minimize the number of times the primary container is opened, because impurities, especially oxygen and water, can be introduced. If a compound will be used several times, aliquot the required amounts to separate storage vials.

Shielding. If the compound came in a shielding container, store it in that container. Otherwise, you must provide a shielded container. Use a monitor to be sure the samples are adequately shielded.

Time. Every compound stored for more than 6 months should be checked for purity. If this is beyond your capacity to do, throw it away and order a new vial.

DISPOSAL

Radioactive waste must be carefully separated into classes that make long-term storage and disposal safe: Both *personal* and *environmental* safety are dependent on the safe disposal of radioactive waste.

There are many factors to consider when planning the disposal of radioactive waste in the lab, and this will already have been organized by the EHS and departmental EHS officer. The guidelines listed below for the disposal of radioactivity may be different at your institution.

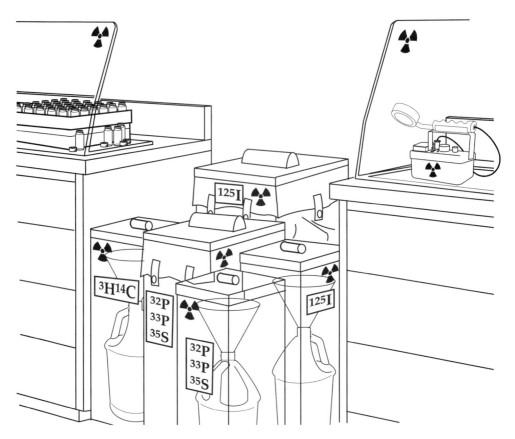

FIGURE 9.

One area of the lab will be dedicated to the disposal of radioactive material. Radioactive material is segregated by isotope (short half-life or long half-life), by chemical nature (aqueous or organic), and by phase (solid or liquid). Biohazard material and scintillation vials are handled separately: Biohazard material must be sterilized before disposal, and scintillation vials are usually disposed of capped and filled with material.

One place in the lab will be designated for radioactive waste. Here, waste will be segregated and stored until removal by EHS. This is done at regular intervals, or when EHS are called. Lab personnel are responsible for replacing containers and bags that they have filled, pH-ing liquid waste, and keeping the area neat and safe.

A suggested order of priority of disposal is:
1. Biohazard
2. ^{125}I waste
3. Half-life
4. Solid versus liquid
5. Aqueous versus organic
6. Scintillation vials
7. Manufacturer's containers

All radioactive waste containers must be labeled, and every piece of radioactive trash must be accounted for. The amount of radioactivity in must equal the amount of radioactivity out.

All **biohazard material** must be disinfected before disposal as "regular" radioactive waste. Liquid may be treated with bleach, solid may be autoclaved: Check with EHS to see how to treat volatile samples. It is then organized according to the priority list. Biohazard material in scintillation fluid is probably sterile: Check with EHS.

^{125}**I waste** is often held separately from other isotopes with short half-lives: As a γ emitter, it requires different shielding than β emitters. Waste from radioiodinations should be treated with 0.1 M Na thiosulfate to bind free radioiodine.

Radioactive waste is always separated with respect to **half-life**. Institutions can hold short-lived isotopes (<90 days or 120 days, depending on the institution) until the emitted radiation is near baseline, and then dispose of it as nonradioactive waste. The ultimate resting ground for long-lived isotopes in the future is still unknown: They must be stored safely indefinitely, a costly and potentially dangerous proposition.

Solid waste is disposed of in bins lined with plastic bags. When filled, the bag is removed, tagged, and immediately replaced by a new bag in the bin. The radioactive disposal area must never be left without a viable disposal container.

Liquid waste (aqueous) is usually poured into gallon plastic containers, through a funnel that is always left in the current container. This practice is actually contrary to EPA regulation. Nalge is currently marketing a one-piece cap/funnel with a lip so the container can always be kept closed.

Organic waste will go into separate containers, as prescribed by EHS.

Scintillation vials are discarded separately. They may be divided into short-life, long-life, and γ emitters. Don't dispose of loose vials: Be sure they are immobilized in a box or another container.

Do not discard the **lead pigs** in the radioactive trash, as they are not usually contaminated with radiation. They are collected for recycling: Otherwise, lead is considered to be hazardous waste (i.e., chemical waste). Check with EHS for instructions.

Manufacturer's vials—the containers that the radioisotope comes in—are also discarded separately. They will probably be divided into short-lived or long-lived isotopes. Discard manufacturer's containers regularly. They are hazardous to have

> *Policy varies from institution to institution as to the balance between safety and expense. You may be encouraged to wash disposable plasticware so it can be put in the regular trash, monitor paper towels and bench paper before disposing of them in radioactive waste, or disposing only the radioactive areas of bench paper. Follow the rules, but never compromise safety.*

All disposal of radioactivity must be recorded. Don't let records back up! Record use and disposal as you go, and save yourself a lot of trouble.

around, and their presence suggests that the lab may have more isotope than it should.

Cardboard boxes with radioactive markings won't be picked up as regular trash unless all radioactive markings are obliterated.

ALTERNATIVES TO RADIOACTIVITY

Radioactivity has been vital to the development of biology, but the issue of safety has always made the idea of an alternative an attractive one. Also, the fact that long-lived isotopes must be stored indefinitely clearly indicates that the current free and easy use of radioactivity will have to be curtailed.

There are nonradioactive substitutes for most protein and nucleic acid radioactive assays commonly done. In many cases, they actually provide more sensitivity than afforded by radioactivity, and the expense is often less. The main impediment to greater use of nonradioactive detection methods is that most laboratories have already invested so much in equipment and supplies that they are loathe to start anew. People get lazy and busy, and don't always want to try a new technique—the "why fix it if it ain't broke" philosophy.

The two main types of assays that substitute for radioactive techniques are colorimetric and chemiluminescent assays.

Colorimetric assays use an enzyme-tagged recognition molecule and the appropriate soluble chromogenic substrate to label molecules. Many colorimetric assays rely on the high affinity of streptavidan or avidan for biotin. The primary antibody (or DNA) is labeled with biotin, and is recognized by streptavidan that has been coupled to an enzyme such as alkaline phosphatase. Upon addition of an alkaline phosphatase substrate such as bromochloroindolyl phosphate/nitro blue tetrazolium (BCIP/NBT), an insoluble colored reaction product is formed. The product is visible on membrane for transfers, or can be quantitated in a spectrophotometer.

Chemiluminescent assays employ much of the hardware and techniques used for autoradiography. Light is chemically generated, and is detected on film, just as radioisotopes are. The ECL assay (Amersham) for Western blotting is an example of a chemiluminescent assay that uses the horseradish peroxidase-catalyzed generation of light (Fig. 10). After transfer, the membrane is incubated with the antibody of interest, the primary antibody, and nonbinding antibody is washed away. A secondary antibody, conjugated with HRP and directed against the primary, is then incubated with the membrane. HRP catalyzes the oxidation of the substrate luminol, which then emits light: This light is chemically enhanced and is recorded on film. The assay takes minutes to perform, and exposure time is also usually measured in minutes or even

> *If the primary antibody is a mouse antibody, the secondary antibody might be an anti-mouse antibody, made in rabbit. This secondary antibody would be called "HRP-conjugated rabbit anti-mouse antibody."*

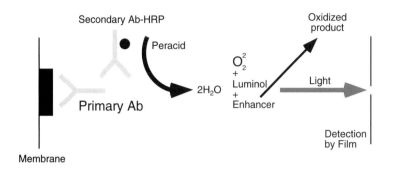

FIGURE 10.
The ECL assay: An example of the use of a nonradioactive detection system.

seconds. ECL can be used with streptavidan-peroxidase reagents for biotinylated antibodies.

Fluorescein label/anti-fluorescein antibody and digoxigenin label/anti-digoxigenin antibody are other systems often coupled to the enzyme-catalyzed generation of light. See Party and Gershey (1995) for a listing of colorimetric and chemiluminescent substitutes for radioactive assays. Many of these are made by radioisotope manufacturers.

RESOURCES

Amersham Life Sciences, Inc. 1992. *Guide to autoradiography.* Arlington Heights, Illinois.

Amersham Life Sciences, Inc. 1996. Catalog. Arlington Heights, Illinois.

Brown T.A., ed. 1991. *Molecular biology LabFax.* Chapter 3, *Radiochemicals.* BIOS Scientific Publishers, Blackwell Scientific Publications. Oxford, England.

Clark D.P., and Russell L.D. 1997. *Molecular biology made simple and fun.* Cache River Press, Vienna, Illinois.

Gerhardt P., Murray R.G.E., Wood W.A., and Krieg N.R., eds. 1994. *Methods for cellular and molecular bacteriology,* Chapter 21, *Physical analysis.* American Society for Microbiology, Washington, D.C.

Gershey E.L., Party E., and Wilkerson, A. 1991. *Laboratory safety in practice: A comprehensive compliance program and safety manual.* Van Nostrand Reinhold, New York.

Haugland R.P. 1996. *Handbook of fluorescent probes and research chemicals,* 6th edition. Molecular Probes, Eugene, Oregon.

Heidcamp W.H. 1995. *Cell biology laboratory manual.* Gustavus Adolphus College, St. Peter Minnesota. Appendix H: Radioactive tracer.
    http:/www.gac.edu/cgi-bin/user/~cellab/phpl?appds/appd-h.html

Holt M.S. 1990. *Appendix:Using the X-Ray Film Processor* (Kodak M35 X-OMAT).
    http://hdklab.wustl.edu/lab_manual/12/12_7.html
    In *Donis-Keller Lab, Lab Manual,* posted 1995.
    http://hdklab.wustl.edu/lab_manual/index.html

Howard G.C. 1993. *Methods in nonradioactive detection.* Appelton and Lange, Norwalk.

Molecular Dynamics. 1996. Brochure 9630. *PhosphorImager SI.* Sunnyvale, California.

Party E. and Gershey E.L. 1995. A review of some available radioactive and non-radioactive substitutes for use in biomedical research. *Health Phys.* **69:** 1–5.

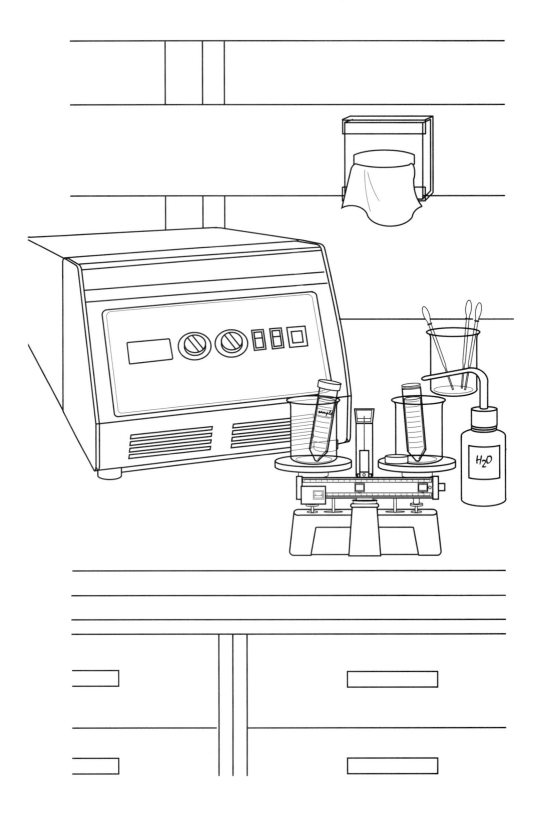

14

Centrifugation

HOW FAST, WHICH ONE, what speed, what temperature? The main use of the centrifuge is to separate biologically important substances, and very few experiments can be done without at least one spin in a centrifuge. Centrifuges are used to concentrate purified proteins, wash DNA, and pellet cells; there are specialized tubes, rotors, and centrifuges for just about any job. The centrifuge supplies the driving force, and the rotor dictates the functional specialization of centrifugation. You will probably use whatever centrifuge someone points you to, but know that, by choosing your centrifuge, rotor, and tubes carefully, you can get that sample just where you want it.

BACKGROUND	345
Centrifugation	346
Centrifuges	349
Rotors	351
WORKING RULES	353
HOW TO SPIN	355
How to determine centrifuge speed	357
Centrifuge tubes	358
Removing supernatants	363
Washing pellets	365
Spinning infectious or dangerous samples	366
GRADIENTS	367
CENTRIFUGE AND ROTOR MAINTENANCE	368
RESOURCES	371

The ubiquitousness of the centrifuge in the laboratory should not cause you to become casual with it. It is an important and complicated instrument that can ruin samples and cause personal injury if used carelessly.

BACKGROUND

A centrifuge is a device for separating particles from a solution. In the biological research lab, these particles are usually cells, organelles, or large molecules, such as DNA.

Centrifugation

There are two main kinds of centrifugation procedures: **Preparative**, the isolation of specific particles; and **analytical**, the measuring of the physical properties of a sedimenting particle.

Most of the centrifugation done in a molecular or cell biology lab is preparative centrifugation, and most of the routine preparative centrifugation done is differential centrifugation.

The *g*-force and revolutions per minute (rpm) listed are approximate: They are dependent on the centrifuge model and rotor used.

 ### Differential centrifugation (pelleting)

Theory: Samples are spun at a given speed, resulting in a supernatant and a pellet fraction. The sample is isolated by sedimentation velocity that, at constant centrifugal force, is proportional to the size of the particle and the difference between the density of the particle and the liquid.

Disadvantages: The pellet is a mixture of all the sedimented components, not all of which are desired.

Rotor used: Fixed, swinging bucket.

Examples: Pelleting bacteria or cells from growth medium, collecting precipitated DNA.

 ### Density gradient centrifugation

• **Rate-zonal centrifugation**

Theory: Separates particles having a similar buoyant density but differing in shape or particle size. Sample is layered on top of a gradient of sucrose

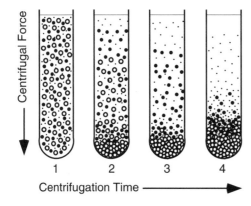

FIGURE 1.

Differential centrifugation (pelleting). (Redrawn, with permission, from Griffith 1986; Beckman Instruments.)

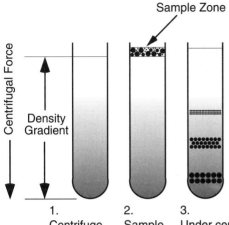

Sample Zone

1.
Centrifuge
tube filled
with density
gradient
solution

2.
Sample
applied
to top of
gradient

3.
Under centrifugal
force, particles
move at different
rates depending
upon their mass

FIGURE 2.

Rate zonal separation in a swinging-bucket rotor. (Redrawn, with permission, from Griffith 1986; Beckman Instruments.)

or other viscous medium: The particle density is higher than the liquid density, so the particle will ultimately pellet. Centrifugation must be stopped when the particle(s) has been separated, but before all particles have reached the bottom of the tube.

Rotor used: Swinging bucket or specially designed zonal rotor/centrifuge.

Examples: Isolation of ribosomal subunits on a 15–40% (w/v) sucrose gradient.

- **Isopycnic (Isodensity) density gradient centrifugation**

Theory: Like equilibrium density gradient centrifugation, used to separate particles on the basis of buoyant density. Sample is mixed with gradient material such as cesium chloride to provide a density equal to the average density of the particle. This homogeneous suspension is spun and a gradient formed during the spin. (Cesium chloride has a low viscosity, and it is difficult to make preformed gradients with it.) Particles cease sedimenting when they reach their buoyant density.

Rotor used: Swinging bucket, vertical, fixed angle. Fixed angle and vertical are preferable, since the shorter path length allows a shorter spin. For subcellular particles, 18–72 hours at 100,000–200,000g are needed.

Examples: Isolation of plasmid DNA in a cesium chloride gradient.

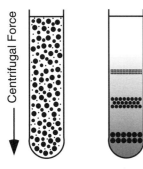

1. Uniform mixture of sample and gradient
2. Under centrifugal force, gradient redistributes and sample particles band at their isopycnic positions

FIGURE 3.

Isopycnic separation with a self-generating gradient. (Redrawn, with permission, from Griffith 1986; Beckman Instruments.)

- **Equilibrium density gradient centrifugation**

  Theory: Used to separate particles on the basis of buoyant density instead of sedimentation velocity, equilibrium density gradient centrifugation is actually a variant of isopycnic centrifugation, done with a preformed gradient instead of a self-generated one. The sample is centrifuged in a density gradient of a medium of density higher than the density of the cells or particles until an equilibrium is reached, at which each particle has

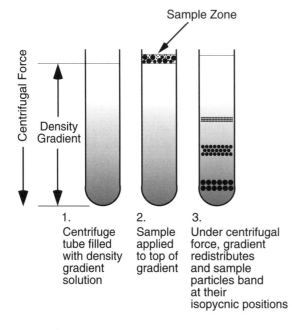

1. Centrifuge tube filled with density gradient solution
2. Sample applied to top of gradient
3. Under centrifugal force, gradient redistributes and sample particles band at their isopycnic positions

FIGURE 4.

Equilibrium density gradient centrifugation. (Redrawn, with permission, from Griffith 1986; Beckman Instruments.)

migrated to a point in the gradient where it has the same density as the surrounding solution.

Rotor used: Swinging bucket, fixed angle, vertical.

Examples: Isolation of lymphocytes on a Ficoll gradient.

Centrifuges

There are descriptive terms for types of centrifuges, but these are not strict definitions, and one centrifuge may fit into several categories. In the lab, centrifuges are generally called by the manufacturer's name.

High speed and ultracentrifuges are built with refrigeration units, needed because of the heat generated by high-speed spins. The other centrifuges are available in both refrigerated and non-refrigerated models.

- **Benchtop centrifuge.** Also known as a multipurpose centrifuge. It is not necessarily on a benchtop, and is often found under a bench.

  Uses: Pellet cells and bacteria, phenol extractions.
  g-Force and rpm: Fixed angle 17,000g/14,000 rpm. Swinging bucket 3,800g/4800 rpm.
  Rotors: Fixed angle, swinging bucket, microplate.
  Tube volumes: 2.0 ml–180 ml.

- **Clinical centrifuge**

  Uses: Serum, urine, cell, and blood sedimentation.
  g-Force and rpm: 4600g/6000 rpm.
  Rotors: Fixed and swinging bucket.
  Tubes: A variety of usually glass tubes, hematocrit capillaries to 75 ml.

- **Microfuge**

  Uses: Mini-phenol extractions and ethanol precipitations. Cell, at low speed.
  g-Force and rpm: Fixed angle 16,000g/13,000 rpm. Horizontal angle 13,000g.
  Rotors: Fixed, some rare swinging bucket.
  Tubes: Eppendorfs, 0.5 ml–2.0 ml.

- **High-speed centrifuge.** Also known as a high-performance centrifuge.

  Uses: Large-volume ethanol precipitations, pelleting bacteria, spin columns, protein precipitations.
  g-Force and rpm: Newer models can achieve 75,000g.
  Rotors: Fixed, swinging bucket.
  Tubes: Polyallomer, Pyrex.

- **Ultracentrifuge**

  Uses: Virus concentration, membrane and subcellular fraction isolation, DNA and RNA isolation.
  g-Force and rpm: 800,000g/100,000 rpm
  Rotors: Fixed angle, swinging bucket.
  Tubes: Nitrocellulose, polyallomer.

- **Benchtop ultracentrifuge**

  Uses: Membrane preps, virus isolation, subcellular fractionation. CsCl DNA plasmid isolations in 30 minutes.
  g-Force and rpm: 625,000g/120,000 rpm
  Rotors: Fixed angle, swinging bucket.
  Tubes: Nitrocellulose, polyallomer.

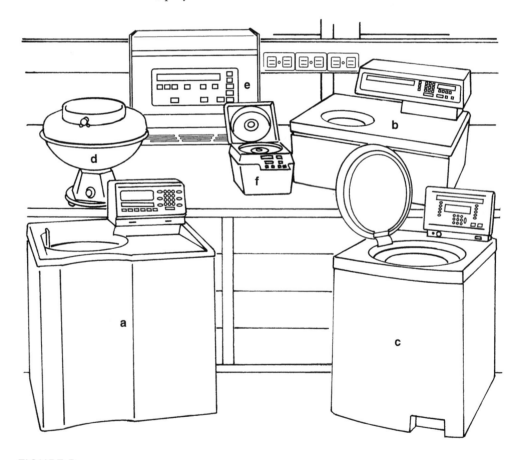

FIGURE 5.

Commonplace centrifuges are the ultracentrifuge, floor (*a*) and bench (*b*) models; the high-speed (*c*); clinical (*d*); general purpose (*e*); and microfuge (*f*).

Rotors

There are four main types of rotors: the fixed angle, swinging bucket, continuous flow, or zonal. Only the fixed-angle and swinging-bucket rotors are standard laboratory equipment: the other two are for very specialized use.

 ### Fixed angle

Uses. Sample concentration. This is the workhorse of the lab.
Description. Sample is held at a given angle to the rotation plane.
Advantages. Works the fastest. Substances have an increased relative centrifugal force and are sedimented faster than in a swinging-bucket rotor. Few moving parts, so few mechanical failures.
Disadvantages. Materials are forced against the side of the centrifuge tube, and then slide down the wall of the tube, leading to abrasion of the particles along the tube wall.
Examples. Sorvall SS-34, or the Beckman JA-20, near vertical rotor (NVR) (Beckman), vertical rotor for high-speed spins.

 ### Swinging bucket (also known as horizontal rotor)

Uses. Material separation. Used often in clinical work to gently separate cells.
Description. Sample is allowed to swing out on a pivot onto the plane of rotation.
Advantages. Materials must travel down the entire length of the centrifuge tube and through the media (often viscous) within the tube: This is gentler to the sample, and allows the formation of gradients and layers. Buckets can be exchanged in the rotor, so different sizes and shapes of tubes can be used. Less likely to cause aerosols.
Disadvantages. Longer apparent centrifugal force, takes longer time to precipitate than for fixed angle. There are many moving parts, which are prone to failure with extended use.
Examples. SW 55 Ti (Beckman).

 ### Continuous flow

Uses. Separation of particles or cells from large volumes of fluid: For example, pelleting liters of bacteria, monoclonal antibody production.
Description. Designed with inlet and outlet ports for separation of large vol-

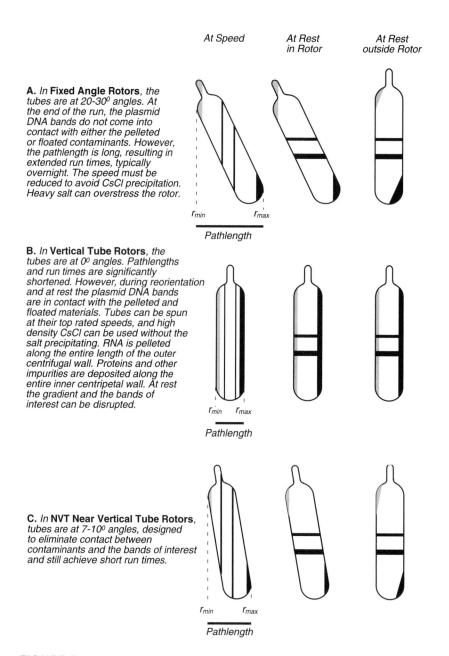

At Speed   At Rest   At Rest
                 in Rotor   outside Rotor

A. *In* **Fixed Angle Rotors**, *the tubes are at 20-30º angles. At the end of the run, the plasmid DNA bands do not come into contact with either the pelleted or floated contaminants. However, the pathlength is long, resulting in extended run times, typically overnight. The speed must be reduced to avoid CsCl precipitation. Heavy salt can overstress the rotor.*

r_{min} r_{max}

Pathlength

B. *In* **Vertical Tube Rotors**, *the tubes are at 0º angles. Pathlengths and run times are significantly shortened. However, during reorientation and at rest the plasmid DNA bands are in contact with the pelleted and floated materials. Tubes can be spun at their top rated speeds, and high density CsCl can be used without the salt precipitating. RNA is pelleted along the entire length of the outer centrifugal wall. Proteins and other impurities are deposited along the entire inner centripetal wall. At rest the gradient and the bands of interest can be disrupted.*

r_{min} r_{max}

Pathlength

C. *In* **NVT Near Vertical Tube Rotors**, *tubes are at 7-10º angles, designed to eliminate contact between contaminants and the bands of interest and still achieve short run times.*

r_{min} r_{max}

Pathlength

FIGURE 6.

Relative positions of the components of a plasmid prep after centrifugation through CsCl in three rotor types. The Near Vertical Tube Rotor (*C*) is the best choice for gradient centrifugation. Black areas represent pelleted material, gray shaded areas are floating components, and black lines indicate bands. (Redrawn, with permission, from Beckman Instruments.)

umes. As volume is slowly and continuously added from outside the centrifuge, the pellets in the tubes grow larger and larger. Different systems can handle 10 to 100 liters an hour.

Advantages. Large volumes can be used.

Disadvantages. Centrifuge must be adapted with inlet and outlet ports. Cleaning and maintenance take time. Many parts which can be lost or broken. Generates aerosols.

Examples. Sharples™ (for cream separation), Z-60 (Beckman).

 ## Zonal

Uses. Large-scale separation of particles on density gradients; can separate liters of solution and pounds of cells or tissue samples.

Description. Cell suspensions and density media can be pumped into the rotor through specialized ports, and the speed can be altered to selectively disgorge cells of different densities.

Advantages. Large volume handling.

Disadvantages. Fairly complicated for unskilled worker.

Examples. Centrifugal elutriator, CF-32 Ti (Beckman).

WORKING RULES

- Don't spin radioactive, biohazard, or infectious material in any centrifuge until you have checked that you are *using the appropriate and designated centrifuge* for those materials.

- *Balance all tubes and tube holders, caps and tops, shields and trunnions.* Don't merely balance the tubes—balance the entire assemblance of removable parts. Be careful that matched sets of trunnions, shields, and adapters are not mixed: Trunnions and shields usually have the weight stamped on them. If you use a balance tube, fill it with material similar to that of the material you are spinning: Water is fine for spinning bacteria out of media, for example, and for most spins, but not to balance cesium chloride.

- If there is a *sign-up sheet,* be meticulous about recording the necessary information. This information is needed to keep track of rotor usage, since many high speed and ultracentrifuge rotors will be down-rated (judged incapable of performing safely at the highest speeds) after a certain number of usage hours have been reached.

> *Not everyone may be careful when working with biohazard material in the centrifuge, and the rotor and the inside of the centrifuge may be contaminated. Use gloves when you are loading or cleaning a centrifuge.*

> *If trunnions, shields, and tubes are not inscribed with their weights by the manufacturer, mark matching sets with paint or colored Sharpies.*

- *Clean up every time* you use any centrifuge, including microfuges. Wipe down the inside of the centrifuge. Remove buckets from swinging-bucket rotors, rinse with distilled water, and dry, inverted. Rinse out the entire fixed-angle rotor.

- *Know the speed limitations of each centrifuge and rotor and do not pass them.* Remember that swinging-bucket rotors cannot go as fast as fixed-angle rotors, so don't make presumptions. If the centrifuge sounds labored when running, you have probably surpassed the recommended speed.

- *Use appropriate tubes and tube holders.* This is particularly important during high-speed spins, when more stress is put on the tube. Tubes should be neither loose nor tight in the holders or rotor. Many tubes and tube holders require adapters.

- *Cover tubes.* Use closures made for the tubes, or wrap the top with parafilm. Do not use aluminum foil, which detaches or ruptures and doesn't contain aerosols.

- *Fill tubes 1–2 cm from the top.* If you fill too much, you will get leaks even from screw-top tubes. If you fill too little, the tube may collapse.

- *Do not use a tube if it is cracked* or compromised in any way. Dispose of it immediately, don't try to save it for slow spins, etc. Check even wrapped disposable tubes for cracks. A tube with a minuscule crack may hold liquid without leaking before a spin, and will only break with the force of the centrifugation.

- *Always run all buckets of a swing-out rotor.* Open and inspect all buckets before and after use—one tube left in an apparently unused bucket can unbalance the centrifuge. Be sure the individual buckets are seated properly and swing freely.

- *Spin infectious material only in enclosed tubes, with covered containers.* Centrifuges generate aerosols, and infectious particles can be dangerously dispersed, even without an overt spill. Heat-sealed tubes should be used for highly toxic or pathogenic materials.

- *Don't forget the cover of the rotor!* Most fixed-angle, and some swinging-bucket, rotors have a lid that fits over the top of the rotor. If you find out you have left it off after your run has started, stop the centrifuge and put on the cover.

- *Close the lid on refrigerated centrifuges between runs to avoid condensation.*

- *Remove samples from the centrifuge immediately.* Never let samples sit after a run. The pellet could become dispersed, and the tubes might be moved by someone who needs the centrifuge. Also, it is extremely seedy to allow an ultracentrifuge run to go extra time because you don't want to come in when the run is ready.

HOW TO SPIN

No matter what the sample or the centrifuge, the basic steps of centrifugation are the same.

1. Choose tubes appropriate to the volume and the nature of what you will spin. Use as few tubes as possible, so find tubes as close to your volume as possible. If you are spinning a liter of bacteria, don't choose 20 x 50-ml tubes if you can choose 4 x 250-ml bottles. Choose tubes of a composition appropriate to your sample. Know the speed at which you will spin (step 2). Most tubes are suitable for low-speed spins, but you must be more particular about tubes for high-speed spins.

   > *Fill tubes to within 2 cm of the top.*

2. Choose a centrifuge and rotor appropriate to your sample and what you want done with it. Steps 1 and 2 actually must be decided at the same time. Know how fast the sample must be spun. Should the sample be refrigerated? Most should. Heat is generated during a centrifuge spin, and this can damage biological samples.

   > *Rotors are often kept in a cold room, the better to keep the samples cold after they are loaded into the rotor.*

3. Balance the tubes. Each tube must be spun with a tube of exact weight across from it. This is true for every rotor and every centrifuge, including microfuges, and for low-speed spins.

How to balance tubes

Only tubes across the rotor from each other need to be of the same weight.

Microfuge tubes. Adjust by volume, not weight: Add the same volume to each pair of tubes.

Ultracentrifuge tubes. Weigh tubes individually on a mettler balance. Tare the balance with a beaker, and weigh one tube at a time.

Benchtop and high-speed centrifuges. It is most convenient to use a pan balance, and balance tubes against each other.

If the sample is sterile, balance by eye as well as you can, and adjust the pairs by adding 70% alcohol or water to the space between the tube and bucket or adapter.

Use the same medium as your sample to balance lone tubes.

---

4. Put the tubes in the centrifuge, always in the same orientation. If the tube has an asymmetry, such as a lip on the closure, always put every tube in the holder in the same way, lip facing in or out. This way, you will always know where to look for the pellet.

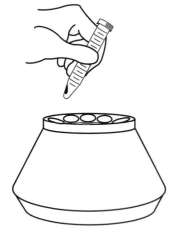

FIGURE 7.

Maintain the tube at the angle of the spin, to avoid perturbing the pellet.

5. Check and recheck that every tube has a balance placed correctly across from it. Especially when you have a lot of tubes, it is easy to forget a balance when loading the rotor. Check when you add the tubes to the rotor, and check again before you screw on the lid.

> *Missing balance tubes and incorrectly balanced tubes cause most centrifuge mishaps.*

6. Put the cover on the rotor. Although samples will usually be safe, you must use the lid every time. Keep it near the centrifuge so you can't forget to put it on. Screw it finger tight.

7. Close the lid of the centrifuge. You will hear a click with most centrifuges. And, unless the lid is properly closed, most centrifuges will not start.

8. Adjust the settings of the centrifuge. All settings must be checked, every time.

   Speed: Turn to 0. If it is a high-speed spin, start at 1000 and turn slowly up to the desired rpm once the centrifuge has been turned on. Some new centrifuges will calculate rpm if the *g* force is entered.
   Temperature: Cold for cells and bacteria, room temperature for phenol spins.
   Brake: Generally, on for pelleting, off for gradients. Check the protocol.
   Timer: Set for the amount of time you need to spin. The actual centrifugation time will be slightly longer because the rotor, even with a brake, will not stop immediately.

> *Do not stop a rotor manually! Not only can this cause injury to yourself, but it can be damaging to the motor shaft and to the brakes. Wait for the rotor to come to a complete stop by itself.*

9. Always wait for the centrifuge to come to full speed before you walk away. If there are any problems, such as unbalanced tubes, the problem usually

announces itself before full speed is reached. Don't be alarmed by a slight and momentary shudder as the centrifuge picks up speed, and the motor reaches its vibration point, as this is normal. But turn off the centrifuge immediately if you hear loud thunks or if a vibration continues.

10. Remove the tubes very slowly and carefully, so you don't disturb the pellet or band. Maintain the angle of the tube as you take the tube from the rotor. Note the position of the pellet, and mark the position of the pellet on the tube with a sharpie, if you are worried about finding the pellet. Have a bucket of ice or tube holder ready to hold the tubes.

11. Remove the supernatant. This can be done by decanting or aspiration.

12. Wash the pellets. (This is not always necessary. It usually improves the purity of the pellet, but do it only if specified.) To the pellet, add approximately half a tube of wash liquid. Cover and vortex until the pellet is resuspended. If the pellet remains fixed, use a sterile pipet to dislodge it from the side of the tube, and vortex again. Fill the tube, balance, and vortex again before spinning.

13. Remove the pellets. After removing the last wash liquid, resuspend the pellet in a small (2–5X the size of the pellet) volume of resuspension or wash fluid, and remove to a smaller tube.

14. Clean up. Wash tube holders, the rotor, and the inside of the centrifuge. Dispose of disposable centrifuge tubes in the appropriate trash (usually biohazard) and put glassware to soak (after rinsing with 10% bleach for biohazard material) or wash.

> *Although ultracentrifuge use basically requires the same steps, there are many other steps that are integral to safe use. For example, you might have to choose acceleration and deceleration times, or pump a vacuum to a certain level before achieving speed. Have someone demonstrate the ultracentrifuge before you use it!*

How to Determine Centrifuge Speed

When choosing a centrifuge for your samples, the speed you require is the main consideration. The volume of your sample is the second consideration.

Speed will be given as either gravitational force (*g*) or revolutions per minute (rpm). *g*-Force is also called RCF, or relative centrifugal force. The gravitational force is the force exerted during centrifugation. Protocols usually give centrifuge speed in *g*, which is a constant. Typical centrifuge speeds are 500*g* for mammalian cells, 3000*g* for bacteria, but this, of course, will vary.

> *For the most part, the kind of centrifuge you need is the one that is available. Labs tend to adapt protocols to centrifuges that are accessible: Centrifuges are expensive, and are generally used until they die.*

The rpm is dependent not only on the force exerted during centrifugation, but also on the type and size of the rotor and the centrifuge model.

△ **Calculating** *g.* You can calculate the *g* force from the rpm, and vice versa, by using this formula:

$$g = 1.12 \times 10^{-6} \times \text{radius (mm)} \times \text{rpm}^2$$

Measure the radius from the center of the rotor to the tip of the tube. For a fixed-angle rotor, how to do this is obvious and simple—just measure to the middle of the cavity. Most manufacturers give three radius measurements: the maximum, minimum, and average radius, or the distances from the center of rotation to the bottom, top, and middle of the sample tube. For most uses, the radius measurement won't matter, and you can use either the tip or middle of the tube measurement.

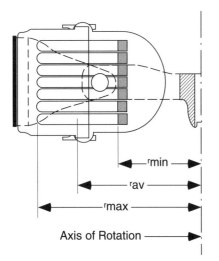

rmin

rav

rmax

Axis of Rotation

FIGURE 8.

To measure the radius for a swinging-bucket rotor, hold the tube out to approximate its position during centrifugation and measure from the tube to the rotor center. (Redrawn, with permission, from Beckman Instruments.)

The radius measurement can also be used to calculate the rpm or *g* from a nomogram (see Fig. 9). Use a ruler to draw a line from the radial distance to either the RCF or rpm, to find the unknown RCF or rpm.

Centrifuge Tubes

Considerations for choosing tubes

- Volumes can range from microliters to liters. The object is to try to use as few containers as you can. Fewer bottles means fewer manipulations, and this usually means a bigger yield.

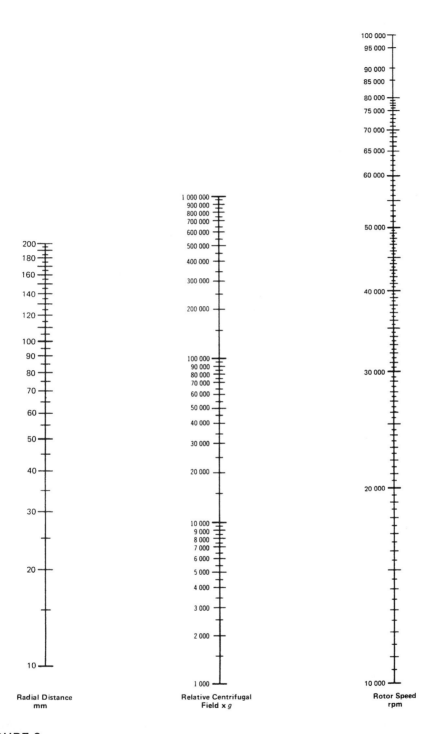

FIGURE 9.

Nomogram for computing relative centrifugal forces. (Reprinted, with permission, from Corning Science Products, Corning, New York.)

- Is your sample aqueous or organic? Is it biohazard material? The composition of the sample will influence the composition and the style of the tube.

   Aqueous samples will be fine in most plastics and glass. Organic materials are safe only in certain plastics, and in glass. Phenol extractions, for example, are usually spun in glass or in an inert material such as polypropylene.

   Special precautions must be taken for biohazard material. The top should be a screw or snap cap: The tube should never be left open.

- Temperature can affect the integrity of the tube. Clear polyallomer and Teflon FEP (not shown on chart) should be spun at maximum RCF only in a refrigerated centrifuge. Refrigerated centrifugation is not recommended for translucent polypropylene.

- Corex tubes (trademark Corex, from Corning Glass Works) are much stronger than regular glass tubes and are more resistant to heat, chemicals, and scratching. They are often used for collecting precipitated nucleic acids. They can be used at speeds up to 15,000–18,000, and may shatter above 18,000 rpm.

- Not all tubes can withstand all speeds. For low-speed spins, this doesn't matter. But as a tube is spun above approximately 5000g, it can shatter or crack from the centrifugal force. Never spin a tube above 5000g unless you are sure it is appropriate for that speed.

- Tubes may be round-bottomed or conical. For most cases, this doesn't matter. In a conical tube, spun in a swing-out rotor, the pellet will be a button on the bottom of the tube, and it is easier to remove the supernatant without disturbing the pellet. If you are spinning cells that don't like to be spun very hard and would therefore leave a soft, more diffuse pellet, this may be of some advantage. But swung in a fixed-angle rotor, the pellet in a conical tube may still be smeared along the side and on one side of the tube.

> *If you spin conical tubes, you will need an adapter, a rubber piece that conforms to the shape of the tube but is the same size as the holder or hole in the rotor. Some adapters just fit on the bottom of the tube. Without the adapter, which reduces centrifugal stress on the tube, the tube may shatter during the run.*

Bottles are used for larger volumes. These are round-bottomed, conical, and flat-bottomed. As for tubes, there is an advantage to using conical bottles for bacterial or cell pellets. And also, as for tubes, adapters should be used with conical bottles. Adapters should be used for flat-bottomed bottles as well.

Microwell plates may be spun in a swing-out rotor in microplate carriers, or in a rotor that has been adapted for microplates. The carriers can hold a standard size microplate, and adapters can be used for smaller plates.

TABLE 1. A Quick Reference Chart to Tube Materials and Their Properties

Type	Optical property	Puncturable	Sliceable	Reusable	Sterilization methods	Chemical resistance[a]
Ultra-Clear Thin-walled Standard tubes Quick-seal tubes	Transparent	Yes	Yes	Yes No	Cold sterilization only, but *not* with alcohol.	Good tolerance to all gradient media *except* alkaline ones (>pH 8). Satisfactory for most weak acids and a few weak bases. Unsatisfactory for DMSO and most organic solvents, including all alcohols.
Polyallomer Thin-walled Standard Quick seal	Translucent	Yes	Yes	Yes	All types can be autoclaved on a test tube rack at 121°C.	Good tolerance to all gradient media, including alkaline ones. Satisfactory for most acids, many bases, many alcohols, DMSO, and some organic solvents.
Polycarbonate Thick-walled Tubes Bottles	Transparent	No No No	No No No	Yes Yes	Cold sterilization recommended, but *not* with alcohol. Can be autoclaved at 121°C but tube life can be reduced	Good tolerance to all gradient media *except* alkaline ones (>pH 9). Satisfactory for some weak acids. Unsatisfactory for all bases, alcohols, and most organic solvents.
Polypropylene Tubes Bottles	Translucent	No	No	Yes Yes	Can be autoclaved at 121°C.	Good tolerance to all gradient media, including alkaline ones. Satisfactory for many acids, bases, and alcohols. Unsatisfactory for most organic solvents.
Stainless steel Tubes	Opaque	No	No	Yes	Can be autoclaved. Dry thoroughly before storage.	Good tolerance to many organic solvents. Marginal with many gradient media and salts. Unsatisfactory for most acids and many bases.
Polyethylene Tubes	Translucent	No	No	Yes	Can be autoclaved at 121°C.	Good tolerance to a wide range of chemicals. Suitable for use with strong acids and bases. Unsatisfactory for most organic solvents.
Corex/Pyrex Tubes Bottles	Transparent	No	No	Yes Yes	Can be autoclaved at 121°C.	Good tolerance to a wide range of gradient media. Corex has greater resistance to alkalis and acids.

(Reprinted, with permission, from Beckman Instruments.)

[a]Chemical resistances are described in general terms, and are not meant to express or imply any guarantee of safety based on these recommendations or resistances. If there is any doubt about a particular solution, it should be tested under actual operating conditions to evaluate the performance of a tube material. High vapor pressure inflammable solvents should not be handled in close vicinity to centrifuges because of possible ignition by sparking switches, relay contacts, or motor brushes.

- Caps must fit tightly, to minimize contamination of the inside of the centrifuge from the aerosols generated during the spin. Of course, no biohazard material must be spun without caps. But even seemingly innocuous material can mess the centrifuge and cause problems if not removed promptly.

Cover Corex tubes with a square of parafilm, not aluminum foil or cotton plugs. If a snap-cap is available for ultracentrifuge tubes, use it.

Heat-sealed tubes have only a nipple opening, and are used to spin hazardous substances in high speed and ultracentrifuges. The tubes are sealed shut before the run. These tubes are used for spinning hazardous substances such as cesium chloride gradients: The only downfall to their use is that the tube must be sliced or pierced to remove the contents, procedures which can also be hazardous.

> *Can disposable tubes and bottles be reused? Generally, yes. Can they be autoclaved? Generally, yes. However, tubes not designed for repeated autoclaving will break down, and you don't want that to happen during a run. If you reuse disposables, use them only for two or three low-speed spins, and then discard them.*

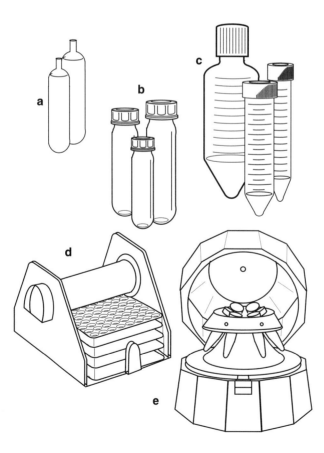

FIGURE 10.

Quick seal tubes (*a*) are heat-sealed and provide containment for biohazard material. Oak ridge style tubes (*b*), made of polyallomer, Teflon FEP, or polysulfone can be used for ethanol precipitations of large volume. Polypropylene 15-ml and 50-ml conical tubes and 250-ml bottles are excellent for pelleting cells (*c*). Microplate rotors or carriers (*d*) allow the microplates used for cell culture, biochemical assays, and DNA sequencing to be spun in an all-purpose centrifuge. A mini-centrifuge (*e*) only spins to a maximum of approximately 2,000*g*, but it can pellet cells and samples for electrophoresis.

Removing Supernatants

There are several ways to remove supernatants, with advantages and disadvantages to each.

- **Pouring off the supernatant (decanting)**

    Advantage: Quick.
    Disadvantage: Creates aerosols, may dislodge pellet.

- **Aspirating the supernatant**

    Advantage: Gentle, doesn't disturb pellet. Not messy, fewer aerosols.
    Disadvantage: Slow for large volumes.

⌂ Decanting supernatants from tubes and bottles

1. Set up an Erlenmeyer flask to use as a receptacle for the supernatant. If you will be spinning biohazard material (such as supernatants from cells or bacteria), add bleach to the bottom of the flask. Add an amount of bleach that is 10% of the volume you will be spinning and pouring.

2. Carry the bottle to the hood or bench where you will be working. Carry the bottle or tube at the same angle you have pulled it out of the rotor. There are tube racks that will maintain this angle.

3. Pour, keeping the pellet on top. If the pellet is firm, pour in one motion. Add wash liquid immediately, as many pellets should not be left to dry out. If you see the pellet starting to break up, stop pouring immediately. Try to aspirate the fluid around the pellet. If you are going to wash the pellet, don't try to remove supernatant at the risk of disturbing the pellet: You will have better luck after washing.

4. Allow the supernatants to incubate with the bleach for at least 30 minutes before pouring them down the drain.

⌂ Decanting supernatants from microplates

The entire plate should be quickly inverted: Partial inversion would allow dripping to occur from well to well. If there are cells or a reaction immobilized on the bottom of the wells, the plate may be quickly and sharply inverted onto a piece of paper towel on the bench.

> *There are automated microplate washers that can wash and remove liquid from all the wells. These are particularly useful for ELISAs.*

Aspirating supernatants from tubes and bottles (See Chapter 9 for more on aspiration.)

1. Attach a pasteur pipet into the tubing of the aspirator. Turn on the aspirator, and adjust so it is pulling only a gentle vacuum.

    You can protect the tip of the pasteur pipet by slipping a 100-µl pipettor tip over the end.

2. Hold the open tube at an angle, with the pellet on the upper side.

3. Insert the tip of the pasteur pipet or tube just below the meniscus on the lower side of the tube.

4. Move the tip toward the base of the tube as the fluid is withdrawn, using gentle suction to avoid drawing the pellet into the pipet tip. Keep the tip away from the pellet.

5. Aspirate the walls of the tube to remove any adherent drops of fluid. With practice, you will be able to gently shake and cajole every drop of fluid away from the pellet by tilting and shaking the tube. You can then carefully aspirate the drops. It is usually desirable to remove as much of the supernatant as possible.

    If you are aspirating with a pipet and a bulb or pipettor, be careful not to blow air into the supernatant. This could disturb the pellet.

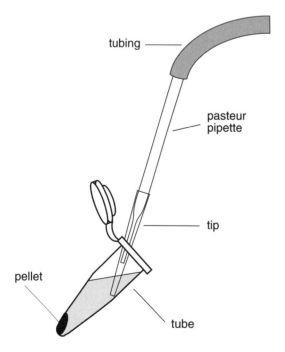

tubing

pasteur pipette

tip

pellet

tube

FIGURE 11.

Avoid the pellet as you aspirate closer toward the bottom of the tube. (Redrawn, with permission, from Sambrook et al. 1989.)

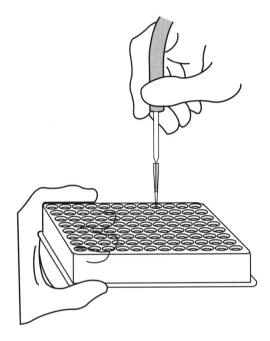

FIGURE 12.

Keep the microplate tilted toward you at an angle of about 30°. As you aspirate, bring the tip straight down, and you will avoid contact with the bottom of the well.

 Aspirating supernatants from microplates. You can quickly move from well to well with an aspirator, removing supernatants or medium. Tilt the plate toward you so the tip, if it contacts the well, will strike the side of the well and not the bottom where cells and reaction products will be concentrated.

Washing Pellets

- Washing the pellet will remove impurities, such as unwanted solvent or culture medium. It should be regular practice to wash pellets.

- The quality of the final preparation is helped by multiple washes. For cells or bacteria, one wash may suffice to spare the cells the trauma of another wash:

If no pellet is formed or is very loose:
- The spin may not have been fast enough or long enough.
- The suspension fluid is very thick. For example, cells may take much longer to sediment in serum than in culture medium.
- There may not be enough material to spin down.
Try to spin longer and faster. Attempts to remove medium around a loose pellet, and add a less dense medium such as a buffer may work. But the efficiency is low, recovery is low, and this should only be done to preserve a very precious material.

However, you must take into account the use the cells will have. If you need them for an enzymatic reaction, it is probably necessary to wash twice.

- Yes, you must *resuspend* the entire pellet in the wash fluid before you centrifuge! If you don't, washing will not be effective. The impurities will be trapped inside the pellet as well as outside, and you might as well do nothing as merely wash the outside of the pellet.

- After you have resuspended the pellet in the wash solution, which is usually a buffer of neutral pH, spin at the same speed at which you originally pelleted the material. But spin for half the time as for the original spin.

> *If the pellet is loose, or must be actually dried, it can be subjected to vacuum drying in a Speed-vac (see Chapter 12).*

Spinning Infectious or Dangerous Samples

Centrifugation is one of the riskiest procedures to perform with hazardous material. Aerosols are generated, and there is always a risk of tube breakage.

- Always use tubes you are sure of. Check carefully for cracks or chips; discard any tube that doesn't look prefect. Although disposable tubes can actually be reused, this isn't the time to do it.

- Use canisters with covers.

- Open the rotor in a hood.

- Open the tubes in a hood.

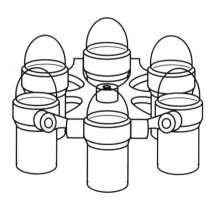

FIGURE 13.

Many buckets or canisters on trunnion-type swinging-bucket rotors have covers and O-rings that will contain biohazardous or dangerous materials.

GRADIENTS

Gradients are used to separate complex solutions and isolate a particular molecule.

 Common density media. Density media have different densities, viscosities, concentrations, and osmolarities. Some cells cannot tolerate some media and may suffer a loss in viability or function, so you should always ask around before using a particular medium for your cells.

- **Percoll™.** A synthetic colloidal suspension of polyvinyl pyrrolidone-coated silica. Designed for sedimentation centrifugation. In a fixed-angle rotor, it will spontaneously form linear gradients. Good for organelle and cell isolation.

- **Ficoll™.** A sucrose polymer, made by Pharmacia. Tends to be less viscous than other media at high density. Used for cell isolation.

- **Metrizamide (Nygaard).** A nonionic derivative of metrizoate. Used for cell isolation.

- **Sucrose.** Sucrose solutions are used to isolate organelles, and are seldom used for cells.

- **Cesium chloride.** A salt used for isopycnic separations, most commonly for the isolation of plasmid DNA.

 Making gradients. Gradients can be made by hand, by centrifugation, with a pump, or with a gradient maker. Discontinuous gradients, or step gradients, are often made by hand, since all one needs to do is to gently layer the lesser density media upon the more dense. An alternative method is to use a long-needled syringe to add layers of increasing density to the bottom of the tube.

Continuous gradients, with a smooth range of densities, can be made by centrifugation. For example, a gradient is formed during the centrifugation of cesium chloride, when isolating plasmid DNA. A gradient maker, which mixes the density media with diluting medium and pumps the increasingly less concentrated solution into a tube, can be used to make a linear or (with programmable models) step gradient.

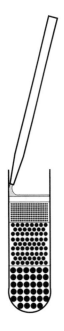

FIGURE 14.

To make a step gradient, use a syringe or pipet to slowly layer the less dense solution upon the more dense. Allow the solution to gently run down the side of the tube just above the surface, so it won't disturb the gradient.

 Removing cesium chloride bands. If you run a gradient at all, it may well be to isolated plasmid DNA by centrifugation through CsCl. Have someone walk you through the entire procedure before you attempt any part.

After the cesium chloride band has been removed from the tube, the ethidium bromide (EtBr) must be removed from the DNA. This is usually done by extraction with organic solvents, and protocols are available in most molecular biology manuals.

You should check with EHS about the disposal of EtBr. It is not okay to merely dump some bleach into the EtBr. In most labs, the EtBr solutions are decontaminated in the lab, and the EtBr is then disposed of in hazardous waste.

CENTRIFUGE AND ROTOR MAINTENANCE

 Centrifuge maintenance. Safe use of the centrifuge (as described earlier in the chapter) is the best way to maintain the centrifuge.

- **Wash any spills inside the centrifuge immediately.** Use water and a mild detergent. If it is a refrigerated centrifuge, don't allow the wash fluid to freeze: Dry well with paper towels after washing.

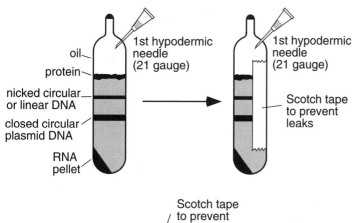

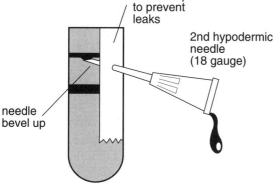

FIGURE 15.

Collection of plasmid DNA from CsCl gradients containing ethidium bromide. (Redrawn, with permission, from Sambrook et al. 1989.)

- **Call a serviceperson if the "Brushes" light comes on.** Brushes, part of the motor, become worn and must be replaced periodically.

- Don't panic immediately if the centrifuge doesn't start. Various safety devices work to ensure that a centrifuge shouldn't run until all settings are correct. If a centrifuge won't start, check that:

  1. The centrifuge is plugged in, and the control panel lighted (if it can be).

  2. The speed is set. Sometimes people turn the rpm to 0 when they are finished, and that is what you are getting—0 rpm.

Many labs have an equipment service plan for all centrifuges (not including microfuges). Basically, this is an insurance plan: The department or laboratory pays a company a set sum, and the company is responsible for payment for all breakdowns. Some service contracts will even cover maintenance. Before you call the manufacturer or a serviceperson to fix a problem centrifuge, check whether you have a service plan.

3. The centrifuge is at the correct temperature. If the temperature is set at a particular temperature, and it hasn't yet been reached, it may wait until that temperature is achieved.

4. The door is closed and the lock engaged.

Rotor Maintenance. Rotors are subjected to a great deal of force, and seemingly minor flaws can become major at high *g*-forces. Once the integrity of the structure is broken, the rotor can very quickly fail. Preventive maintenance is the only way to avoid problems.

*   *Observe the speed and sample density ratings for each rotor.* Centrifugal force can cause stress of the metal, making it stretch and change in size, and inappropriate speed is the major culprit. Every ultracentrifuge rotor has a maximum speed, and it is part of the rotor name: For example, the SW28 can achieve a maximum of 28,000 rpm. However, it is recommended that the SW28 not be used above 25,000. Check the manufacturer's manual to find the recommended speed for all rotors.

*   *Don't use a rotor past the time covered by the warranty.* Warranty times are based on a certain number of runs or hours of use, or to a certain period of time, after which the company considers use to be unsafe. Usually only high-speed and ultracentrifuge rotors are warrantied in this way.

*   *Have the rotor inspected periodically,* according to the manufacturer's suggestion.

*   *Keep the cavities and buckets of the rotor clean.* Moisture, chemicals, or alkaline solutions such as cesium chloride and other salts can cause metal surfaces to corrode. Rotors should be cleaned after every use.

    > *Never clean the cavities and buckets with an ordinary bottle brush, with sharp wire ends. These brushes can damage the rotor. Use plastic-coated brushes only.*

Cleaning rotors

1. Remove the buckets from swinging-bucket rotors. The body of the rotor should never be immersed in water, as the hanger mechanisms are hard to dry and may rust. The entire fixed-angle rotor can be rinsed, but should not be immersed in water.

2. Rinse each bucket or cavity with water. Be very careful when inverting fixed-angle rotors. If there has not been a spill, rinsing is usually sufficient.

3. If radioactive counts are not removed, or there has been a spill in a bucket, wash the bucket with a mild detergent. Ask the dealer to recommend a detergent. Most solutions used for radioactive decontamination are highly alkaline, and should not be used on a rotor.

4. Rinse with distilled or deionized water.

5. Air dry the buckets or fixed-angle rotor upside down, resting on a paper towel.

6. Store the rotor in a dry place. All fixed-angle rotors should be stored upside down, with lids or plugs removed. Swinging-bucket rotors should be stored with the buckets in place, but with the bucket caps removed.

RESOURCES

Centrifuge. 1996. GenChem Pages. Department of Chemistry, University of Wisconsin-Madison.
http://genchem.chem.wisc.edu/labdocs/catofp/centrifu.htm

Centrifugation. Nalgene Centrifuge Ware, Sigma catalog, p. 2067, 1996. Sigma-Aldrich, Milwaukee.

Collins C.H., Lyne P.M., and Grange J.M. 1991. *Microbiological methods,* 6th edition. Butterworth-Heinemann, Oxford.

Freshney R.I. 1994. Physical methods of cell separation. In *Culture of animal cells. A manual of basic technique,* 3rd edition. Wiley-Liss, New York.

Gerhardt P., Murray R.G.E., Wood W.A., and Krieg N.R., eds. 1994. *Methods for general and molecular bacteriology.* American Society for Microbiology, Washington, D.C.

Gershey E.L., Party E., and Wilkerson A. 1991. *Laboratory safety in practice: A comprehensive compliance program and safety manual.* Van Nostrand Reinhold, New York.

Griffith, O.M. 1986. *Techniques of Preparative, Zonal, and Continuous Flow Ultracentrifugation.* Applications Research Department, Spinco Division, Beckman Instruments, Fullerton, California.

Heidcamp W.H. 1995. *Cell biology laboratory manual.* Gustavus Adolphus College, St. Peter, Minnesota.
http://www.gac.edu/cgi-bin/user/~cellab/phpl?index-1.html

Rotor Safety Guide. 1987. Spinco Division of Beckman Instruments, Inc. Palo Alto, California.

Sambrook J., Fritsch E.F., and Maniatis T. 1989. *Molecular cloning: A laboratory manual.* Cold Spring Harbor Laboratory Press, Cold Spring Harbor, New York.

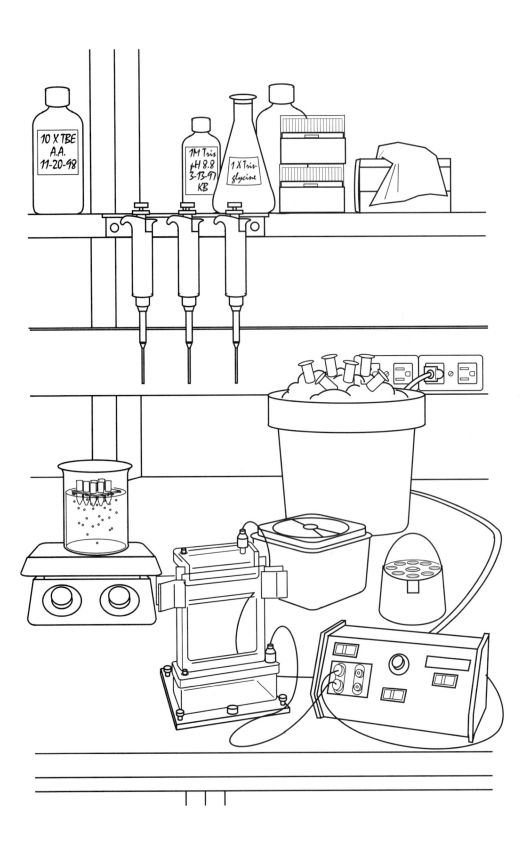

15

Electrophoresis

ELECTROPHORESIS, THE SEPA-RATION of charged molecules in an electrical field, is an essential technique in any lab. With electrophoresis, molecules in a mixture are separated from each other on the basis of size, shape, or charge. It is the first step for dozens of procedures, such as DNA sequencing and Western blots. Electrophoresis is automated in some labs, but in most labs, electrophoretic separation of DNA, RNA, and protein is done manually. Pouring a gel (the matrix

BASIC RULES	373
GENERALITIES	374
SPECIFICS	380
DNA gels	380
RNA gels	390
Protein gels	392
TRANSFERRING GEL CONTENTS	
TO MEMBRANES	397
RESOURCES	401

through which the molecules are separated) will probably become routine.

Whether your sample is a plasmid mini-prep or a purified protein, the steps for performing electrophoresis will be similar. Once you have run one gel, all other gels will be familiar.

BASIC RULES

- **Turn the power OFF** before manipulating a gel box.

- **Make sure the gel has solidified** before loading and running it.

- **Record what you loaded immediately.** As you load the wells, keep the tubes in the rack in the order in which they were loaded: Don't throw them away as you are working, only move the used tubes to another row. Use this order to check against your protocol or to write down the contents of each lane.

- **Wear gloves** if you are touching gels or gel buffer. The buffer may contain ethidium bromide (EtBr), a strong mutagen, and there might be traces of acrylamide powder around.

- Don't melt agarose with EtBr (or any lab stuff, actually) in a microwave used for food: **be sure the microwave you use has been okayed for EtBr use.**

- **Don't leave your gel to dry up in the gel box.** As soon as you have finished with the gel, dispose of the buffer and rinse out the gel box with distilled water.

- **Put the leads on correctly.** Black is –, the anode. Red is +, the cathode. Check the leads into the power supply, and the leads on the gel box, and check again. Unbelievable as it sounds, everyone makes this mistake, just once, and the samples migrate upward until halted.

  > *Watch the samples for a minute or two after you turn on the power supply to the gel, to be sure they are migrating in the proper direction.*

GENERALITIES

Sample preparation

- The sample must be actually dissolved in the sample buffer (also known as loading buffer), or it will not move through the gel. Too concentrated a sample can lead to artifacts.

- Sample buffers contain salts needed to maintain the sample, glycerol to add the weight needed to sink the sample in the well, and a tracking dye that allows you to monitor the progress of the electrophoresis.

- Sample buffers can be frozen in aliquots.

- Samples are loaded after buffer has been added to the gel.

- Tracking dyes in the sample buffer are used to indicate when the run should be terminated. The two most commonly used dyes are bromophenol blue (BPB) and xylene cyanol FF.

Standards/markers

- Molecular weight standards should be run. These can be used to monitor the progress of the run and to analyze the results.

- Use standards appropriate to the size of the molecular species you are interested in.

- Hang a Polaroid or a picture of a gel with the molecular weight markers you often use. Label the bands with the sizes. You will refer to these constantly.

- Standards are available unlabeled or labeled. Label can be fluorescence, luminescence, or radioactivity. If labeled markers aren't available, the stained gel can be compared with the labeled blot afterward.

- Load the standards into the same lane on every gel. It is easiest to always load your markers into the first lane. Knowing your standards are always in a particular lane gives you a point from which you can always orient yourself, should you drop the gel or just become confused.

- Whenever possible, positive and negative controls should be run.

Format

- Agarose gels are usually run horizontally, acrylamide gels are run vertically. Submarine gels are a type of horizontal gel in which the gel lies flush on the bottom of the chamber.

- Gels can be made in a variety of sizes. Sequencing gels do need to be large, but for most screening and transfers, even for 2-D gels, mini sizes will work fine as long as you are not trying to distinguish between bands of similar molecular weights.

- Capillary electrophoresis uses narrow-bore capillaries to perform automated and high-efficiency separations of DNA, proteins, or other small molecules. Separation is coupled to detection and analysis, in a similar way to chromatography instrumentation. This is only found in specialty labs.

The gel

- Acrylamide versus agarose. Although gels can be run on paper, cellulose acetate, starch, or other matrixes, acrylamide and agarose gels are the only ones most investigators run. Both are porous gels, acting as molecular sieves (the higher the percentage of acrylamide or agarose, the smaller the pores), and theoretically, either could be used to separate DNA, RNA, or

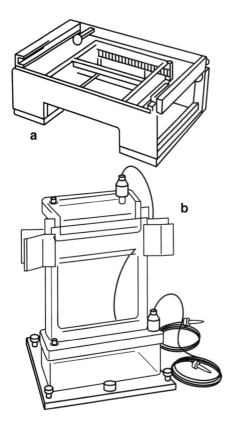

FIGURE 1.

Gel box formats. Horizontal boxes (*a*) are used for agarose gels; vertical boxes (*b*) are used for acrylamide gels.

protein. But acrylamide, at low percentages, is very floppy and difficult to handle: It is usually used only at high percentages to analyze proteins and small oligonucleotides.

• Low percentage agarose gels are relatively rigid and easy to handle, and are used to separate large molecules such as DNA and RNA, and very large proteins and protein complexes.

• The concentration of the gel should be appropriate to the size of the fragment of interest.

• Precast gels are available from many companies. They are expensive, costing a few dollars per gel, and can be stored at 4°C for months. But if you run gradient gels, or run gels infrequently, it is well worth it. There are also multi-gel casting systems, used to make up to 10 gels at a time.

- Cut off the same corner of the gel every time. This gives you an orientation point in case the gel is dropped or turned, and for setting up the gel for transfers.

Buffers

- Most running buffers are made or purchased as concentrated stock, and are diluted at the time of the run.

- Each buffer will have a characteristic voltage at a particular amperage. Get to recognize the characteristics of each buffer, so you will recognize when something is wrong.

Power

- Power output can be in several modes: constant voltage (mV), constant current (measured in amperage, or amps), or constant power (watts, or W). Many models allow you to program a run for automatic crossover between modes, so you can use the optimum voltage (which can change during the run) without exceeding the power capacity.

- Not all power supplies are the same, and you cannot merely plug your electrophoresis apparatus into any available power supply. Know what amperage or voltage you need, and identify the power supply that will provide that.

- Most labs have at least one power supply for sequencing gels (which require high wattage), electrophoretic transfers (which require high current), and one for agarose and acrylamide gel electrophoresis (which use a wide range of voltages). There are few power supplies that can satisfy all three needs.

- Samples in denaturing protein gels and DNA and RNA gels will run from the cathode (negative) to the anode (positive). Use the red lead for the anode (+), and the black for the cathode (–).

- You can run multiple gels on the same power supply, but don't do it without asking the other user, as electrophoretic conditions may be changed.

- If the power supply has a timer and will terminate a run automatically, use it; otherwise, set a timer to remind yourself to check the gel. Especially if

TABLE 1. Effects of Currents

Current (mA)		Effects
AC	DC	
≤1	5	Causes no sensation
1–8		Sensation of shock, not painful
8–15		Painful shock; individual can releaase grasp
15–20	75	Muscular control lost; cannot release grasp
20–50		Muscular contractions; hard to breathe
50–100	300–500	Possible ventricular fibrillation
100–200		Certain ventricular fibrillation
≥200		Severe burns; muscular contractions so severe that heart may stop

Current is not entirely dependent on the voltage, but on the resistance of the body. In general, the body's resistance to electrical shock is minimal, and voltages of 45 to 60 mA have proven fatal. (Reprinted, with permission, from Gershey et al. 1991.)

you are looking at a molecule of low MW, it is easy to run the samples off the gel and into the buffer.

- Electrophoresis units are built very safely, and there is little to worry about if you obey the Big Rule: Make sure power is OFF to electrophoresis apparatus before you touch anything! Don't "just add a little more buffer" to your mini-gel, or shift the box an inch over, or quickly load one more well, or ever put the lid on the unit, *until the power is off.* Period.

 ## Fixing

- Whether or not a gel needs to be fixed depends on the application. Gels that will be stained must usually be fixed, whereas gels that are used for transfers are not fixed.

Drying

- By removing the water from a gel, the matrix is made thinner. Dried gels give a sharper band after autoradiography.

- Drying a gel will take less than an hour in a gel-dryer. The gel-dryer can be heated, making the drying process more rapid.

Staining

- DNA and RNA gels are stained by the addition of dye to the sample or buffer before the electrophoresis run. They can be stained afterward, as well, but it is less convenient.

- Protein gels are stained after electrophoresis.

Documentation

- Polaroid pictures of gels stained with EtBr and 35 mm photographs of protein gels are the most common documentation.

- Digital documentation and analysis systems are growing in presence. No film is used, and the data can even be set up for presentations.

- Documentation of transfers will depend on the system and experiment. For example, autoradiography and chemiluminescence results can be recorded on X-ray film, and the signal quantitated with a densitometer.

Determining molecular weight. The molecular weight of proteins can be determined by SDS-PAGE, and of DNA and RNA by agarose gel electrophoresis. There is a linear relationship between the logarithm of the molecular weight of a molecule and its R_f (effectively, the distance traveled). A standard curve of the distance migrated against the $\log_{10}$ MW of the standards can be plotted and the R_f of the sample—and hence, the molecular weight—can be extrapolated from the graph.

1. Make a gel of a concentration that will best resolve molecules of the approximate size. Always run molecular weight standards, of a range encompassing the approximate size of the molecule in question.

2. Run the gel so the dye front almost runs off the end of the gel.

3. Stain the gel, and take a picture. If samples are radiolabeled, you can either use radiolabeled standards or compare the gel with the autoradiography film.

4. Measure the distance from the well to each band of standard. Take the $\log_{10}$ of each number, and plot it on regular (non-log) graph paper, on the y axis. The x axis is the distance traveled (cm are probably easiest to translate.) You should have a straight line for much of the distance of the standards.

5. Plot the distance migrated for the sample. Extrapolate to the standard line and determine the molecular weight.

> *Computer programs available on the WWW (and many calculators) can be used to extrapolate the molecular weight of an unknown from a standard curve. The advantage to plotting the curve manually is that you can be sure if the value of your protein falls into the linear (and valid) part of the standard curve.*

SPECIFICS

DNA Gels

DNA gels are run to separate, identify, or purify DNA fragments. Sequencing gels, used to run and analyze DNA sequencing reactions, are not described here. There are as many ways to pour a sequencing gel as there are lab members, and all of them work. Get someone to demonstrate one method, and stick with it until you can get it to work.

 Sample preparation

- 6x loading buffer is typical: 30% (v/v) glycerol, 0.25% (w/v) bromophenol blue, 0.25% (w/v) xylene cyanol, in distilled water. Store at –20°C.

> *Electrophoresis is usually halted when the BPB dye front is 3/4 of the way to the bottom for agarose gels.*

- Sample buffer and DNA are heated at 60°C for 5 minutes.

 Standards/markers

- In agarose gels, marker dye BPB will co-migrate with DNA molecules of approximately 600 bp, and xylene cyanol with DNA molecules of approximately 4000 bp. The exact migration is dependent on the quality and concentration of agarose.

TABLE 2. Migration of Marker Dyes

	% Polyacrylamide	Bromophenol blue[a]	Xylene cyanol[a]
In polyacrylamide gels			
	3.5	100	460
	5.0	65	260
	8.0	45	160
	12.0	20	70
	20.0	12	45
In denaturing polyacrylamide gels			
	5.0	35	130
	6.0	26	106
	8.0	19	70–80
	10.0	12	55
	20.0	8	28

(Adapted, with permission, from Maniatis et al. 1982.)
[a]The numbers are the approximate sizes of fragments of DNA (in nucleotide pairs) with which the dyes would comigrate.

- BPB and xylene cyanol can also be used for marker dyes in DNA acrylamide gels. See Table 2.

- There is an endless supply of DNA standards available. Most of them are pieces generated from the enzymatic digestion of a known piece of DNA. These standards yield fragments of nonuniform sizes, making it easier to quickly estimate the size of an unknown, and provide a control for gel-to-gel variability. You can make your own, but it isn't usually worth the trouble.

- Molecular rulers are DNA ladders, with sizes of regular intervals. These are best for precise measurement of the molecular weight of the sample DNA. Most contain a visually distinct reference band.

- Have your own supply of the DNA standards you use most often. Two useful sets of DNA size markers in bp are:

  > Lambda cut with *Hin*dIII: 23,130, 9416, 6557, 4361, 2322, 2027, 564, 125
  > φX174 cut with *Hae*III: 1353, 1078, 872, 603, 310, 281, 271, 234, 194, 118, 72

Format

- *Medium gel boxes versus mini-gels.* Mini-gels can be used to monitor the progress of restriction digestions, or to check the quality of plasmid preps, two of the most common uses of DNA gels. The main advantages of mini-gels over medium gels is that the gel is finished running much sooner (less than an hour, compared to 3–4 hours) and they require less DNA. Southern blots are better done as larger size gels, since the signal may be weak and more DNA can be run in a larger format.

- *Preparative versus analytical gels.* An analytical gel is run to gather information. In a preparative gel, the DNA of interest is removed from the gel: Preparative gels are often larger, to accommodate a larger amount of sample. A preparative gel may have only one huge well at the top of the gel.

Resolving agent

- Agarose or acrylamide: resolving power versus range of separation!

- Agarose (good range of separation) is used standardly, good for 200 bp to 50 kb, and is run as a horizontal gel. DNAs up to 10,000 kb may be run in pulsed-field gel electrophoresis.

- Use polyacrylamide (good resolving power) for separating small fragments of DNA from 5 to 500 bp. It is set up as a vertical gel. Alkaline agarose gels are used to hydrolyze DNA and analyze the individual DNA strands. A common reason to run an alkaline agarose gel is to check the size of first and second DNA strands synthesized by reverse transcription in the first step in making cDNA. The addition of base to hot agarose would hydrolyze the agarose, so the gel is prepared in a neutral solution and is equilibrated in freshly made alkaline electrophoresis buffer before running.

- Low-melt agarose has been chemically modified to gel and melt at lower temperatures (it gels at 30°C and melts at 65°C), and resolves better than normal agarose but not as well as acrylamide. Perform the electrophoresis run in the cold room to prevent melting of the agarose. Low-melt agarose is useful for preparative gels, since there are a number of ways to recover DNA from low-melt agarose.

- Use the appropriate concentration of agarose. See Table 3.

TABLE 3. Concentration of Gels Used for Electrophoresis of DNA

A	Agarose (%)	Effective range of separation of linear DNA molecules (kb)
	0.3	60–5
	0.6	20–1
	0.7	10–0.8
	0.9	7–0.5
	1.2	6–0.4
	1.5	4–0.2
	2.0	3–0.1

B	Acrylamide (%)	Effective range of separation (nucleotides)
	3.5	100–1000
	5.0	80–500
	8.0	60–400
	12.0	40–200
	20.0	10–100

(Modified, with permission, from Maniatis et al. 1982.)
(A) Choose the concentration of agarose that gives good separation of the size of DNA molecules you are analyzing.
(B) If the DNAs you are interested in are smaller than 1 kb, an acrylamide gel should be used.

⚗ Buffer

- The same buffer is used to make the gel as to actually run the gel.

- If you mix the agarose in water instead of buffer by mistake (and this is one of the most common mistakes made), there is little electrical conductance and the DNA will move slightly or not at all. Discard the gel and make a new one.

- The most common buffers for DNA are TAE (Tris-acetate-EDTA) and TBE (Tris-borate-EDTA). TPE is also used less frequently.

- Gels prepared and run with different buffers look different. For example, double-stranded linear DNA fragments migrate approximately 15% faster through TAE than through TBE or TPE. Resolution of supercoiled DNA is better in TAE.

TABLE 4. Commonly Used Electrophoresis Buffers

Buffer	Working solution		Concentrated stock solution (per liter)	
Tris-acetate (TAE)	1x:	0.04 M Tris-acetate 0.001 M EDTA	50 x	242 g Tris base 57.1 ml glacial acetic acid 100 ml 0.5 M EDTA (pH 8.0)
Tris-phosphate (TPE)	1x:	0.09 M Tris-phosphate 0.002 M EDTA	10x:	108 g Tris base 15.5 ml 85% phosphoric acid (1.679 g/ml) 40 ml 0.5 M EDTA (pH 8.0)
Tris-borate[a] (TBE)	0.5x:	0.045 M Tris-borate 0.001 M EDTA	5x:	54 g Tris base 27.5 g boric acid 20 ml 0.5 M EDTA (pH 8.0)
Alkaline[b]	1x:	50 mN NaOH 1 mM EDTA	1x:	5 ml 10 N NaOH 2 ml 0.5 M EDTA (pH 8.0)

(Reprinted, with permission, from Sambrook et al. 1989.)

[a]A precipitate forms when concentrated solutions of TBE are stored for long periods of time. To avoid problems, store the 5x solution in glass bottles at room temperature and discard any batches that develop a precipitate. TBE was originally used at a working strength of 1x (i.e., a 1:5 dilution of the concentrated stock) for agarose gel electrophoresis. However, a working solution of 0.5x provides more than enough buffering power, and almost all agarose gel electrophoresis is now carried out with a 1:10 dilution of the concentrated stock. TBE is used at a working strength of 1x for polyacrylamide gel electrophoresis, twice the strength usually used for agarose gel electrophoresis. The buffer reservoirs of the vertical tanks used for polyacrylamide gel electrophoresis are fairly small, and the amount of electric current passed through them is often considerable. 1x TBE is required to provide adequate buffering power.

[b]Alkaline electrophoresis buffer should be freshly made.

- *Recommendation:* Use TBE. It has the highest buffering capacity.

- If EtBr was mistakenly omitted from the gel, it should be added to the running buffer.

Power

- Applied voltage. The effective range of separation in agarose gels decreases as the voltage is increased. To achieve maximum resolution of a DNA fragment greater than 2 kb, run gels at 5 V/cm or less (for cm, approximate the distance between electrodes). 5–10 V/cm is good for most gels. 100 V will be approximately 50 mA for some buffers.

- If you want the gel to run overnight, the total voltage should be 20–25 V. You can turn it higher in the morning.

- Running a gel at constant power rather than constant voltage or current will prevent large voltage spikes or excessive heating from occurring.

- Run low-melt agarose gels more slowly than a regular gel, to avoid generating heat.

Staining

- Add EtBr to the gel mixture after it is melted. Add 1 µl of 10 mg/ml EtBr to every 10 ml of agarose solution.

- It is not usually necessary to add EtBr to the gel buffer, or to stain the gel after electrophoresis: EtBr in the gel mixture is enough to see most bands.

Analysis

- DNA in a gel is visualized on an UV transilluminator.

- Lay the gel (use gloves) on a piece of plastic wrap and carry the gel to the UV transilluminator. You may carry the gel/plastic wrap on the base or tray, but put only the gel/plastic wrap on the UV box: The tray will absorb too much light, and you may not see weakly stained bands.

- In gels with DNA not treated with RNase, tRNAs will often be seen as diffuse bands on the bottom of the gel.

- Why are there so many DNA bands? Even uncut plasmid DNA may appear on a gel as more than one band. Superhelical circular (uncut), nicked circular (partially cut), and linear (completely cut) DNA migrate through agarose gels at different rates: One prep of incompletely digested DNA may show three different bands.

- It is difficult to predict which band is which (since agarose concentration, current strength, and buffer type are some of the influences), but usually, superhelical DNA moves like a compact bullet through the gel and runs the fastest, with linear and then nicked DNA following.

 ## Making gels

Agarose gels

- DNA gels are made just before the gel will be run. A prepared gel can be either stored in running buffer or wrapped in plastic wrap overnight in the refrigerator.

- Use diluted 10X stock buffer and agarose to prepare the gel. Either make just what you need, in an Erlenmeyer flask, or make enough gel for several gels in a glass bottle. The agarose will solidify, but the contents of the bottle can be melted again in a microwave. Store agarose/buffer "solutions" at room temperature.

- Agarose comes in various grades: the purer (and more expensive), the fewer contaminants of proteins, salts, and other polysaccharides you will find. It is also available for the isolation of differently sized nucleic acids. If you must recover the DNA, use the purest agarose you can afford, as contamination can inhibit enzyme reactions and is a major impediment to successful cloning. FMC BioProducts is a source of high-quality agarose.

The microwave

Hazards: EtBr, a teratogen, is often included in agarose mixtures (although it should be added after melting) and may be splattered on the inside of the microwave. Protective gloves should always be worn. Overheated agarose mixtures may suddenly boil over, so always remove agarose with tongs and/or heat-protective gloves. A wad of paper towels should not be used.
Remarks: No metal (No stir bars!). No food in any but a dedicated food microwave, no reagents in a food microwave. Put paper towels under anything you microwave, to make a boil-over easier to clean.
Alternatives: Heater stir plate.

To microwave

1. Put the top very loosely on the bottle. Air must be able to escape, or the bottle could explode. If you are using a flask, use a large one to reduce the chance of boiling over. You can leave off the top, or cover the top loosely with plastic wrap (not aluminum foil!).

2. Put the microwave on high. Freshly made agarose mixture will take longer to heat than solidified agarose. 100-ml volumes will take 3–5 minutes, larger volumes will take approximately 6–10 minutes.

3. After a minute, stop the microwave, grab the bottle with a gloved hand, and rotate to swirl the contents. A homogeneous mixture will heat more quickly and evenly.

4. Put the bottle back in the microwave. Stop it again after a minute, and swirl.

5. Replace the bottle in the microwave and heat until it just starts to boil.

6. Using tongs or heat-resistant gloves, remove the bottle.

7. Let the agar cool until the bottle can almost be touched. Swirl well before pouring. If you see that part of the agarose mixture has started to solidify, microwave it briefly again.

Yes, you can reuse gels. Some investigators have been known to keep a pet gel for checking reactions, running the current samples out of the gel before reloading. The gel must be stained with every new run, and using an old gel doesn't really save much time or money.

Acrylamide gels

- Polyacrylamide gels must be carefully polymerized by the mixing of monomeric units of acrylamide, an initiator of polymerization, and a catalyst, as well as the appropriate salts or buffer.

The percentages of acrylamide and BIS are different in sequencing gels and protein gels. If you used prepared acrylamide:BIS solutions, be sure you have grabbed the correct one.

- *Acrylamide and bis* (N,N′-methylenebisacrylamide) are the monomeric units that form the gel matrix. Buy the premade solutions!

- *Ammonium persulfate* initiates gel polymerization. Gel recipes call for a 10% ammonium persulfate solution, which should be made in water. Most protocols tell you to make it up fresh, every time. However, a 10%

solution can be stored for weeks at 4ºC without a noticeable loss of activity. Make 10 ml of maximum and discard it either when a gel won't polymerize or whenever it makes you feel better.

- *TEMED* (N,N,N′,N′-tetramethylethylenediamine) is the catalyst. It comes in a brown bottle, and is stored in a brown bottle, usually in the cold. It is always added last, just before the gel is poured.

> *Unpolymerized acrylamide is a neurotoxin. Wear gloves, even when handling polymerized acrylamide, as there may be monomers in the area.*

- In addition, polyacrylamide sequencing gels have gel buffer (TBE) and urea added. The urea is a denaturant and makes the formation of hairpin loops in the DNA reactions less likely.

- The glass plates for acrylamide electrophoresis should be washed before and after every electrophoresis run. After a run, wash the plate in warm, soapy water, using a soft brush or rag that won't scratch the glass. Rinse well in distilled water, and place upright to dry.

- Water or dust can lead to patchy polymerization. Before a run, use Windex or another glass cleaner to wash the plate. Use a soft brush to scrub. Rinse well in distilled water, and dry the plate fairly well with a paper towel and completely with a Kimwipe. A last rinse with 70% ethanol before using a paper towel can help clean and speed up the drying. Add ingredients in order: Acrylamide:BIS, water, buffer, APS, TEMED. Mix well by swirling, and pour immediately.

- It is not necessary to degas the acrylamide solution before polymerization. (Acrylamide solutions used to be placed under a vacuum, to remove air bubbles: Polymerization is inhibited by O_2.)

Loading tips

Set up the gel box

> *Remember that the samples have glycerol in them, and will sink into the wells.*

- Place a black piece of paper under the gel box. A dark background makes the wells more visible.

- Fill the tank with enough buffer that the gel is just covered.

- If there is an overhead light, turn it on and direct the light onto the gel.

Load the pipettor with the sample

- Use an automatic pipettor.

- The tips that fit on the 10–200-μl pipettors are fine for most wells. For very small (under 10 μl) wells, the long tips used for sequencing gels can make the job easier.

- With just the tip in the sample, aspirate the sample slowly and deliberately into the tip. The sample may be viscous because of the glycerol, and rapid aspiration will leave sample in the tube and air bubbles in the tip.

- After loading the tip, touch the tip gently on the edge of the tube or with a Kimwipe to remove drops on the outside of the tip. Don't allow capillary action to drain the sample.

> *If sample is not limiting, it is helpful to follow the 10% plus rule: For each sample, make 10% more volume and content than you need. For example, if you intend to load 1.0 μg in 5 μl, make up 1.1 μg in 5.5 μl. Several microliters can be lost in pipetting, and this can be crucial if you are comparing amounts. Making a bit extra takes this worry away, and makes the pipetting job easier, as you don't have to suck up every last drop.*

Load the well with the sample

- Maintain a bit of pressure on the pipettor, so the sample is slightly bulging out of the bottom of the tip.

> *Maintaining positive pressure on the sample while loading prevents bubbles or buffer from entering the tip as you position the pipet.*

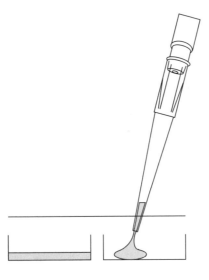

FIGURE 2.

Maintaining positive pressure on the sample while loading prevents bubbles or buffer from entering the tip as you position the pipettor over the well. Keep pressure in the tip while removing the pipettor as well.

- Put the tip into the buffer, just above the well, maintaining positive pressure. The tip of the tip (!) can be just into the well.

- Very slowly and steadily, push the sample out. If your tip is above the well, the sample will sink into the well. Fill by allowing the sample to sink, not by pushing into the well.

- As soon as the last drop has left the tip, push the pipettor to the second stop, slowly raising the pipettor tip straight up and out of the buffer as you do so.

> *Holding a last bit of air in the tip will prevent inadvertent suction from disturbing the sample.*

How to load a vertical gel

- In a vertical gel, the wells are found between two glass plates. In a very thin gel, a pipettor tip will not even fit between the plates. Remember the glyc-

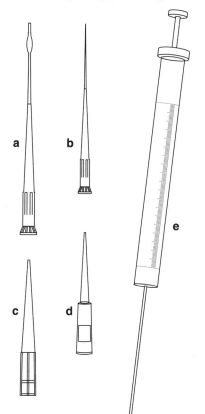

FIGURE 3.

Flat-tipped (*a*) and extended round tips (*b*) are very useful for loading vertical gels, as the tips can fit between the glass plates. Tips with a wide orifice (*c*) make it easier to load viscous DNA samples. Tips with an aerosol barrier (*d*) prevent carryover, and are used for radioactive samples. Microliter Hamilton syringes (*e*) are an easy way to load all gel samples: The syringe should be rinsed out with running buffer between samples. Of course, standard pipettor tips can be used for loading gels.

erol! If you position the tip above the well, the sample will sink into the well.

- Always flush out the wells of a vertical acrylamide gel before loading samples. This removes unpolymerized polyacrylamide and water that may be on the bottom of the well, and which effectively makes the well smaller. Use a 25- or 50-ml syringe, with an 18 gauge needle. Aspirate the running buffer, and flush the wells strongly but carefully to remove water.

- It can be hard to see the wells, but once you have loaded one well, the rest are easier to see. If you are having trouble and have an extra lane, load one well with sample buffer containing BPB.

RNA Gels

RNA gels are used to analyze RNA by Northern blotting. mRNAs comprise only about 5% of total RNAs, and are not visible on EtBr-stained gels: Therefore, a particular mRNA must be detected with a labeled probe.

 Sample preparation

- RNA samples must be denatured before and during the electrophoresis run; otherwise, molecular weight cannot be accurately determined. This is done with formaldehyde and formamide. It can also be done with glyoxal and DMSO or methyl mercury (not recommended).

- Sample buffer for MOPS gels: 0.75 ml of deionized formamide, 0.15 ml of 10x MOPS, 0.24 ml of formaldehyde, 0.1 ml of deionized RNase-free water, 0.1 ml of glycerol, 0.08 ml 10% (w/v) of bromophenol blue. Store in small aliquots at –20°C or make fresh every time.

- Add 25 μl of sample buffer to 5 μl of RNA. You may have to concentrate your RNA.

- Samples in sample buffer are heated to 65°C for 15 minutes. Add 1 μl of 1 mg/ml EtBr to each sample and mix well. You do not need to add EtBr to the buffer.

- Load 5–20 μg of total RNA for a medium size gel, 1–5 μg in a mini-gel.

- You will usually get a cleaner and stronger signal with 3 µg of mRNA than with 5–20 µg of total RNA.

Standards/markers

- Yes, you do need standards for RNA gels.

- Many people use the ribosomal RNAs of the sample itself as a rough marker, and this is usually sufficient. Eukaryotic ribosomal RNAs are 28S and 18S (approximate sizes 5300 and 2000 bases): Prokaryotic ribosomal RNAs are 23S and 16S (approximate sizes 3566 and 1776 bases for *E. coli*).

- RNA standards are commercially available. DNA standards don't run well in formaldehyde gels, and shouldn't be used. Defined templates for in vitro RNA synthesis can be used to make defined-length RNA transcripts, needed if the size of an unknown RNA must be tightly defined.

- BPB and xylene cyanol can be used as tracking dyes. As in DNA electrophoresis, the exact position will depend on the agarose quality and concentration (see Table 5).

Format

- RNA gels are run just like DNA gels. *You do not need separate boxes and equipment to run RNA gels!* Just wash the gel box before and after use.

Buffer

- 10x MOPS/EDTA buffer contains 0.2 M MOPS [3-(N-morpholino) propanesulfonic acid], 50 mM sodium acetate, 10 mM EDTA adjusted to pH 7.0. Autoclave for 15 minutes. A slight yellow color appearing over time is normal. Use at 1x for electrophoresis.

- MOPS buffer (and other RNA buffers) are very low in ionic strength. During electrophoresis, a pH gradient may be generated along the length of the gel, resulting in hydrolysis of the gel. This may only be a problem during long electrophoretic runs and can be avoided by recirculating the buffer with a peristaltic pump or by occasionally pipetting buffer from one end to the other.

The gel

- RNA must be run under denaturing conditions. MOPS-formaldehyde gels are the safest and best bet.

- Formaldehyde gels must be poured and allowed to solidify in a fume hood. Hot formaldehyde vaporizes and is dangerous to breathe. Get directions before you do this.

- Agarose gels with formaldehyde are more fragile than standard agarose gels and must be manipulated carefully.

- 1% or 1.2% gels are generally good for most Northerns.

Power

- Power requirements are similar to DNA agarose gels. For a medium size gel, 100 V (approximately 50 mA) will take 3–4 hours to run.

Staining

- With the inclusion of EtBr in the sample buffer, further staining is not necessary.

Analysis

- The ribosomal subunits should be discrete. Unless the gel has been overloaded, the subunits should not be smeared, which would indicate degradation.

- mRNA, if visible at all on a gel, will look like a smear.

Protein Gels

Most protein gels run are sodium dodecyl sulfate polyacrylamide gel electrophoresis (SDS-PAGE) gels run in reducing conditions.

Sample preparation

- A reducing agent, either 2-mercaptoethanol or dithiothreitol, is included in the sample buffer for denaturing gels. This reduces disulfide bonds in

TABLE 5. Tracking Dye Mobilities for RNA Formaldehyde Gels

	Formaldehyde gels	
	xylene cyanol	bromophenol blue
SeaKem® Gold Agarose		
1.0%	6300	660
1.5%	2700	310
2.0%	1500	200
SeaKem GTG® and LE Agarose		
1.0%	4200	320
1.5%	1700	140
2.0%	820	60[a]
SeaPlaque® and SeaPlaque GTG Agarose		
1.0%	2400	240
1.5%	800	80[a]
2.0%	490	30[a]

[a]Nucleic equivalent for dye migration determined by extrapolation.

proteins, ensuring that they maintain the random-coil configuration necessary for the determination of molecular weight. Use stock reducing agents in a fume hood.

- Keep sample buffer at –20ºC in small aliquots. The glycerol concentration is high enough to prevent freezing, so you don't have to worry about damage caused by freeze-thawing. When you can no longer smell the reducing agent in the tube, it is time to get a new tube of sample buffer.

- For SDS-PAGE: 2**x** buffer is 4% SDS, 20% glycerol, 10% 2-mercaptoethanol (or 100 mM dithiotheitol) 0.004% bromophenol blue, and 0.125 M Tris-HCl. pH should be approximately 6.8.

- Samples must be boiled (or heated at 95ºC) in the sample buffer for 5 minutes just before being loaded. Use a floating tube rack if you heat the samples in a beaker or water bath: In a pinch, you could poke holes in a piece of styrofoam. Chill the tubes on ice after boiling. Hold each tube firmly when opening it, in case all the pressure hasn't yet dissipated, to prevent the lid from popping open.

- If you boil samples with the lids closed, the lids will pop open, and the entire tube can spectacularly explode into the air. This can be avoided in several ways. You could wait until the samples have just started to boil, and then gently open the tube to release the pressure. Or you could use a pin and poke a hole in the lid of each tube, but this shouldn't be done with radiolabeled samples. There are racks used to boil samples that clamp a lid on the microfuge tubes, preventing the caps from opening. The best alternative is the use of individual plastic clamps that slide onto the lids of microfuge tubes and prevent them from opening.

 Standards/markers

- Standards are available in high, low, and broad ranges. They are available unstained or prestained: Prestained is more convenient. Store standards at $-20°C$, unless otherwise noted.

- Rainbow standards (Amersham) are very useful (and pretty), since each protein is stained a different color. They are expensive, but it is incredibly easy to monitor the progress of electrophoresis when the identity of each marker protein is clear.

- The covalent binding of dyes to the markers produces variation in the molecular weights of the proteins. For precise molecular weight determinations, use calibrated molecular weight standards.

- Biotinylated standards can be incorporated into horseradish peroxidase (HRP) or alkaline phosphatase detection procedures for immunoblots. Other markers are designed to be used for silver or other staining.

- Most markers are designed for SDS-PAGE gels. If you are running native (nondenaturing) gels, you must get markers designed for that.

 Format

- Polyacrylamide gels are always poured between glass plates. The plates are held apart by spacers. Spacers come in different thicknesses, and are matched to a comb of the same thickness.

- Continuous vs. discontinuous. A continuous gel system has a resolving gel with the same buffer used at the anode and cathode. A discontinuous gel has two parts: a stacking gel (a large-pored gel) overlaid over the resolving gel. In a discontinuous system there is a different buffer used at the anode and cathode. Resolution is much better in a discontinuous system.

- 2-D (2-dimensional) gels are used to more precisely characterize proteins. The samples are run twice, called the first and second dimensions. The first dimension is an isoelectric focusing gel (IEF), usually run as a tube gel, to determine the pI of each protein. This tube gel will then be placed

Protein (kD)						
(Tris-glycine)						
7.5%	10%	12%	15%	4-15%	4-20%	10-20%

(Figure showing protein molecular weight marker positions across gel concentrations)

7.5%: 200, 116, 97.4, 66, 45

10%: 200, 116, 97.4, 66, 45, 31, 21.5

12%: 200, 116, 97.4, 66, 45, 31, 21.5, 14.5

15%: 200, 116, 97.4, 66, 45, 31, 21.5, 14.5, 6.5

4-15%: 200, 116, 97.4, 66, 45, 31, 21.5, 14.5

4-20%: 200, 116, 97.4, 66, 45, 31, 21.5, 14.5, 6.5

10-20%: 200, 116, 97.4, 66, 45, 31, 21.5, 14.5, 6.5

FIGURE 4.

Protein molecular weight markers. The positions of proteins of 200, 116, 97.4, 66, 45, 21.5, 14.5, and 6.5 kD are shown after electrophoresis through gels of different acrylamide concentrations, using Tris-glycine buffer. (Redrawn, with permission, from Bio-Rad Laboratories, Hercules, California.)

onto a slab gel for the second dimension, and the proteins are separated according to molecular weight.

- Tube gels versus slab gels. Tube gels were once used for general electrophoresis. They are now used only for the first dimension of 2-D gels.

 The gel

- 38:1 w:w ratio of acrylamide to BIS is the usual ratio of stock solution used to make protein gels. The amount of the 38:1 mix is varied when making the gel, to get a gel of various concentrations of acrylamide.

- Gradient or nongradient gels. Nongradient gels are of a single percentage acrylamide, and provide the best separation of a single band from surrounding bands. Use single percentage gels to look at two bands close in molecular weight. Gradient gels are used to resolve high and low molecular weight bands on the same gel.

- Denaturating or nondenaturing gels. Since proteins are amphoteric compounds, their net charge will be determined by the pH in which they are suspended: Depending on the pKa of the protein and the pH of the medium, a particular protein will be attracted to the cathode or anode. Therefore, under nondenaturing conditions, the electrophoretic separation of proteins is determined by both the size and the charge of the proteins. Under denaturing conditions, separation is determined only by size.

- SDS-PAGE. SDS is an anionic detergent that denatures proteins and gives them a negative charge. When run under denaturing conditions, charge is no longer a factor and the electrophoretic migration of a protein is only dependent on the molecular weight.

Buffers

- Most protein gels use a glycine-SDS buffer (196 mM glycine/0.1% SDS/50 mM Tris-HCl, pH 8.3). Make at least 2 liters of 10X buffer, and store it at room temperature.

- Tricine buffer is used for peptide and small protein electrophoresis (2–80 kD).

Power

- Run at 25–30 mA (200 V). Electrophoresis is usually halted when the dye front reaches the bottom of the gel.

- Run proteins more slowly through the stacking gel, at below 50 V. Once your samples are at the stacking gel/resolving gel interface, you can up the voltage to 200 V.

⚗ Staining

- Gels are stained after electrophoresis by incubation with staining solutions, followed by multiple washes to remove excess stain.

- The most common stain is 0.2% Coomassie Brilliant Blue, in 45:45:10% methanol:water:acetic acid for 2–3 hours at 37°C, with agitation. Destain with 25:65:10 methanol:water:acetic acid.

- Silver staining is a more sensitive stain and is used for proteins that stain weakly or not at all with Coomassie. It is also more complicated to use.

TRANSFERRING GEL CONTENTS TO MEMBRANES

The gel is a thick but fragile matrix, making it difficult to subject to handling or incubations. If hybridization of the gel contents is to be done, the material in the gel is induced to move from the gel onto a piece of nitrocellulose filter or nylon membrane. This is called the transfer.

Once transferred, the filter can be incubated with a probe, to see whether the probe can hybridize to a molecule on the filter. The probe is labeled with radioactivity or other indicators so it can be detected. The hybridization of the filter with the probe is referred to as blotting.

The first use of blotting, which was to detect specific nucleotide sequences in DNA separated by electrophoresis and transferred to nitrocellulose, was described by a man named Southern. Hence, this kind of blot was called a Southern blot. As dif-

Southern blot: DNA on the filter is probed with DNA.
Northern blot: RNA on the filter is probed with DNA or RNA.
Western blot: Protein on a filter is probed with antibody.
Southwestern blot: DNA on a filter is probed with protein.
Middle eastern blot: Poly(U)-derivatized paper is probed with mRNA.

ferent kinds of templates and probes were used, they were lightheartedly given other directional names.

There are three ways in which biological material is transferred from the gel to a filter or membrane:

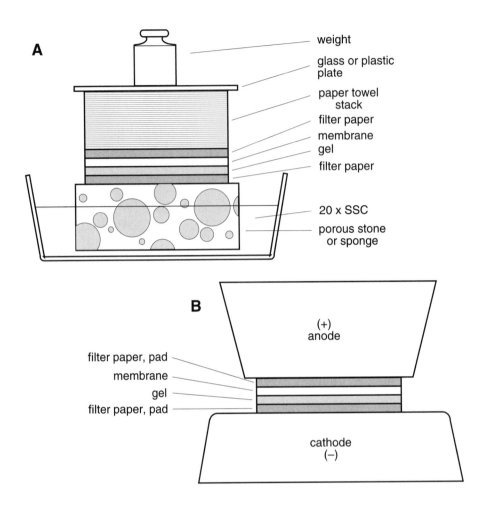

FIGURE 5.

(*A*) Capillary transfer of molecules relies on the movement of salt solution, which is pulled from the basin through the gel and membrane and into the wad of paper towels, and carries the DNA or RNA with it. Vacuum transfer is set up in the same way. (*B*) Electrophoretic transfer depends on the movement of negatively charged DNA, RNA, or protein from the gel to the membrane, in its attempt to reach the anode. In wet blotting, the entire system is immersed in one transfer buffer, whereas in semi-dry blotting, filters are wet with separate anode and cathode transfer buffers to facilitate the current.

- *Capillary transfer.* Used for DNA and RNA.

- *Vacuum transfer.* Used for DNA and RNA.

- *Electrophoretic transfer.* Used for DNA, RNA, and protein. There are two main apparatuses to do this, both of which use current to move molecules from the gel toward the anode, and onto a membrane. These are dry blotters or semi-dry blotters, in which the current is carried only through filter papers soaked in anode and cathode buffers, and wet blotters, in which the gel and membrane are immersed in a transfer buffer. This type of transfer requires a power source capable of very high amperage.

Membranes

- Membranes are available in rolls or in precut sizes. Unless everyone in the lab only runs one size gel, buy the roll.

- Wear gloves when you cut or handle any membrane. Grease or oil from your fingers can impede transfer.

- Pick up membranes with a clean, flat-edged forceps. Sharp or pointed tweezers can tear the membrane.

- Your choice for a transfer membrane is mainly between nylon (various kinds) and nitrocellulose (regular or strengthened with cellulose acetate for easier handling).

- Nylon is best for nucleic acids. It is durable, binds nucleic acid well, and can be stripped and reprobed multiple times. Nylon tends to have more background staining, and so requires a higher concentration of blocking agents during hybridization. Cationized nylon works best for nucleic acids, as binding does not depend on the ionic strength of the buffer. Nucleic acids cannot be electrophoretically transferred to nitrocellulose.

- Nitrocellulose is best for some proteins, nylon for others. Nylon has a higher binding capacity in general, but there are a few proteins that don't bind well at all. Essentially, both work, although lab workers will swear by one or the other. Use what is used in the lab for your particular molecule. If you must use nitrocellulose, use strengthened nitrocellulose. If you are starting anew, try a PVDF (polyvinylidene difluoride) nylon such as Immobilon-P (Millipore) for Western blotting.

- Protocols for nitrocellulose and nylon are very different: In fact, protocols are different for different types of nylon.

- You do not usually have to worry about pore sizes. 0.45 μm is the standard. Smaller sizes are available for specialized use.

RESOURCES

Brown T.A. 1994. *DNA sequencing. The basics.* IRL Press at Oxford University Press, New York.

Darling D.C., and Brickell P.M. 1994. *Nucleic acid blotting. The basics.* IRL Press at Oxford University Press, New York.

Flowgen Hints and Tips. The electrophoresis of RNA. 1997.
http://www.philipharris.co.uk/flowgen/hints6.html

FMC BioProducts. 191 Thomaston Street, Rockland, Maine 04841
http://www.bioproducts.com

Gershey E.L., Party E., and Wilkerson A. 1991. *Laboratory safety in practice: A comprehensive compliance program and safety manual.* Van Nostrand Reinhold, New York.

Harlow E. and Lane D. 1988. *Antibodies. A laboratory manual.* Cold Spring Harbor Laboratory Press, Cold Spring Harbor, New York.

Kaufman P.B., Wu W., Kim D., and Cseke L.J. 1995. *Handbook of molecular and cellular methods in biology and medicine.* CRC Press, Boca Raton, Florida.

Life Science Research Catalog 1997. Bio-Rad Laboratories, Hercules, California.
http://www.bio-rad.com/

Maniatis T., Fritsch E.F., and Sambrook J. 1982. *Molecular cloning: A laboratory manual,* 1st edition. Cold Spring Harbor Laboratory, Cold Spring Harbor, New York.

Rybicki E., and Purves M. 1996. SDS Polyacrylamide gel electrophoresis. Dept. Microbiology, University of Cape Town, SA.
http://www.uct.ac.za/microbiology/sdspage.html

Sambrook J., Fritsch E.F., and Maniatis T. 1989. *Molecular cloning. A laboratory manual,* 2nd edition. Cold Spring Harbor Laboratory Press, Cold Spring Harbor, New York.

Sigma Catalog. 1997. Sigma-Aldrich Corporation, St. Louis, Missouri.

Southern E.M. 1975. Detection of specific sequences among DNA fragments separated by gel electrophoresis. *J. Mol. Biol.* **98**: 503–517.

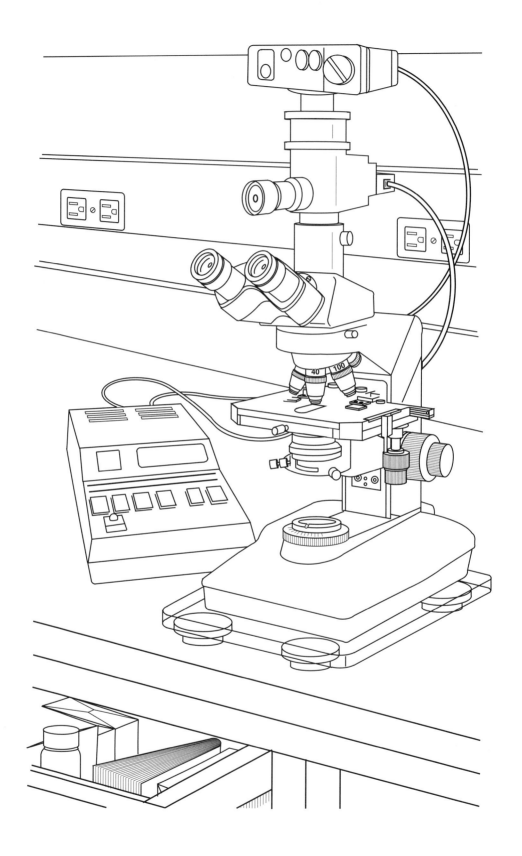

16

The Light Microscope

OST PEOPLE USE THE MICRO-
SCOPE only to view a slide and take a
picture. Once a week, they plop down,
look at a slide, wipe the lens quickly,
and walk away. Unless someone in the
lab has been designated as the microscope person, and all others are forbid-
den to alter anything on the microscope, you should know (besides basic
operating procedures) how to align the
lights and lens to maximize the light
for high-resolution microscopy, how to
clean the lens, and how to replace the
light source.

It is well worth becoming comfortable with a microscope. With it, you
can monitor cells and bacteria for contamination, essential even if *E.coli* is
the only organism you know. It is
indispensable for morphological and
functional studies.

BACKGROUND

BACKGROUND	403
Kinds of microscopy	404
USING THE LIGHT MICROSCOPE	409
Working rules	409
Parts and usage of the compound light microscope	410
Using immersion oil on the objective lens	413
Using immersion oil on the condenser lens	413
Achieving maximum lighting and resolution	414
Koehler illumination	415
SLIDES AND STAINS	417
Making a cell smear	418
Fixing the specimen	419
Staining the specimen	420
FLUORESCENCE MICROSCOPY	420
PHOTOGRAPHY	422
Steps for photography	423
What film should be used?	424
SHARED INSTRUMENT FACILITIES	426
RESOURCES	427

**The main purpose of the micro-
scope** is usually considered to be magnification, an apparent increase in size. This
it does. But more importantly, the microscope provides *resolution*, the minimum distance between two dots that can be discerned.

The two players in providing resolution and magnification are *light* and the *lenses* used to manipulate the light. Most of the microscope is a framework to maintain the all-important lenses. However, different qualities of the lens improve the quality of resolution versus magnification. Resolution does not depend on magnification, as shown in the following formula:

$$\text{Resolution} = 0.61 \times \frac{\text{light source wavelength}}{\text{numerical aperture (N.A.)}}$$

The *numerical aperture* (N.A.) is a measure of the light-gathering capacity of a lens or, more technically, a geometrical calculation of the angle of light transmitted through a particular lens, and through the medium between the specimen and the front of the objective lens (the refractive index). Each objective lens is rated with a N.A., and that number is inscribed on the lens. The higher the number, the better the resolution the lens is capable of providing.

The *refractive index* (n) is a measure of how much light is transmitted versus refracted. A higher n results in greater light gathering by the lens, and so, better illumination and image intensity. Oil has a much higher refractive index than air (1.5 vs. 1.0) but the apparent value of the numerical aperture can be increased by the use of immersion oil only if the N.A. of the lens is higher than 1.0.

The maximum resolution for the light microscope is 200 nm, using light of the shortest visible wavelength (approximately 426 nm) and immersion oil.

The factors influencing total *magnification* are more simple. Total magnification is the product of the objective magnification and the eyepiece magnification.

To be seen, the image through the microscope must have a high degree of *contrast* with its surrounding medium. Contrast can be provided by changes in the degree and angle of light through the lens, and this is done by controlling the light intensity of the illumination source, changing the light coming through the condenser lens with a diaphragm, or phase rings. It can be done by filters, which filter light of particular wavelengths and can be placed over the illumination source. Contrast can also be enhanced by sample staining.

Kinds of Microscopy

Lens, filters, and illumination can be manipulated to magnify and resolve and enhance a variety of images. The kind of sample you have, and the documentation you need, determine what method you choose. Try not to be limited by the equipment at hand: In many cases, the addition of a few components can transform your system. Some of the most common microscopic methods are described below.

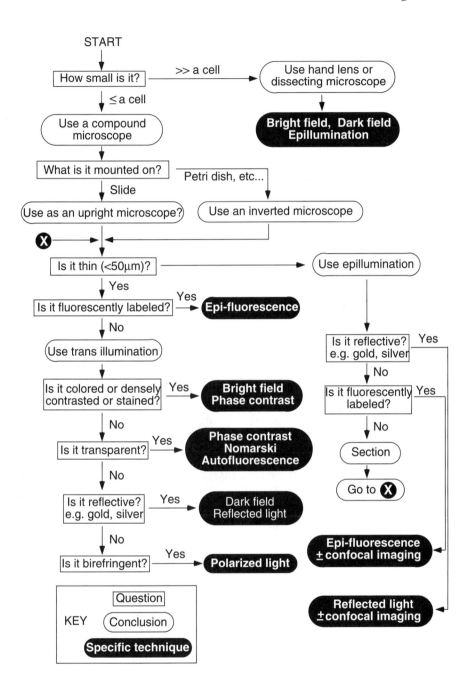

FIGURE 1.

Flow chart for the selection of microscope observation method. (Redrawn, with permission, from Rubbi 1994.)

Light microscopy

 ### Bright-field microscopy

Use: View living and fixed tissue, cells, and microorganisms.
Advantages: Readily available, easy.
How it works: This is standard light microscopy, with the microscope aligned to achieve the maximum lighting possible (Koehler illumination).
Appearance: Gray or dark images against a white background.
When you need this: If you work with any prokaryotic or eukaryotic organisms.
Requirements: Any light microscope, with the minimum of 10**X** and 40**X** objective lenses, a 10**X** ocular, and a light source.

 ### Dark-field microscopy

Use: Looking at wet mounts of unstained specimens and detecting very small structures by reflected and diffracted light.
Advantages: Low-contrast or unstained specimens can be seen.
How it works: Specimen is illuminated so only the light diffracted by objects in view (and not the background) will be seen. A black background is imposed behind the sample.
Appearance: Field of bright, luminescent objects against a dark background.
Requirements: Light microscope with a dark-field stop. Stop is placed in the filter holder below the substage condenser, and directs light around the stop and to the specimen. If you have no disc, tape a dime or cut-out cardboard circle into the filter below the condenser. Move the condenser to a position where light can move in a ring around the coin or circle. At high magnification, a dark-field objective with an iris is needed, along with a special dark-field condenser.

 ### Phase-contrast microscopy

Use: Induces contrast in wet mounts, unstained and unmounted specimens.
Advantages: No fixation or staining needed to visualize a sample.
How it works: It incorporates two light filters (or annuli) that complement each other. The first filter blocks all light except from the perimeter; the second filter blocks all light from the perimeter, in a mirror image of the first. Therefore, all direct light is blocked and only indirect refracted and diffracted light goes to the specimen.
Appearance: Many dark and light gray colors.
Requirements: Two filters must be mounted on the microscope: one below the condenser, and the other within the body of the objective.

Nomarski imaging (differential interference contrast [DIC])

Use: Visualize transparent and internal structures.

Advantages: Samples don't have to be fixed and stained, so living tissue and cells can be studied.

How it works: Phase changes that occur when light passes through a sample (light goes slower through regions of high refractive index) are converted into amplitude changes and greater contrast is achieved.

Appearance: A 3-D look.

Requirements: Special objective lens.

Fluorescence microscopy

Use: Labeling/visualization of discrete parts of a cell or bacteria.

Advantages: Can see parts of a cell or organ not visible by regular light.

How it works: Samples are labeled with one or more fluorescent molecules, and the excitation and emission light of the fluorescent molecules is regulated by filters to provide color and contrast.

Appearance: Bright colors, usually against a dark background.

Requirements: An excitation light source, optical filters appropriate to the fluorescence of the stains used, and, ideally, special objective lens.

Inverted microscopy

Use: Checking morphology of living cultures in flasks and dishes. In situ staining of adherent cells in dishes.

Advantages: Long working distance.

How it works: Like a compound microscope, but with the condenser located above the objective, giving a large stage for flasks and dishes.

Appearance: Dark and light grays.

When you need this: Essential for doing tissue culture work.

Requirements: Inverted microscope. A long-working-distance phase-contrast condenser and phase-contrast objectives are necessary for contrast. A 40X or higher objective is also needed to discern contamination.

Confocal microscopy

Use: Determine cellular localization of organelles, cytoskeletal elements, and macromolecules; trace specific cells through a tissue; three- and four-dimensional reconstruction.

Advantages: Shallow depth of field virtually eliminates out-of-focus flare, reducing background.
How it works: Laser scans fluorescently stained specimen. Successive images can be compiled to reconstruct a 3-D image.
Appearance: Similar to ordinary fluorescence image, with more resolution.
When you need this: Colocalization studies, if the background is complex; for example, colocalization of a bacterium within a cell and a cellular protein.
Requirements: Confocal microscope, computer.

Electron microscopy

Electron microscopy uses electrons, rather than light, as an illumination source. Its wavelength is only about 0.04 nm, about 10,000 times shorter than that of visible light. Since the light source wavelength is much smaller than for visible light, the achievable magnification and resolution are much greater than for light microscopes. The setup and theory of magnification are the same for electrons as for light, but the technology is different. An electron gun generates electrons that travel through a vacuum. Instead of glass lenses, electromagnets are used to focus the electron beam, and glass lenses are only used to magnify the image.

The preparation of the samples is complicated, and electron microscopy is usually farmed out to a specialty lab, or is done at a shared instrument facility.

 ### Transmission electron microscopy (TEM)

Use: View internal structures closely.
Advantages: Great resolution, since electrons are the light source (resolution improves with shorter wavelength). Can be combined with immunological labeling for localization studies.
How it works: A tungsten filament generates electrons, which are focused by electromagnets to a fixed, sectioned, and stained specimen. The image is captured on film or a phosphorescent screen. Immunoelectron microscopy can be done with antibodies, and gold or other metal staining.
Appearance: Black and white cross sections.
Requirements: Transmission electron microscope.

 ### Scanning electron microscopy (SEM)

Use: View external structures closely.
Advantages: Great resolution, since electrons are the light source (resolution improves with shorter wavelength). Resolution not as great as TEM.

How it works: Specimen is scanned with a focused beam of electrons, producing secondary electrons as beam hits. These are detected and converted onto a TV screen.

Appearance: 3-D view of outside of cell.

Requirements: Scanning electron microscope.

USING THE LIGHT MICROSCOPE

Working Rules

- **Check with the in-charge person** to be sure you can use the microscope. Even if you are adept at microscope use, ask her to run you through the use of the microscope, and to explain the lab use and maintenance rules, resources, and default microscope settings.

- **Keep the working area scrupulously clean.** Don't bring food, coffee, or cultures near the microscope. Never prepare samples or stain slides near the microscope.

- **If there is a sign-up list, sign up every time.** Don't forget to sign off! Keeping track of microscope usage is particularly important for fluorescence and electron scopes, as bulb and filament wearout can be predicted.

- **Don't fiddle with knobs.** Knob-fiddling is what puts microscopes out of alignment. Unless you are actually aligning the scope, leave all knobs, except the focus knob, alone!

- **Return the microscope to its usual settings** when you are finished. Remove extra lenses, micrometers, and everything that will prevent the next user from using the standard microscope setting.

- **Turn off** the microscope when you are finished.

- **Clean oil immersion lenses** every time you use them. (see p. 414.)

- **Cover the microscope** after every use or at night, whichever is the custom.

> *Exceptions to the turn-off rule may be fluorescent microscopes, when someone else is waiting to use it (turning the bulb on and off shortens bulb life), electron microscopes (usually the beam is turned down, not off, between users), and confocal microscopes.*

> *Don't use Kimwipes to clean microscope lenses! Kimwipes can scratch the lens, as can tissues or paper towels. Use only lens paper.*

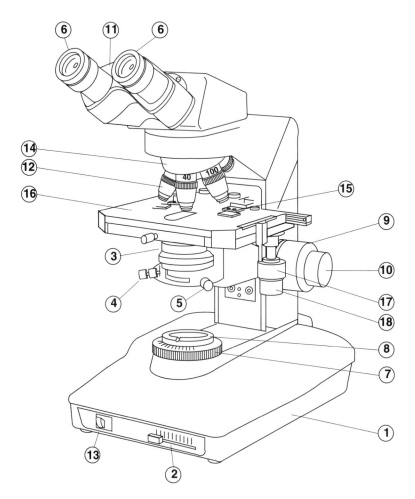

FIGURE 2.

(See facing page for legend.)

Parts and Usage of the Compound Light Microsope

Learning to identify the various parts of the light microscope and understand their function is necessary for proper operation, and therefore, clear observation of your cultures, recording of your experiments, and publication of your data. The more you know, the better you can see, and the better you can photograph what you see (see Fig. 2).

Types of illumination. *Halogen light* (or quartz light) is very intense: It has a high color temperature, which means that the resulting light is very white. Halogen light is the best type of lighting for microscopy. *Tungsten light* (or incandescent

FIGURE 2.

The compound light microscope. **Key:** (1) *Base.* The stable bottom of the microscope. (2) *Brightness control dial.* Controls light intensity. (3) *Condenser.* Used to obtain a bright, even viewfield, and influence resolution, contrast, depth of focus, and brightness. (4) *Condenser aperture diaphragm control ring.* The aperture diaphragm is attached to the condenser lens and is used to reduce scattered light by restricting the diameter of the light beam. It controls resolving power, contrast, and depth of focus. Setting the aperture at 70–80% maximum opening will reduce resolving power and brightness, but increase the contrast and the depth of focus. (5) *Condenser centering screw.* Centers the illumination condenser. (6) *Eyepiece.* Contains the ocular lens. (7) *Field diaphragm control ring.* The field diaphragm is used to restrict the illumination range. It is not used to adjust the light intensity. (8) *Field lens.* The light source lies directly below the field lens. (9) *Focus, coarse.* Turn away from yourself to lower lens, toward yourself to raise it. (10) *Focus, fine.* Turn away from yourself to lower lens, toward yourself to raise it. If it is turned too far down, turn it back toward yourself about half its range and refocus with the coarse control. (11) *Interpupillary distance scale.* Shows how much distance between each eyepiece: Set until right and left viewfields become one. (12) *Objective lens.* Lens that forms the primary image. The quality of the objective lens determines the resolving power of the microscope. (13) *Power switch.* Turns the light on and off. Turn it off when the microscope isn't in use. (14) *Revolving nosepiece.* Objective lenses are screwed into the revolving nosepiece. Any openings without an objective lens should be covered with a screw-in cap. Usually, objective lens are screwed into the nosepiece in such an order that magnification of the lens increases as the nosepiece is rotated clockwise. (15) *Slide holder.* Holds a slide snugly if the slide is seated in, not on, the holder. (16) *Stage.* Area on which the sample sits for observation. (17) *Stage y-axis travel knob.* Rotation of the knob moves the stage up or down. (18) *Stage x-axis travel knob.* Rotation of the knob moves the stage left or right.

light) has a lower color temperature, so it gives a yellowish light. However, it is cheaper to use than halogen light.

- **Changing the bulb.** The only rule is to *make sure there is a replacement bulb* when you need one! Even if you are not "in charge" of the microscope, you may be stuck when the bulb blows in the middle of a picture-taking session. Find out where the replacement bulbs are kept. If there are none, order two immediately (more than two, and other labs will just "borrow" yours when their bulb blows). Either find out what you need from the manual, or open the bulb casing, remove the bulb, and read the specifications on the stem of the bulb.

- **The objective lens.** Each objective lens will be labeled with the N.A. (the higher the N.A., the more resolution), the type, and the magnification.

  CF Achromat, CF Plan Achromat, and *CF Plan Apochromat* are, in order, names for types of objectives of increasing quality. The CF Achromat is good for general observation, but resolution and contrast are corrected well only in the center of the lens. The CF Plan Achromat has been corrected also at the periphery, and this lens is good for photomicrography. The CF Plan Apochromat has been further corrected to give the best color reproducibilty and the flattest field, making it ideal for photomicrography and close observation.

  Phase contrast objectives can be used for other types of observation. Phase contrast objectives have a phase plate attached and coated in the back focal plane, but most of the light gathered by an objective doesn't encounter the plate and is available for non-phase use with only a slight lessening of the image quality. Bright-field observations are generally just fine.

- **Measurement.** The are several *mechanical aids* that can be used to size light microscopy samples. *Calibrated slides* like hemocytometers (see Chapter 10) and Petroff Hausser chambers (see Chapter 11) are usually used for enumeration, but the grids can be used for a rough estimation of the size of the sample. Ocular micrometers (placed in the eyepiece) allow comparison of grids or circles of known size with the sample under view. Ocular micrometer images will not photograph, of course: If you need a very accurate measurement and/or a permanent record of the measurement of the sample, the calibrated standards of a *stage micrometer* would be appropriate to use.

You should always be aware of size when looking at a sample, and you should gain a feeling for the "right" size of things. A comparison of your unknown sample with remembered known samples will help assure you that things are as they should be.

Sizes of typical biological samples:

Prokaryotic cell (*E. coli*), 0.4 x 2 μm
Budding yeast (*S. cerevisiae*) 2–4 μm
Human red blood cell, 7.2 μm
Tissue culture eukaryotic cells, 10–100 μm
Nucleus, 5–25 μm
Mitochondrion, 1–10 μm
Lysosomes and peroxisomes, 0.2–0.5 μm

You may wear your glasses when you use the microscope. Glasses are only necessary if they correct for astigmatism, not for distance.

The use of immersion oil

Immersion oils cover the oil immersion lens and sample, providing a refractive index similar to glass. For maximum resolution, immersion oil can be added to the condenser lens, where it can contact the bottom of the slide. This is usually not necessary, and should not be routine, as it is quite a messy undertaking. Never use mineral or other oils.

General purpose immersion oil comes in Type A and Type B. Type A, with a lower viscosity, is preferred. Some labs mix A and B. For routine work, it won't matter. There are specialty immersion oils, such as low-fluorescence and high viscosity oil.

Add oil slowly to avoid making bubbles.

When it is said "Observe under oil immersion," it is meant oil only on the objective lens.

PROTOCOL

Using Immersion Oil on the Objective Lens

1. After locating the desired area of your specimen under 40X, swing the 40X objective out of the way. Be sure not to get any oil on the 40X lens!

2. Add one very small drop to the area of the slide under light; you only need enough oil to make a "seal" between the sample and the lens.

3. Swing the oil immersion objective lens into place.

4. Use the fine focus to make the specimen clear.

5. When you are finished, swing the oil immersion objective to the side.

6. Wipe the lens clean with lens paper.

> *Solvents such as xylene or ether can be used to remove immersion oil. But solvents can dissolve plastic and most are hazardous chemicals; some labs don't use solvents at all to clean immersion oil. Microscope users wipe all oil off with lens paper and rely on the microscope serviceperson to clean the lens during microscope maintenance visits.*

PROTOCOL

Using Immersion Oil on the Condenser Lens

> *Use high-viscosity oil to minimize dripping oil.*

1. If your slide is on the stage, remove it.

2. Place a drop of oil on the top lens of the condenser, and then lower the condenser below stage level to allow access to the bottom of the slide.

3. Place a drop of oil on the underside of the slide below the area you are interested in.

4. Set the slide down on the stage with the drop in the middle of the hole, and clamp it into place.

5. Raise the condenser so that drop meets drop and until the top condenser is fully covered with oil.

6. Place a drop of oil over the specimen and focus with the objective.

7. Adjust the condenser to give Koehler illumination and observe.

8. When you are finished, lower the condenser before picking up the slide.

9. Clean the top of the stage, as usual; the objective lens, as usual; the underside of the stage; and the condenser lens. Remove the condenser lens to clean it. Remove excess oil with lens paper. Clean the lens with fresh lens paper moistened with xylene, or a solvent recommended by the manufacturer of the lens.

Cleaning the microscope

- Brush off visible dust with a soft brush or with canned air. The field lens usually gets quite dusty.

- *Objective lens.* For smudges, wipe in a circular motion with lens paper. If xylene can be used in your lab, moisten lens paper *slightly* and wipe the lens after excess oil has been removed with lens paper alone.

- *Ocular lens.* The upper lens in the eyepiece becomes greasy from eyelashes and fingers. Wrap a piece of lens paper around your finger and wipe. To do the edges of the lens, wrap the lens paper around the tip of a wooden stick and move it gently around the perimeter of the lens. (Most labs have a microscope cleaning kit buried in a drawer. This is where you will find thin wooden sticks.)

- *Stage.* Oil from microscope slides can sometimes get smeared on the stage, but solvents usually used for cleaning immersion oil would ruin the stage. Wipe as much excess oil away as you can, using dry lens paper; do a final wipe with lens paper slightly moistened with alcohol.

Achieving Maximum Lighting and Resolution

This protocol will obtain an evenly lit field of view against which the detail of the specimen will be plainly recognizable and will light the specimen with as wide a cone of light as possible in order to achieve maximum resolution of fine detail.

This illumination method was devised by a German named Koehler in 1893 as the one nearing the ideal and has been taken as the accepted standard for aligning a light microscope. Everyone who uses a light microscope should be able to do this.

PROTOCOL

Koehler Illumination (Adapted, with permission, from Nikon Inc.)

1. Prepare the microscope head.

   a. Turn on the light and set it to a comfortable intensity level with the brightness control switch.

   b. Rotate the 10x objective into position.

   c. Rotate eyepiece diopter ring to 0′ position.

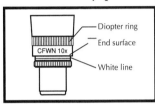

FIGURE 3.

Ocular. (Reprinted, with permission, from Nikon Inc.)

   d. Adjust interpupillary distance so both right and left images merge into one.

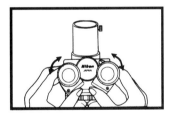

FIGURE 4.

Eyepiece. (Reprinted, with permission, from Nikon Inc.)

2. Focus for your eyes.

   a. Place a specimen on the stage.

   b. Using the coarse knob, focus the 10x objective. Adjust with fine focus on the smallest detail possible.

   c. Position the 40x objective and fine focus.

   d. If you have a 4x or 20x objective, focus with it and refocus at 40x.

   e. Select your working objective.

3. Set the condenser focus.

   a. Using the field diaphragm control ring, close the field diaphragm to its smallest size.

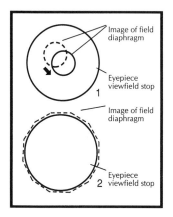

FIGURE 5.

Field diaphragm image. (Reprinted, with permission, from Nikon Inc.)

b. Bring the image of the field diaphragm into focus with the condenser focus knob.

c. Using the condenser centering screws, bring the field diaphragm image to the center of the field of view.

d. Diaphragm must be centered before clearing from the field of view.

e. Centering must be checked for each objective.

4. Center the illumination. (This step is not required for newer microscopes, with pre-centered illumination systems.)

   a. To focus and center the illumination remove the diffuser.

   b. Close the aperture diaphragm on the condenser.

   c. Use a filter (the ND or a blue filter) as a mirror to observe the filament image on the underside of the condenser. (For reflected light systems, remove an eyepiece and look at image at the back of the objective.)

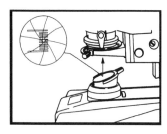

FIGURE 6.

Filament image. (Reprinted, with permission, from Nikon Inc.)

   d. Focus the filament image until it becomes sharp.

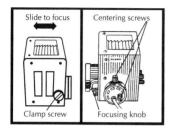

FIGURE 7.

Lamphouse. (Reprinted, with permission, from Nikon Inc.)

   e. After illumination is focused and centered, replace the diffuser.

5. Control contrast and depth of field.

   a. Remove one eyepiece. Look down the tube at the back of the objective.

   b. Adjust the aperture diaphragm so that it is just inside the opening (about 25% less than full aperture).

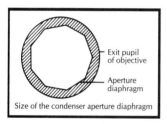

FIGURE 8.

Condenser aperture diaphragm. (Reprinted, with permission, from Nikon Inc.)

Quickie usage. Once the microscope has been aligned, you can rapidly examine your samples.

1. Remove the cover and place it out of the way.
2. Turn on the microscope. You should see, when you turn the light control on toward maximum, the light turn on.
3. Turn the objective lens out of the way.
4. Place the slide on the stage.
5. Focus with the 10X or 20X objective.
6. Switch to a higher objective.

SLIDES AND STAINS

You should always have available the supplies needed to allow you to microscopically look at all of the organisms you work with.

Tissue culture cells can often be looked at in situ with an inverted microscope. For other cultures, it is necessary to remove a sample from the culture to a slide, and either look at it as a wet mount, or fix and stain the sample and then view it.

A wet mount allows you to see living organisms. A stain is done to provide information about the internal structure or chemical properties of the cells or bacteria.

A wet mount is a suspension of cells, placed on a slide, and covered with a coverslip: The cells are viewed directly, without fixation or staining. This is a quick method, and is the easiest way to monitor the health or the density of the culture.

PROTOCOL

Making a Cell Smear

Before you can stain and fix cells or bacteria, a suspension must be spread evenly on the slide. You can add a drop of well-suspended cells to a slide and smear it with the loop or the tip of a pipet, but it is difficult to get an even spread. This can be best done with a Cytospin, a centrifuge that will spread and flatten the specimen on a microscope slide. Smearing can also be done with the aid of another microscope slide.

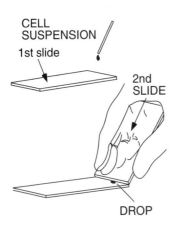

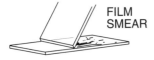

FIGURE 9.

Making a cell smear with a slide. (Redrawn, with permission, from Freshney 1994.)

Procedure

1. Add a drop of cell or bacteria suspension to the end of a microscope slide. Smears work best if the cell suspension contains serum.

2. Take another microscope slide, and place it, end up, into the drop and against the slide. Allow the drop to seep along the edge of the second slide.

> *Keep a small tube of expired serum in the refrigerator, to be used for smears. Either suspend a cell pellet in a drop of serum, or add a drop of serum to the cell suspension.*

3. Push the second slide along the length of the first slide, maintaining a 45° angle. Keep the motion smooth and constant.

4. Lift and discard the second slide. Allow the smear to air dry before fixing and staining.

PROTOCOL

Fixing the Specimen

Many stains and procedures have their own required fixatives. Solvents such as methanol can be used to fix cells and bacteria, as can protein cross-linkers such as glutaraldehyde and paraformaldehyde. In the absence of any other instruction, use methanol.

Procedure

1. Cover the sample area with methanol. This is best done in a small jar (Coplin jar) or a beaker. If you don't have a jar, pipet methanol onto the slide. Use fresh anhydrous methanol, as methanol will absorb water from the air and this will inhibit staining.

2. Remove methanol after 5 minutes.

3. Replace with fresh methanol. Leave for 5 minutes and remove.

4. Air dry.

PROTOCOL

Staining the Specimen

- Staining gives contrast to cells. Always have at least one stain to look at your cultures. It should be a stain that can give you as much information as possible about your cultures or your experiment. There are stains that are used just for particular organelles, for cell types, and in response to certain chemical reactants.

- A Gram stain kit is ideal for bacteria, as it is ready to use, very rapid, and the reagents will last for many months. The crystal violet stain in the Gram stain can be used to stain yeast, although morphology won't be preserved as it would for yeast stains made to penetrate the tough yeast cell walls. Auromine will also stain most bacteria, but won't differentiate among bacteria as will the Gram stain.

- Wright's stain and Giemsa stain are designed to differentiate among blood cell types, but they will stain most eukaryotic cells and are very simple to use.

- Methylene blue will stain everything! You won't be able to make out any detail in cells or bacteria, but you will sure know that they are there.

FLUORESCENCE MICROSCOPY

Fluorescence is a type of luminescence for which the absorption of light by a molecule is followed by the short-term emission of light. The wavelength of the emitted fluorescence is usually of a longer wavelength than the absorbed (or excitation) light (a phenomenon known as Stoke's Law), and this difference can be further enhanced with filters to selectively pass light of a defined color. Great contrast can therefore be achieved. The use of different fluorochromes allows more than one labeled molecule to be visualized in the same sample.

 Uses

- The major use of fluorescence microscopy is immunofluorescence. Antibodies labeled with fluorescence bind to their specific antigen, and the fluorescent label allows visualization of the presence, localization, and amount of the antigen.

> *Immunofluorescence can be direct or indirect. In direct the specific antibody is conjugated to a fluorochrome and is used to stain the specimen. In indirect, the specific antibody is allowed to bind to the antigen and the bound antibody is itself recognized by a fluorescently tagged antibody.*

- Molecules other than antibodies can be fluorescently tagged, and the application will depend on the molecule. In addition, living cells can be loaded with fluorescent molecules. Examples of physiological processes that can be studied with fluorescent labeling and microscopy are changes in pH, calcium, membrane potential, and the lateral mobility of lipids in membranes.

- Samples may be stained with more than one color, so two or three molecules labeled with different colors can be visualized. There can be problems with background with multiple staining, in that one stain may "bleed through" into the range supposedly specific for a particular fluorochrome. Many labs only use fluorescein as a green marker, and rhodamine as a red marker, but many, many more options are available. The Molecular Probes catalog gives a good discussion of fluorescent choices.

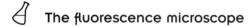

The fluorescence microscope

- A fluorescence microscope is a compound light microscope, with modifications for epifluorescence, or incident light. The objective is both the condenser lens and the objective lens of the system, containing the chromatic beam splitter that separates excitation light from emitted light. Some fluorescence microscopes use filters in combination with a bright-field microscope, but this does not give the differentiation of signals possible with epifluorescence.

- Filters—usually interference filters—give specificity to the system. Each fluorochrome requires a set of excitation and emission filters to enhance its particular signal. These are not trivial in price, and most labs have only a few sets.

- The light sources are high-pressure vapor lamps filled with mercury or xenon gas, and different light sources are recommended for different wavelengths.

- Most microscopes allow you to switch to bright-field or phase, so a non-fluorescent image of the sample can be compared with the fluorescent image.

- Cameras are commonly found on fluorescence microscopes. The use of excellent film requiring little light makes fluorescence photography relatively straightforward.

△ **Tips**

- Protect the light source. The illumination sources for fluorescence are more expensive, and have a limited life. Turning the lamp on and off should be avoided, as should leaving the light on. Most lamps need to warm up before use. Check the requirements for your lamp. There will usually be a sign-up sheet, and/or a sheet to log in lamp usage.

- Sample preparation is susceptible to artifacts. Fixation and staining are simple, but small details such as the type or temperature of the fixative or the container used to stain the sample can make a major difference in result. Each cell sample and each antibody will have its own particular needs. Speak with someone who not only has done immunofluorescence, but has done it with the same cells and, hopefully, the same antibody.

- The filters used for fluorescence microscopy are different from and in addition to the filters used to generate fluorescent light of a particular wavelength.

- When taking pictures, you will usually have to move quickly, because fluorescent samples are subject to bleaching (a decrease in fluorescence during excitation). The addition of oxygen radical scavengers such as DABCO (diaminobicyclo octane) to the sample mounting medium is effective in reducing the fading.

- Find out what filters you have before you decide on stains. It is certainly cheaper to buy a stain than a filter. However, there may be applications for which only certain stains will do, and then you must make the investment or look around your institution for a fluorescence microscope you can use.

PHOTOGRAPHY

Data must be recorded. Unless you are using the microscope just for routine checking of morphology and for contamination, you will probably need to document what you see. Also, counting or measuring samples in a photograph (and/or with the aid of a computer) rather than on the microscope is usually a much easier task.

Steps for Photography (Adapted, with permission, from Nikon Inc.)

> *Check for dust and foreign matter in the optical system before taking pictures. The microscope should be set up on a vibration-free table. Don't touch the microscope or table when taking pictures.*

Procedure

1. Make sure the microscope is set up for maximum illumination and resolution.

2. Set the ocular viewfinder.

   a. Without a specimen on the stage, focus on photo mask reticle. Start by unscrewing ocular and focus, turning slowly clockwise.

   b. Look away, then recheck.

3. Focus the specimen.

   a. Place a clean specimen on the slide.

   b. Focus on the specimen and compose the subject.

   c. Recheck focus through the ocular viewfinder. Always make the last focus movement up against gravity.

4. Set the voltage and filter.

   Automatic systems: Set the ASA only. Some microscopes will not even require this.
   Manual systems: Check the manufacture's chart for suggested film, filter, and voltage settings.

5. Set the exposure.

   Automatic systems: The exposure time will be determined once the sample is viewed, according to the ASA and the available light: When sufficient exposure has occurred, the shutter will close.
   Manual systems: Bracket your exposures because specimens vary greatly in their ratio of dark area to light. Compensate for different lighting conditions: For bright-field, the setting is usually within ±1/3 of exposure adjustment. For dark-field and fluorescence, the setting is usually between −1 and −2 of exposure adjustment. Use a light meter to determine the exposure. Experience is the only way you will get your exposure settings correct.

6. Adjust the aperture and field.

   a. Readjust the aperture diaphragm on the condenser for best results with the particular specimen.

   b. Close the aperture to approximately 75% of full aperture. Closing the aperture further will give more contrast and depth of field at the expense of resolution.

   c. Set the field diaphragm just outside of the film format in photo mask reticle.

   d. Recheck.

   e. Press exposure button to expose film.

What Film Should Be Used?

Use Kodak film. It is dependable film, and you can get plenty of technical advice. Of course, ask whomever shows you the microscope and photographic system about the film he or she recommends. Older systems, with less bright illumination and without automatic exposure meters, relied much more heavily on film choice, as most manipulation of image was done by film and filter choice. It is much easier now to capture the image you see, and you generally will not have to worry about daylight colors and filters and stopping up and down.

Format: 35 mm film

Black and white

   • Black and white film can be used to document color as well as black and white samples. It is less expensive than color film and can give as much information. If color is not needed to get across your point, use black and white film.

   • Kodak Technical Pan Film (TP). A high-contrast film, good for general photomicrography, as well as interference and phase contrast photomicrography.

   • Kodak T-MAX 400 Professional Film (TMY). A faster film than TP, good for photographing dimly lit subjects. Use for fluorescence or dark-field photomicrography, or for photomicrography of live biological specimens.

Color slide film

- Use color slide film for presentations and seminars.

- Kodak Ektachrome 64T Professional Film (EPY). Good for general use with tungsten-halogen or ordinary tungsten lamps. Excellent for bright-field microscopy of stained tissue.

- Kodak Ektachrome 160T Professional Film (EPT). Use with tungsten illumination.

- Kodak Ektachrome P1600 Professional Film (EPH). Designed for low-light photography. Use for singly or doubly labeled fluorescence specimens.

Color print film

- Prints are usually only useful for photographs for publication. Prints can also be made from slides, with a minimal (to most eyes) loss of quality.

- Kodak Pro 100 Professional Film (PRN) (or 400 or 1000, for photography with lower light).

> *Speed ratings are given in ISO or EI, for Kodak films. The higher the number, the less light is required. Most films have an ISO rating: EI ratings are used when the standard conditions used for testing exposure don't apply to the film use. The numbers very approximately are comparable.*

Filters

Filters are used to enhance or slightly alter the color inherent in the film. Most of the effects of filters are personal preferences.

- Neutral density filter absorbs light evenly through the visible spectrum. It therefore lowers the intensity of light without changing color.

- Daylight blue filter absorbs some yellow to red light from the microscope lamp, giving light of better color to daylight film.

- Tungsten color films generally require no filter.

- A green filter gives additional contrast to black and white film. It can be used when taking a black and white picture of a stained sample.

> *For color daylight film, voltage should be set to film specifications and color balance.*

Storage

Film, especially professional film, should be stored below 55°F. The package of film must be warmed to room temperature before it is opened. Film can be kept in the freezer, but the refrigerator is ideal, since you won't have to wait as many hours for the film to warm up.

Processing

Although color film is almost unvaryingly sent away to be developed, many labs develop black and white films themselves, and send the negatives only to be printed. Developing film is a simple matter, but because unevenness in development can be a problem, be sure to follow developing directions carefully.

How to Tell if You Have a Good Picture

- Does it demonstrate the point of the experiment?

- Does it document a problem or minor point of the experiment?

- Is it pretty? Is it clear?

SHARED INSTRUMENT FACILITIES

Certain microscope systems, such as electron microscopes, confocal microscopes, and fluorescence activated cell sorters (FACS), are very expensive to purchase and maintain and are beyond the financial reach of many investigators. These tend to be found in shared instrument facilities, meaning that the department, institution, or group of investigators shares in the costs.

The good side of this is that an individual researcher can test a theory or procedure without a huge expenditure. There is usually a highly skilled person in charge of the microscope who can take care of minor problems and help you to understand what is going on.

The bad side is that you may have to wait for quite a long while for your turn. These facilities are run in different ways: You may be required to do anything from turning over your unfixed samples to the facility to running the equipment yourself.

Always check with the microscopist several weeks before you plan to do the experiment. Find out when he or she can do your samples, and how the samples must be prepared.

RESOURCES

Care and Use of the Light Microscope. Department of Anatomy and Cell Biology, Emory University School of Medicine, 1995.
http://www.emory.edu/EMORY_CLASS/CELL_BIOLOGY/Microscope.html

Fisher Scientific. FAQ- Microscopy.
http://www.fisher1.com/faq/micro.html

Freshney R.I. 1994. *Culture of animal cells. A manual of basic technique,* 3rd edition. Wiley-Liss, New York.

Haugland R.P. 1996. *Handbook of fluorescent probes and research chemicals,* 6th edition. Molecular Probes, Eugene, Oregon.

Heidcamp W.H. 1995. *Cell biology laboratory manual,* Chapter 1, *The microscope.* Gustavus Adolphus College, St. Peter, Minnesota.
http://www.gac.edu/cgi-bin/user/~cellab/phpl?index-1.html

How to use a microscope and take a photomicrograph. Nikon Inc., Instrument Group.
1300 Walt Whitman Road
Melville, New York 11747-3064
(516) 547-8500
Fax (516) 547-0306
For film and filter types, setting up for photomicrography, setting up a microscope
http://www.pharm.Arizona.edu/centers/tox_center/swehsc/exp_path/m-i_onw3.html

Lacey A.J., ed. 1989. *Light microscopy in biology. A practical approach.* IRL Press at Oxford University Press, New York.

Matsumoto B., ed. 1993. *Cell biological applications of confocal microscopy. Methods Cell Biology,* Volume 38. Academic Press, New York.

Molecular Probes Web site
http://www.probes.com/probes/
Information on matching of filter sets with fluorophores.

Murray R.G.E. and Robinow C.F. 1994. Light microscopy. In *Methods for general and molecular bacteriology* (ed. Gerhardt P. et al.), chapter 1, pp. 7–20. American Society for Microbiology, Washington, D.C.

Omega Optical
1-(800) 254-2690
http://www.omegafilters.com/fforfstart.html
Filters for Nikon, Zeiss, Leitz, and Olympus.

Pawley J.B., ed. 1995. *Handbook of biological confocal microscopy,* 2nd edition. Plenum Press, New York.
For the advanced user.

Rawlins D.J. 1992. Light microscopy. BIOS Scientific Publishers, Oxford.

Rubbi C.P. 1994. *Light microscopy. Essential data.* BIOS Scientific Publishers, John Wiley and Sons, New York.

Stanier R.Y., Adelberg E.A., and Ingraham J.L. 1986. *Microbial world,* 5th edition. Prentice-Hall, Englewood Cliffs, New Jersey.

Glossary

Absorbance: The amount of light not passed through a substance.

Accession number: A coded identifier provided by a database for an individual DNA sequence.

Acid: A substance that gives up a proton and so may have a positive charge associated with it. An acid has a pH below 7.

Acrylamide: A synthetic polymer that forms a matrix used for electrophoresis.

Additive effect: The effect of treatment A and the effect of treatment B give the same effect, just greater in quantity, suggesting that A and B work through the same pathway.

Aerobe: An organism that grows in the presence of oxygen.

Aerosol: A gaseous suspension of fine or liquid particles.

Affinity: Strength of the binding between ligand and receptor.

Agar (or agar agar): A complex polysaccharide used as a gelling agent to prepare solid or semisolid microbiological medium. Agar consists of about 70% agarose and 30% agaropectin. Agar will melt at temperatures above 100°C and will gel at 40–50°C.

Agarose: A non-sulfated linear polymer consisting of alternating residues of D-galactose and 3,6-anhydro-L-galactose. It is extracted from seaweed and is widely used as the resolving agent in electrophoresis.

Alkaline phosphatase: Enzyme that can produce a chromogenic reaction product, used as a reporter gene or to detect antibody binding.

Alpha particle: A species formed by radioactive decay, consisting of two protons and two neutrons.

Amphoteric: Able to act as an acid or a base.

Amplification: (1) The increase in copy number of a plasmid by inhibition of chromosome replication while allowing plasmid replication to continue. (2) The increase of the number of copies of a gene either by duplication in the chromosome or by cloning into a plasmid vector. This is normally referred to as gene amplification.

Ampoule: A small glass or plastic vial.

Anhydrous: Free of water. Often used to describe a solid having no water of crystallization or a solvent from which traces of water have been removed.

Anion: A negatively charged ion.

Anionic detergent: Detergent in which the hydrophilic function is fulfilled by anionic groups. Fatty acids and SDS are examples.

Annealing: The formation of double-stranded DNA from single-stranded DNA.

Anode: The positively charged electrode to which anions are attracted.

Antibiotic: A substance able to kill or inhibit the growth of certain microorganisms.

Antifungal, antimycotic: A substance that kills fungi.

Antiseptic: An agent that kills or inhibits microbial growth but is not harmful to human tissue.

Antiserum: A serum containing antibodies.

Apoptosis: Programmed cell death.

Artifact: A result caused by other than the desired manipulation.

Aseptic technique: Manipulation of sterile instruments or culture in such a way as to maintain sterility.

Aspirate: To remove liquid or gas by suction.

Assay: To examine by experiment; qualitative or quantitative analysis.

Atomic weight, atomic mass: The average weight of an atom of an element; the total mass of protons and neutrons in an atom.

Attenuation: (1) Reduction in the virulence of a pathogen; usually an attenuated pathogen is still capable of immunizing. (2) A process that plays a role in the regulation of enzymes involved in amino acid biosynthesis.

Autoclave: Steam sterilizer.

Autoclave tape: Heat-sensitive tape that usually spells the word "Sterile" only after being autoclaved.

Autoradiography: Detection of radioactivity in a sample, for example, a cell or gel, by placing it in contact with a photographic film such as an X-ray film.

Auxotroph: A mutant that has a growth factor requirement.

Axenic: Culture containing a single type of cell.

Bacillus: A bacterium with an elongated, rod shape.

Background: An effect present at constant level among treated and untreated groups.

Bactericidal: Capable of killing bacteria.

Bacteriostatic: Capable of inhibiting bacterial growth without killing.

Badge: Pocket dosimeter.

Bake: To expose to high temperatures to dry.

Band: (1)After gel electrophoresis and staining, an individual fragment or peptide seen as a rectangular piece in a lane. (2) Individual areas in a gradient after separation of a complex mix.

Basal medium: An unsupplemented medium that allows the growth of many types of microorganisms which do not require any special nutrient supplements; e.g., nutrient broth.

Base: A substance that accepts a proton, and so may have a negative charge associated with it. A base has a pH above 7. Alkaline = basic.

Baseline: A line used as reference, minus treatment or manipulation.

Becquerel (Bq): 1 Bq = one disintegration per second. A standard unit of radioactivity.

Bench paper: Plastic-backed absorbent paper, which comes in individual sheets or a roll.

Beta particle: A particle formed by radioactive decay, equivalent to an electron.

Biochemicals: Biological substances.

Biohazard: A biological substance that is potentially harmful. For disposal, this means anything living or anything that has touched anything living.

Biosafety cabinet (biohazard cabinet): Hood or cabinet equipped to protect the worker from the material she is working with. There are three main classifications of biosafety cabinets, to be used with organisms posing different levels of risk.

Blank: Reference solution. In spectroscopy, a solution containing all components except the absorbing species of interest.

Bleaching (fading): A decrease in fluorescence during excitation.

Blotting: The transfer of the DNA, RNA, or protein in a gel to a filter (a piece of nylon or nitrocellulose).

Blue-white selection: Color screening system to determine whether or not a plasmid is carrying an insert. Insertion of a foreign gene into the polylinker of reporter gene *lacZ* (coding for β-galactosidase) inactivates β-galactosidase and colonies remain white. Plasmids not carrying an insert produce β-galactosidase, which can hydrolyze chromogenic substrate X-gal and make the colony appear blue.

Blunt ends: Ends of a DNA molecule that are fully base-paired.

Bomb: Nitrogen cavitation bomb, which disrupts biomatter by nitrogen.

Box: Container for gel electrophoresis.

Boyle's Law: The volume of gas is inversely proportional to the pressure.

Bremsstrahlung. A kind of radiation created when beta rays interact with and are slowed down by solid material.

Brownian (salutary) motion: Not to be confused with motility; the small back and forth or circular motion of a microbe or cell in suspension.

Brushes: Part of a motor completing a circuit. In the centrifuge, brushes are subject to wear and must be replaced.

Budding: (1) Asexual reproduction (usually by yeasts) beginning as a protuberance from the parent cell that grows to become a daughter cell. (2) Release of an enveloped virus through the plasma membrane of an animal cell.

Buffer: A solution whose pH resists change following addition of small amounts of an acid or a base.

Calibrate: To check, adjust, or systematically standardize the graduations of a quantitative measuring instrument.

Capillary action: The spontaneous movement of a liquid into thin tubes or fibers, determined by adhesive and cohesive forces and surface tension.

Carcinogen: A substance that causes the initiation of tumor formation. Frequently a mutagen.

Cathode: The negatively charged electrode toward which cations are drawn.

Cation: A positively charged ion.

Causality: The relationship between something that produces an effect and the effect.

Caustic: Any strongly alkaline material that produces either corrosion or irritation to living tissue.

Cell wall: The layer or structure outside the cytoplasmic membrane; it supports and protects the membrane and gives the cell shape.

Chaotropic agent: A chemical or mixture that will disrupt a cell.

Chase: To follow a treatment with a period without treatment, to analyze the timing of the effect of the active substance in the treatment.

Chelate: To bind a metal ion to a multivalent ligand. This usually effectively reduces the ion's participation in other reactions.

Chemical: A substance produced or used in a chemical process.

Chemical reactivity: The ability of a material to chemically change, possibly resulting in explosion hazards or the liberation of toxic fumes.

Chemiluminescence: The emission of light as a side product of a chemical reaction.

Chi square: A theoretical sampling distribution used to test whether a sample was drawn from a given population.

Chromatography: The separation of a mixture into its components by passing the fluid over a non-mobile absorbant and isolating the components by differential absorption and elution.

Chromogenic: Capable of a color change.

Clone: (1) A population of cells all descended from a single cell. (2) A number of copies of a DNA fragment to be replicated by a phage or plasmid.

Cloning vector: A DNA molecule that is able to bring about the replication of foreign DNA fragments.

Cold: Slang for nonradioactive.

Colony: A clone of bacterial cells on a solid medium that is visible to the naked eye.

Colony forming unit (cfu): Any entity (usually a viable single cell) that can form a colony on an agar plate.

Comb: A piece of plastic used to make wells in gels.

Competence: The ability of a bacterium to take up DNA and become genetically transformed.

Complex buffer: A buffer with more than one ingredient.

Complex medium: A medium whose precise chemical composition is unknown. Also called undefined medium.

Concatemer: A DNA molecule consisting of two or more separate molecules linked end to end to form a long linear structure. Usually a cloning artifact.

Consensus sequence: A nucleic acid sequence in which the bases present in given positions are those bases most commonly found when many experimentally determined sequences are compared.

Consistent: Successive results agree with the first.

Constitutive: Occurs constantly, without a stimulus.

Contact inhibition: The inhibition of continued growth and division of a cell or colony due to physical contact with other cells or colonies.

Contamination: A relative term for having some living thing you don't want growing where you think it shouldn't.

Contrast: In microscopy, exaggeration of dark and light elements.

Control: A standard against which experimental variations can be compared.

Cooling trap (vapor trap): Chamber kept cold; used to prevent volatile substances from being drawn into a vacuum pump.

Copy number: (1) The number of copies of a plasmid per cell. (2) The number of copies of a gene.

Correlation: A correspondence between two entities.

Correlation coefficient: Describes the strength of the linear relationship between two effects.

Corrosive: A chemical that causes destruction of tissue by chemical action at the site of contact.

Cosmid: Cloning vector used to carry large pieces of DNA.

Counts per minute (cpm): The number of B particles detected per minute. cpm = dpm $\times$ efficiency of the counting device.

Culture: A particular strain or kind of organism growing in a laboratory medium.

Curie (Ci): An older but still used standard of radioactivity. Measures the amount of radioactive decay. 1 Ci = 2.22 $\times$ 10^{12} dpm.

Cuvette: A vessel used to hold a sample in a spectrophotometer.

Cytokine: A family of small secreted peptides usually not produced by lymphocytes with a variety of effects on inflammation, chemotaxis, angiogenesis, and T-cell proliferation.

Dalton: Unit of molecular mass approximately equal to the mass of a hydrogen atom.

Data sheet: Materials Safety Data sheet.

Decay: Disintegration of a radioactive atom.

Deductive thought: A hypothesis is proposed, and data are collected to confirm or disconfirm the hypothesis.

Defined medium: A medium whose exact chemical composition is quantitatively known.

Degeneracy: In relation to the genetic code, the fact that more than one codon can code for the same amino acid.

Degrees of freedom: The number of observations minus the number of parameters that must be estimated. For example, if only the standard deviation of a population is estimated, then the number of degrees is one less than the sample number (Carr 1992).

Deionization: The removal of ionic impurities by passing the liquid through an ion exchange resin.

Deletion: A removal of a portion of a gene.

Denaturation: Irreversible destruction of a macromolecule, such as the destruction of a protein by heat.

Denature: To disrupt the secondary or tertiary structure of a protein by physical or chemical means, usually resulting in a loss in biological activity.

Densitometer: Instrument that measures the light transmitted through a solid support such as X-ray film, and therefore allows quantitation of the signal on the film.

Depth of field: The distance through the object along the optical axis within which an object's features appear acceptably sharp.

Desiccation: Drying.

Detergent: Surface-active molecules with polar (water-soluble, hydrophilic) and nonpolar (hydrophobic) domains. They bind strongly to hydrophobic molecules or molecular domains to confer water solubility. Examples include sodium dodecyl sulfate (SDS), fatty acid salts, the Triton family, and octyl glycoside.

Deuterium: The isotope of hydrogen with one neutron in its nucleus.

Dewar flask: Container used to transport and pour liquid nitrogen.

Dialysis: A process in which ions or small molecules in a solution pass through a semipermeable membrane while larger molecules remain behind.

Differential medium: A medium used to differentiate different types of microorganisms on the basis of their differences in reaction to a component of the medium.

Dilution: The addition of a solvent to a solution or mixture to decrease the concentration of a solute or compound.

Dimer: A molecule formed by the combination of two smaller identical units.

Discontinuous electrophoresis (disc electrophoresis): A type of polyacrylamide gel electrophoresis that uses gels of two different concentrations of acrylamide, the one of lower concentration stacked on the one of higher concentration, to better resolve bands.

Disinfectant: An agent that kills microorganisms but may be harmful to human tissue.

Disintegrations per minute (dpm): The number of atoms disintegrating per minute in a radioactive element.

Distillation: The process of boiling a liquid and condensing the vapor to either remove impurities or separate components of a liquid mixture.

Domain: A region of a protein having a distinct function.

Dominant negative: The expression of a mutated form of a gene suppresses the activity of its non-mutated homolog.

Dose-response: The range of effects of a substance ranging through a dose with no effect, the minimum dose needed for an effect, the dose needed for a maximum effect, and the dose needed for a toxic effect.

Double-blind study: An experiment made to test a treatment or drug in which neither the subjects nor the investigators know the identity of the treatments given to any group.

Doubling time: The time needed for a population to double. Also known as generation time.

Download: To retrieve a file via the Internet.

Downstream position: Refers to nucleic acid sequences on the 3′ side of a given site on the DNA or RNA molecule.

Dry ice: Frozen carbon dioxide, called dry because of its tendency to sublime (go from a solid to a gas without first forming a liquid).

Dry run: Experiment performed without one or more components.

Electroelution: To drive a substance out of a matrix with an electric current.

Electrolyte: A substance that dissociates in water to form ions, thus increasing the extent to which the liquid conducts electricity.

Electron volt (eV): The energy acquired by an electron when accelerating along a potential gradient of 1 volt. $1 \text{ eV} = 1.6 \times 10^{12}$ erg. $1 \text{ mV} = 10^6 \text{ eV}$.

Electronic bulletin board: A WWW site where users can post and respond to notices.

Electrophoresis: The separation of molecules based on their mobility in an electric field. High-resolution techniques normally use a gel support such as agarose or acrylamide for the fluid phase.

Electroporation: The use of an electrical current to create transient pores in the cell membrane. Usually used for the uptake of DNA.

Emulsion: A mixture of two normally unmixable liquids (e.g., water and oil) in which one exists as tiny particles within the other.

Enrichment culture: Use of selective culture medium and incubation conditions to isolate microorganisms directly from nature.

Enteric bacteria: A large group of gram-negative rod-shaped bacteria characterized by a facultatively aerobic metabolism. Many are found in the intestines of animals.

Enzyme-linked immunoabsorbent assay (ELISA): An immunoassay that uses specific antibodies to detect antigens or antibodies. The antibody-containing complexes are visualized through enzyme coupled to the antibody. Addition of substrate to the enzyme-antibody-antigen complex results in a colored product.

Epillumination: An illumination mode where the illuminating light reaches the specimen from the objective lens, which thus works both as a condenser and objective.

Epitope: Antigenic determinant.

Ethidium bromide (EtBr): A fluorescent carcinogen that intercalates into nucleic acid molecules and is used to stain and visualize nucleic acids.

Exponential growth: Also known as log growth (for logarithmic); that stage when the cell number of a population doubles within a fixed time period.

Expression: The ability of a gene to function within a cell in such a way that the gene products are formed.

Expression vector: A cloning vector that contains the necessary regulatory sequences to allow transcription and translation of a cloned gene or genes.

Extracellular matrix: A mixture of proteins in the outside of the cell that help the cell attach to a surface on which it can grow.

Extract: To remove a component, such as performing a phenol treatment (extraction) of cells to remove protein.

Facultative: An adjective used to describe an environmental factor that is optional. For example, a facultative aerobe can normally grow in the presence of oxygen but, alternatively, can also grow without oxygen.

Fallacy: A false belief, a notion based on untrue or incorrect reasoning.

Feeder layer: Cells (usually lethally irradiated) grown with the desired cell cultures, providing a growth factor for the desired cells.

Fermenter: A self-contained environment for the culture of one to thousands of liters at a time.

Ficoll: A biologically inert sucrose polymer used as a thickening agent in solutions (such as hybridization mixtures and gradients).

Fix: (1) To preserve tissue or cells for staining or other treatment. (2) To repair, an uncommon lab usage.

Flame: (1) A personal attack over the web. (2) To pass a glass pipet or flask, or metal transfer needle or loop, quickly through a flame.

Flammable liquid: Flammable liquids have a flash point below 37.8°C (100°F).

Flash point: The lowest temperature at which a liquid gives off sufficient vapor to form an ignitable mixture with the air at the liquid's surface.

Fluor: The light-response agent in scintillation fluid.

Fluorescein: A fluorescent molecule used to label antibodies green.

Fluorescein isocyanate: A fluorescent chemical derived from fluorescein used to label proteins.

Fluorescence: The emission of one or more photons by a molecule activated by the absorption of electromagnetic radiation. A molecule absorbs light of one wavelength and emits light of lower energy at a longer wavelength. Detection of fluorescence requires both a beam of light to excite the dye and a photodetector to detect the fluorescent emission.

Fluorescence activated cell sorter (FACS): A machine that sorts particles such as cells or chromosomes according to their fluorescence.

Fluorophore: A protein found in jellyfish that fluoresces green visible light when excited by UV light of 395 nm. It can function as a biological marker when attached to other proteins.

Formula weight: The gram molecular weight of a compound substance. The molecular weight of Na is 22.98, the formula weight of NaCl is 58.43, 22.98 for Na and 35.45 for Cl.

Friend buffers: A series of zwitterionic (both positively and negatively charged) buffers used for all culture and biochemical work. Examples are HEPES, MES, PIPES, and MOPS.

G force: Gravitational force exerted during centrifugation.

G + C ratio: In DNA and RNA from any organism, the percentage of total nucleic acid that consists of guanine plus cytosine bases.

Gamma ray: High-energy radiation emitted during radioactive decay.

Gaussian distribution (normal distribution): The chance of occurrence of two alternative events.

Geiger counter: A device used to measure the amount of radioactivity present.

Gel: An inert polymer usually made of agarose or polyacrylamide, used for separating macromolecules such as nucleic acids or proteins by electrophoresis.

Gelatin: A protein extracted from the connective tissue of animals.

Gene disruption: The use of both in vitro and in vivo recombination to substitute an easily selected mutant gene for a wild-type gene.

Generation time: The time needed for a population to double. The same as doubling time.

Gopher: A menu-driven Internet information system, consisting of files posted by individual servers.

Gram negative: In Gram's stain, a differential bacterial stain, gram-negative cells lose the primary stain after alcohol and retain the pink counterstain.

Gram positive: In Gram's stain, a differential bacteria stain, gram-positive cells retain the purple color of the primary stain, even after alcohol treatment.

Gram's stain: A differential stain that divides bacteria into two groups, gram positive and gram negative, based on the ability to retain crystal violet when decolorized with an organic solvent such as ethanol.

Growth curve: Graphic representation of the increase in cell numbers over time.

Growth rate: The rate at which growth occurs, usually expressed as the generation time.

Half-life: The time it would take for half of the radioactivity in a sample to disappear.

Heteroduplex: A double-stranded DNA in which one strand is from one source and the other strand from another, usually different but related, source.

Hood: Biosafety cabinet or fume hood.

Horseradish peroxidase (HRP): A peroxidase isolated from the horseradish plant, used to label proteins and nucleic acids. The molecule to be labeled is attached to the HRP molecule, and the mixture is exposed to a substrate that changes from clear to colored when it is oxidized by HRP.

Hot: (1) Radioactive. (2) Important and sexy.

Hot room: A room or area used for radioactive work.

Hybridization: The natural formation or artificial construction of a duplex nucleic acid molecule by complementary base-pairing between two nucleic acid strains derived from different sources.

Hybridoma: The fusion of an immortal cell with a single B lymphocyte to produce an immortal lymphocyte that produces a monoclonal antibody.

Hydrophilic: Tending to combine or mix with water.

Hydrophobic: Tending not to combine or mix with water.

Hygroscopic: Absorbing moisture from the air.

Immobilized enzyme: An enzyme attached to a solid support over which substrate is passed and is converted into product.

Immunoblot (Western blot): Detection of proteins immobilized on a filter by complementary reaction with specific antibody.

Immunoglobulin: Antibody.

Incubate: To maintain a sample at certain conditions, not necessarily in an incubator.

Inducible: The ability of a particular protein to be synthesized in response to an external substance (the inducer).

Inductive thought: Examines a collection of evidence and then proposes a theory to account for all of the observed facts.

Infection: (1) Invasion of the body by microorganisms that can then grow. (2) Manipulation of the growth of viruses or bacteria in the lab.

Infectious waste: Waste that is capable of causing disease, containing oncogenic viruses or pathogenic organisms.

Inhibition: Prevention of growth or function.

In-house: In one's own institution.

Inoculating loop, inoculating needle: Plastic or metal rod used to introduce a sample of microorganisms to fresh medium.

Inoculum: Material used to initiate a microbial culture.

In situ: In the original place (Latin). Experimental manipulation done without removing the experimental material to another environment.

Internet: A network of interconnecting computers.

Ion: An atom or covalently bonded set of atoms that carries an overall net charge.

Ion exchange: The replacement of ions by other ions, usually on the surface of a resin designed as a reservoir for ions.

Ionizing radiation: Electromagnetic radiation of sufficient energy to knock electrons from molecules, forming ions.

Ionophore: A compound that can cause the leakage of ions across membranes.

Isoelectric point: The pH at which a molecule's overall surface charge is neutral.

Isoschizomer: Restriction enzymes that cleave in the same target sequence as each other.

Isotope: One or more atoms of an element that differ in the number of neutrons found in the nucleus.

Kinase: An enzyme that adds a phosphate to a protein.

Knockout: Disruption of a gene so that the gene cannot be transcribed.

Koehler illumination: Aligning a compound microscope to achieve the maximum illumination.

Label: (1) To attach an indicator molecule such as radioactivity to a cell or macromolecule. (2) To write the contents, date, and your name on every tube.

Laboratory Safety Department: The institution's group that oversees safety.

Laboratory Safety Officer: A laboratory member who acts as liaison between the members of the lab and the Laboratory Safety Department.

LacZ: Bacterial gene coding for B-galactosidase, used as a reporter gene in eukaryotic transfections.

Lag phase: The period after inoculation of a population before growth begins.

Lambda: Abbreviation for microliter.

Laminar flow: Sterile air blown over a work surface in a cabinet or hood.

Lane: The path of a sample in a gel.

Leukocyte: A white blood cell, usually a phagocyte.

Library: A collection of cloned DNA fragments which in total contain genes from the entire genome of an organism. Also known as a DNA library, gene library, or cDNA library.

Ligand: (1) One of the molecules or metal ions in a complex. (2) The target of a particular antibody. (3) The molecule that binds to a receptor.

Ligase: Enzyme that joins together two pieces of DNA.

Light box: (1) Visible light screen used to look at slides or autoradiographs. (2) Slang for transilluminator.

Linear regression: If two effects have a linear relationship, one can be predicted from the result of the other.

Lipopolysaccharide (LPS): Complex lipid structure containing unusual sugars and fatty acids, found in the outer layer of the cell wall of gram-negative bacteria. LPS has a profound effect on many mammalian cells.

Listserv lists: Special interest groups who sign up by E-mail, and receive relevant postings by E-mail.

Lowry assay: Protein determination method, now supplanted by the BCA assay.

Luciferase: An enzyme that catalyzes light emission in marine bacteria, coded for by the lux genes. Lux genes are used as part of a transcriptional fusion as a reporter gene.

Luminescence: Production of light.

Lysis: Rupture of a cell, resulting in a loss of cell contents.

Lysogen: A prokaryote containing a prophage.

Macromolecule: A molecule with a molecular weight over 1000 daltons.

Manifold: Setup of piping that allows several tanks to be controlled by the same regulator.

Mass spectrophotometer (mass spec): An instrument that measures the mass of ions by accelerating them through electric and magnetic fields.

Materials safety data sheet (MSDS): The description of the properties of a chemical that must be included by the manufacturer or distributor with every chemical sold.

Mechanistic approach: Designing experiments to find how things work.

Medium (plural media): A liquid or solid material that is prepared for the growth, maintenance, or storage of microorganisms or cells.

Meniscus: The curvature of a liquid in a vessel at the liquid/air interface. Volume is measured from the bottom of the meniscus.

Metabolism: All biochemical reactions in a cell, both anabolic and catabolic.

Microaerophilic: Requiring oxygen but at a level lower than atmospheric.

Microcarriers: Plastic globular particles approximately 10 times the size of cells, upon which cells can be cultivated. The particles are kept suspended by the movement of the medium.

Microorganism: A living organism too small to be seen with the naked eye. Includes bacteria, fungi, protozoans, microscopic algae, and viruses.

Milli-Q: Trade name (Millipore) for a water purification system that provides reagent grade water by treatment with a series of resins and filters.

Miscible: Able to dissolve in each other in any proportion.

Mitogen: A substance able to induce mitosis of certain eukaryotic cells.

Mohr pipet: Measuring pipet; has graduations to allow it to deliver a range of volumes.

Molarity: The number of moles of solute in 1 liter of solution.

Mold: A filamentous fungus. A common contaminant in tissue culture.

Mole: A mole equals the gram molecular weight of the solute.

Molecular weight: The sum of the atomic weights of the atoms of a molecule.

Monoclonal antibody: An antibody produced from a single clone of cells. This antibody has uniform structure and specificity. Produced in mouse, hamster, and rat; usually mouse.

Monocyte: Circulating white blood cell that contains many lysosomes and can differentiate into a macrophage.

Motility: The property of movement of a cell under its own power.

Mutagen: A substance that causes heritable genetic damage.

Mutant: An organism, population, gene, or chromosome, etc., that differs from the corresponding wild type by one or more mutations.

Mycoplasma: A group of bacteria without a cell wall, very small (probably the smallest organisms capable of autonomous growth), and most famous as a tissue culture contaminant.

Necrosis: Once considered to be nonspecific cell death, characterized by traumatized membranes and cytoplasmic changes.

Needle: Inoculating needle.

Negative control: Experimental control done to show what the lack of an effect looks like.

Newsgroups: Special interest groups whose topics are posted on the Internet. Newsgroups are similar to Listserv lists, but do not receive the information by E-mail.

Nick translation: A procedure for making a DNA probe in which a DNA fragment is treated with DNase to produce single-stranded nicks, followed by incorporation of labeled nucleotides from the nicked sites by DNA polymerase I.

Nonionic detergent: Detergent in which the hydrophilic head group is uncharged: Hydrophilicity is usually conferred by –OH groups. Examples are the Tritons and octyl glucoside.

Nonsense mutation: A mutation that changes a sense codon into one that does not code for an amino acid.

Normal: A solution having one gram equivalent weight of solute per liter of solution.

Normality: The molarity of a solution multiplied by the number of moles of that substance that occur in a chemical equation.

Northern blot: Hybridization of a single strand of nucleic acid (DNA or RNA) to RNA fragments immobilized on a filter.

Nucleotide: A monomeric unit of nucleic acid, consisting of a sugar (ribose), a phosphate, and a nitrogenous base.

Null hypothesis: The assumption that experimental results are random: A rejection of the null hypothesis means that the results are not due to chance variation.

Nutrient agar: The solid version of nutrient broth for bacteria supplemented with agar.

Nutrient broth: A general purpose liquid basal medium composed of, e.g., beef extract and peptone, which allows many types of organisms to grow.

Obligate: An adjective referring to an environmental factor that is always required for growth; e.g., obligate aerobe.

Oligonucleotide: A short nucleic acid molecule, obtained from an organism or synthesized chemically.

Open reading frame (ORF): The entire length of a DNA molecule that starts with a start codon and ends with a stop codon.

Organelle: A membrane-enclosed body specialized for carrying out certain functions. Found only in eukaryotic cells.

Organic: A species containing carbon. Certain small ions and compounds containing carbon (such as carbon dioxide) are usually considered to be inorganic.

Osmosis: Diffusion of water through a semipermeable membrane from a region of low solute concentration to one of higher concentration.

Oxidation: A process by which a compound gives up electrons, acting as an electron donor, and becomes oxidized.

P value: The letter P stands for the probability of a particular event to occur. The P value is a fraction between 0 and 1.0: 0 means that there is no chance the event would occur, and 1.0 means there is no chance the event would not occur. A probability is usually considered significant at 0.01 to 0.05.

Palindrome: A nucleotide sequence on a DNA molecule in which the same sequence is found on each strand, but in the opposite direction.

Paradigm: Thought pattern through which a person (or field) filters all perspective.

Parafocal: Objectives with very similar focusing distances, so little or no focus adjustment has to be made when changing objective lens.

Passage: Subculture: the transfer of cells, usually with feeding, from one culture vessel to another.

Pathogenicity: The ability of a parasite to inflict damage on the host.

Pellet: The compacted particle matter or cells found at the bottom of a tube after centrifugation.

pH: A logarithmic measure of the concentration of hydrogen ion.

Phagemid: A cloning vector that can replicate either as a plasmid or as a bacteriophage.

Phenomenology: Description without dissection, a necessary step before a mechanistic analysis.

Phenotypic drift: The propensity of an organism to apparently change over time.

Phosphatase: An enzyme that removes phosphates from proteins.

Photobleaching: Dampening of the excitation of a fluorescent molecule by light.

Photon: A quantum of energy from electromagnetic radiation.

Phototube detector: Converts light energy to an electrical signal.

Pig: The outermost container, made of lead, for radioactive materials.

Pilot: Tentative model for further experiments.

Plaque: A localized area of lysis or cell inhibition caused by virus infection on a lawn of cells.

Plasma: The noncellular portion of blood.

Plasma cell: A terminally differentiated B lymphocyte that secretes antibodies.

Plasmid: An extrachromosomal genetic element not essential for growth and which has no extracellular form.

Plate: To dispense cells into a container after splitting.

Plates: Petri dishes, used for bacterial growth on solid medium.

Plating efficiency: The percentage of cells formed that grow into colonies. The term is sometimes used loosely to mean seeding efficiency (the percentage of cells seeded that grow and can be recovered).

Polymerase chain reaction (PCR): A method for amplifying DNA in vitro, using oligonucleotide primers complementary to nucleotide sequences in a target gene and DNA polymerase to copy the target sequence.

Precipitation: (1) The formation of a solid within a solution, often by combination of cations and anions to form an insoluble ionic compound. (2) A reaction between antibody and soluble antigen resulting in a visible mass of antibody-antigen.

Prehybridization (prehyb): To treat with appropriate macromolecules to saturate nonspecific binding before addition of a specific probe.

Primary structure: The precise sequence of monomeric units in an informational macromolecule such as a polypeptide or nucleic acid.

Primer: Short, preexisting polynucleotide chain to which new deoxyribonucleotides can be added by DNA polymerase.

Probability: Likelihood.

Probe: (1) Nucleic acid probe. A strand of nucleic acid that can be labeled and used to hybridize to a complementary molecule from a mixture of other nucleic acids. (2) A short oligonucleotide of unique sequences used as hybridization probe for identifying pathogens.

Prophage: The state of the genome in a temperate virus when it is replicating in synchrony with that of the host, typically integrated into the host genome.

Protease: An enzyme that hydrolyzes the peptide bonds linking amino acids, rendering the protein nonfunctional.

Protocol: Experimental method.

Protoplast: A cell from which the cell wall has been removed.

Pulse: To treat for a discrete and usually short period of time.

Pulsed field gel electrophoresis: The direction of the electric field is changed periodically: Larger molecules of DNA take longer to realign themselves in the new field direction. Thus, different-size pieces of DNA can be differentiated.

Quantum sufficiat (q.s.): A sufficient quantity. Used as "bring to volume," for example, q.s. to 1000 ml.

Quaternary structure: In proteins, the number and arrangement of individual polypeptides in the final protein molecule.

Quenching: In fluorescence microscopy, a reduction in fluorescence due to heavy metal ions.

Radioactivity: The spontaneous release of particulate and/or electromagnetic energy from the nucleus of an atom. These emissions can be visualized and quantitated, and the radioactivity can be used as a label.

Radioimmunoassay: An immunological assay employing radioactive antibody or antigen for the detection of certain substances in body fluids.

Radioisotope: An isotope of an element that undergoes spontaneous decay with the release of radioactive particles.

Radiolabeled: A molecule tagged with a radioactive element.

Radionucleotide: A radioactively labeled nucleotide.

Random priming: A method of labeling nucleic acids by priming in vitro transcription with mixed random primers.

Reagent: A chemical substance known to react in a certain way, used as a component in a chemical reaction.

Recombinant DNA: A DNA molecule containing DNA originating from two or more sources.

Reducing agent: A chemical that disrupts sulfhydryl bonds.

Regulation: Processes, such as induction and repression, that control the rates of synthesis of proteins.

Replacement vector: A cloning vector, such as a bacteriophage, in which some of the DNA of the vector can be replaced with foreign DNA.

Reporter gene: (1) A gene used as an indicator of a successful gene transfer. (2) A gene whose regulation is controlled by the DNA regions under examination.

Reprint request: A request to the author of a paper for a copy of the paper.

Resolution: The minimum distance between two dots that can be discerned.

Retrovirus: Virus containing single-stranded RNA as its genetic material and which produces a complementary DNA by action of the enzyme reverse transcriptase.

Reverse osmosis: Water is forced through a semipermeable membrane, trapping salts and particles and removing them from the water.

Roentgen: Unit of ionizing ability, equal to the number of ionizations necessary to form one electrostatic unit in 1 cc of dry air.

Run: (1) (*noun*) The performance of a timed experiment or technique. One speaks of a centrifuge run, a FPLC run, a lunch run. (2) (*verb*) To perform a timed experiment or technique, for example, to run a gel.

Running buffer: Buffer used to electrophorese a gel.

Safety can: Flammable liquids should be stored in a container that controls flammable vapors. According to OSHA, the can must be leaktight, automatically vent to relieve internal pressure, and automatically close after filling or pouring. A yellow band must be placed around cans containing liquids with flash points at or below 26.7°C (80°F).

Salt: An ionic component that can be formed by replacing the hydrogen ion of an acid with a different cation.

Scintillant: Fluorescent chemical that emits light in response to radioactivity.

Scintillation counter: A machine that records faint light pulses generated by radioactive emissions or by chemical reactions.

Secondary antibody: Antibody that binds to an antibody that is already bound to antigen. Usually used to recognize or label the first antibody.

Secondary structure: The initial pattern of folding of a polypeptide or polynucleotide, usually the result of hydrogen bonding.

Secretion vector: A DNA vector in which the protein product is both expressed and secreted (excreted) from the cell.

Section: To cut or slice a sample for microscopy.

Sediment: To cause particles in solution to settle out of the solution and to the bottom of the container. This can occur by gravity alone or by centrifugation.

Selection: Placing organisms under conditions where the growth of those with a particular genotype will be favored. Antibody selection is the most common.

Selective medium: A medium that allows the growth of certain types of microorganisms in preference to others. For example, an antibiotic-containing medium allows the growth of only those microorganisms that are resistant to that antibiotic.

Semipermeable membrane: A membrane that selectively permits some molecules to pass through while stopping other molecules: For example, solvents may pass through a particular membrane, and proteins may not.

Serology: The study of antigen-antibody reactions in vitro.

Serum: The fluid portion of blood remaining after the blood cells and materials responsible for clotting are removed.

Sharpie: Brand name, used generically, of a permanent marking pen.

Sharps: Any sharp object in the lab, which must be specially and carefully disposed of, such as needles, pasteur pipets, pipetman tips.

Significant: A result is statistically significant when the P value is less than a predetermined value. This does not necessarily mean that the result is important!

Site-directed mutagenesis: The insertion of a different nucleotide at a specific site in a DNA molecule using synthetic DNA methodology.

Slide: A piece of glass or plastic on which tissue or organisms can be immobilized for staining and microscopy.

Smear: Spread cells on a microscope slide, able to be fixed and stained.

Soap: Salt of a fatty acid.

Southern blot: Hybridization of a single strand of nucleic acid (DNA or RNA) to DNA fragments immobilized on a filter.

Specific activity: The radioactivity of an element per unit mass. The higher the specific activity, the more radioactive the molecule.

Spin: To centrifuge.

Split: To reduce the number of cells in a culture.

Spore: A general term for resistant resting structures formed by many prokaryotes and fungi.

Standard: An acknowledged measure of comparison for quantitative or qualitative work.

Standard curve: The plot of the concentration of a known substance against a property of the substance (such as O.D.) that is dependent on the concentration.

Standard deviation: The square root of the variance, it is the measure of the spread of the data.

Standard unit (S.I.): The international system of units (Systeme International d'Unité) based on seven fundamental quantities.

Stationary phase: The period during the growth cycle of a population in which growth ceases.

Sterile: Free of living organisms and viruses.

Sticky ends: Ends of a DNA molecule with short single-stranded overhangs.

Stock: The main source of your reagents in the lab. The lab stocks are the bottles of reagents as they come from the company; your stocks are the solutions you have made up.

Stoichiometry: The relationship among the amounts of reactants and products in a chemical reaction.

Strain: A derivation of a species having specific markers or properties.

Subculture: To split and feed a culture.

Substrate (reaction and culture): (1) The molecule or ion that an enzyme uses as a reactant. (2) Nutrients available to a cell in liquid culture.

Substratum: The growth surface available for the attachment and growth of cells.

Supercoil: Highly twisted form of circular DNA.

Supernatant: After centrifugation, the fluid left above the pellet.

Supplies: Needed items.

Survey: A comprehensive examination showing the extremes or boundaries.

Svedberg value or **Svedberg constant, S value:** A sedimentation coefficient, a particle's velocity in a centrifugal field.

Synergistic effect: The effect of treatment A and the effect of treatment B together give more or a different result than either treatment alone gives, suggesting that A and B work through different pathways.

t-Test: A test that a value lies on a normal distribution curve.

Tare: To obtain the net weight of a material by deducting the weight of the container from the combined weight of the material and the container.

TCA precipitation: The use of TCA to drive a protein or nucleic acid out of solution. This usually destroys the material, and is done for quantitation of the collected material.

Telnet: Remote login, allowing you to browse a distant computer through your own.

Template: A molecular mold or pattern for the synthesis of another molecule.

Teratogen: Substance that interferes with normal embryonic development.

Tertiary structure: The final folded structure of a polypeptide that has previously attained secondary structure.

Theory: A hypothesis assumed for the sake of argument; the still incompletely tested explanation for a set of results.

Titer: (1) Measure of antibody quantity, often given in the form of, e.g., 1/4000. (2) Number of bacteria in a viable count. (3) Amount of phage in a sample, as determined by the number of plaques.

Titration: Two reagents are mixed, one with a known concentration and one with an unknown concentration. There is some way to indicate when the two reagents have reacted essentially completely.

Toxic: A chemical that can be lethal at some doses.

Toxic chemicals: Substances that can cause significant disease in humans.

Tracking dye: Dye of known apparent molecular weight that allows the progress of electrophoresis to be followed.

Trans: (1) Relationship between groups attached to doubly bonded carbon atoms and located on opposite sides of the double bond. (2) Groups located across from one another in a complex. (3) An effect caused by a participant from outside the unit.

Transduction: Transfer of host genetic information via a virus (or bacteriophage) particle.

Transfection: (1) The transformation of a prokaryotic cell by DNA or RNA from a virus. (2) The process of genetic transformation in eukaryotic cells.

Transfer: To move a prescribed fluid volume from one container to another.

Transformation: (1) The transfer of genetic information into a prokaryotic cell via free DNA. (2) A process initiated by infection with certain viruses, whereby a normal animal cell becomes a cancer cell.

Transgenic: Genetically modified plants or animals containing foreign genes inserted by means of recombinant DNA techniques.

Transmittance: The measure of light passing through a substance.

Transposable element: A genetic element that has the ability to move from one site on the chromosome to another.

Transposition: The movement of a piece of DNA around the chromosome, usually through the function of a tranposable element.

Transposon: A type of tranposable element which, in addition to genes involved in transposition, carries other genes, often conferring selectable phenotypes such as antibiotic resistance.

Trial run: An experimental experiment!

Tritium: Hydrogen isotope ^3H, with two neutrons in its nucleus.

Troubleshooting: Figuring out what went wrong and how to fix it.

Trunnion: Swing-out rotor part holding the pins upon which the tube holder swings.

Trypsin: A proteolytic enzyme used to remove anchorage-dependent cells from the substratum. It hydrolyzes peptide bonds on the carboxyl side of arginine and lysine.

Tungsten filament lamp: Used to generate white light (containing all the wavelengths visible to the eye) in spectrophotometers.

Two-hybrid system: System for detecting interactions between proteins in vivo in yeast.

Upstream position: Refers to nucleic acid sequences on the 5′-side of a given site on a DNA or RNA molecule.

UV box: Transilluminator.

Variability: How much observations differ from each other, measured commonly by the range, standard deviation, and the variance.

Variance: A measure of dispersion of the data, the variance is the average squared deviation from the mean.

Vector: A plasmid or virus used in genetic engineering to insert genes into a cell. Or an agent, usually an insect or other animal, able to carry pathogens from one host to another.

Viable: Alive, able to reproduce.

Viable count: Measurement of the concentration of live cells in a microbial population.

Virulence: Degree of pathogenicity of a parasite.

Virus: A genetic element containing either DNA or RNA that is able to alternate between intracellular and extracellular stes, the latter being an infectious state.

Volatility: The tendency of a liquid or solid to pass into the vapor state at a particular temperature.

Warm room: Room heated enough to act as an incubator.

Wash: For a pellet, to remove the supernatant and centrifuge the pellet resuspended in "new" fluid.

Well: The trough in a gel into which sample is loaded.

Western blot: *See* Immunoblot.

Wet mount: Liquid sample on a slide for microscopy.

Wild type: A strain of microorganism isolated from nature. The usual or native form of a gene.

Window: An opening of particular dimensions, such as wavelength, time, or light.

Wobble: The concept that nonstandard base-pairing is allowed between the anticodon and the third position of the codon.

Working distance: The distance from the objective to the coverslip.

World Wide Web (WWW): Through hypertext, the reader can move to another document on the Internet directly.

X-gal: In vitro substrate for β-galactosidase.

X-ray: A high-energy form of light having sufficient energy to ionize inner electrons.

Zwitterion: A molecule with a positively charged end and a negatively charged end. Also known as ampholyte or dipolar ions.

RESOURCES

Brown T.A. 1994. *DNA Sequencing. The Basics.* IRL Press, New York.

Chen T. 1997. *Glossary of Microbiology.*
    http://www.hardlink.com/~tsute/glossary/index.html

Dow J. 1998. *Dictionary of Cell Biology.* Glasgow University/Academic Press.
    http://www.mblab.gla.ac.uk.dictionary/

Life Science Dictionary. 1995–1997. BioTech Resources.
    http://biotech.chem.indiana.edu/search/dict-search.phtml

Rubbi C. P. 1994. *Light Microscopy. Essential Data.* John Wiley and Sons, New York.

Specialty Media Glossary.1998.
    http://www.specialtymedia.com/glossary.htm

Index

A

Acid
    concentration of commercial acids, 142
    disposal, 176
Agarose gel electrophoresis. *See* Electrophoresis
Alarm, equipment
    importance, 38
    response, 38–39
Aliquoting
    commonly aliquoted material, 170–171
    protocol, 171–172
    rationale and indications, 170–171
Ammonium acetate, stock solution preparation,
    143
Ammonium persulfate, stock solution prepara-
    tion, 143
Analysis of variance (ANOVA), 77
ANOVA. *See* Analysis of variance
Antibiotics
    eukaryotic cell culture, 215–217
    selection of plasmid-carrying bacteria strains,
        257–258
Antibody
    applications, 308–309
    monoclonal versus polyclonal, 309
    sources, 308
    storage, 309
    tips for use, 309–310
Aseptic technique
    aspirating, 196
    bottle handling and flaming, 189–190
    experiments requiring, 186
    filter sterilization. *See* Filter sterilization
    gloves, 188
    importance, 185
    mistakes, 190
    pipeting
        disposable pipets, 192
        reusable glass pipets, 190–192
    pouring, 193
    work space organization, 187–188
Aspirator

biohazardous material aspiration, 196
    maintenance, 55–56
    setup, 53–55
    supernatant aspiration, 364–365
Attitude
    courtesy at the bench, 15–17
    first week, 11–14
    long-term, 15
Autoclave
    autoclavable materials, 155
    avoiding substrate breakdown, 157
    function and hazards, 28–29
    operation, 156–157
Autoradiography
    applications, 330
    film autoradiography
        advantages and disadvantages, 331
        exposure protocol, 332–333
        film processing, 334–335
        film types, 332
        fluorography, 332
        intensifying screen, 331
        principle, 331
    isotope selection, 330
    phosphorimager autoradiography
        advantages and disadvantages, 335–336
        exposure protocol, 336
        principle, 335

B

Bacteria culture
    antibiotics for selection of plasmid-carrying
        strains, 257–258
    apparatus, 246–247
    biohazard classification, 245–246
    contamination, 276
    counting methods
        counting chambers, types, 263, 265
        Petroff Hausser counting chamber proto-
            col, 265–267
        viable plate counts, 263–264, 267–270

451

Bacterial culture (*continued*)
  disposal, 176, 248
  growth curve, 250–251
  media preparation
    liquids, 251–252
    plates, 252–254
    slants, 254–255
  picking colonies, 262–263
  reviving cultures
    freeze-dried cultures, 256
    frozen cultures, 256–257
    large inoculum for fussy cultures, 257
    vial opening, 255
  sources of strains, 248–249
  storage
    freezing, 274–275
    long-term storage options, 273–274
    short-term, 273
  streaking
    multiple strains, 261–262
    single strains, 259–260
  turbidity measurement of growth
    generation time calculation, 271–272
    spectrophotometer operation, 270–271
  working rules, 247–248
Base
  concentration of commercial bases, 142
  disposal, 176
Bench
  coverings, 48
  equipment and materials, 22–23, 49–51
  initial setup, 44–45
  maintenance, 55–57
  properties and function, 22–23, 43
  shelf storage, 48–49
Bibliographic management software, 61–62
Bicinchonic assay, 305
Biohazard
  biosafety level requirements of facilities,
    197–198
  classification, 197
Biohazardous waste, disposal, 176
Biosafety cabinet. *See also* Laminar flow hood
  aseptic technique, 198, 200–202
  classification, 198–199
Biuret assay, 306
Blotting. *See* Electrophoresis
Bradford assay, 305–306
Bright-field microscopy, 406

Bromophenol blue, migration in gels, 380
Buffer
  definition, 129
  discarding, indications, 159–160
  disposal, 176
  pH adjustment, 153
  pK_a values of commonly used buffers, 142
  storage, 158–159

C
Calcium chloride, stock solution preparation,
    143
Carbon dioxide incubator
  alarms, 236–237
  Fyrite gas analyzer, 237–239
  gas cylinder, 239–242
  maintenance, 236–237
Cell culture. *See* Bacteria culture; Eukaryotic
    cell culture
Cell disposal, 177
Cell lysis
  detergent lysis, 303–304
  physical lysis methods, 303
  protease inhibitors, 304
Centrifugation
  balancing tubes, 355
  calculation of *g*-force, 357–359
  centrifuge
    maintenance, 368–370
    operation, 355–357
    types, 349–350
  density gradient centrifugation
    cesium chloride band removal, 368
    equilibrium density gradient centrifuga-
      tion, 348–349
    gradient formation, 367
    isopycnic density gradient centrifugation,
      347
    media, 367
    rate-zonal centrifugation, 346–347
  differential centrifugation, 346
  handling of dangerous samples, 366
  pellets
    handling, 357
    washing, 365–366
  preparative versus analytical, 346
  rotor
    cleaning, 370–371
    maintenance, 370

types, 351–353
supernatants
  aspirating, 364–365
  decanting, 363
tubes
  caps, 362
  considerations in selection, 358, 360, 362
  materials and properties, 361
  temperature effects, 360
  working rules, 353–354
Cerenkov counting, 338
Chemical waste, hazardous and nonhazardous
  disposal, 177–179
Chromatography, types, 299–300
Cold room, organization, 30–31
Collaboration, disputes, 102
Colony, picking from plate, 262–263
Communication tips. *See also* Manuscript; Oral
  presentation; Seminar
  getting along in the lab, 102–105
  networking, 106–108
  nonnative English speakers, 104–105
  seminar attendance, 108–109
Compressed gas cylinder. See Gas cylinder
Computer
  basic rules for use, 64–65
  Internet access, 62
  software for laboratory, 61–65
Confocal microscopy, 407–408
Confrontation, mediation, 102–103
Controls
  definition, 73–74
  necessity, 74
  prioritizing, 75
  types, 74–75
Courtesy guidelines, 15–17

D
Dark-field microscopy, 406
Darkroom, organization, 29, 31
Density gradient centrifugation. *See*
  Centrifugation
Department
  facilities and utilization, 4–5
  library, 31
Desiccated reagents
  containers for storage, 166
  desiccant properties, 166–167

desiccators
  opening, 168
  vacuum sealing, 167
Desk
  bay organization and function, 31
  essential items, 58
  filing system, 58–60, 91
  organization, 57
Detergent, removal from samples, 306–308
Dialysis
  principle, 300
  setup and buffer changes, 302
  tubing preparation, 301
Differential interference contrast microscopy,
  407
Dilution. *See* Stock buffer dilution
Dithiothreitol, stock solution preparation, 143
DNA isolation. *See also* Oligonucleotides
  concentration determination by ultraviolet
    spectroscopy, 288–289
  conversion units of DNA measurement, 281
  ethanol precipitation, 286–288
  gel electrophoresis. *See* Electrophoresis
  genome features of common species, 281
  kits, 281
  phenol extraction, 284–286
  plasmid miniprep, alkaline-SDS protocol,
    282–284
DNA synthesizer, overview, 36
Dress code, expectations for laboratory work, 8,
  17
Dry ice, disposal, 179

E
EDTA, stock solution preparation, 143
Electron microscopy
  scanning electron microscopy, 408–409
  transmission electron microscopy, 408
Electrophoresis
  basic rules, 373–374
  blotting
    membrane selection and handling,
      399–400
    transfer methods, 397–399
    types of blots, 397
  buffers, 377
  DNA gels
    agarose gel preparation, 385–386

Electrophoresis (*continued*)
 agarose versus polyacrylamide gel electrophoresis, 381–382
 buffers, 383–384
 formats, 381
 gel box setup, 387
 loading
  agarose gels, 388–389
  vertical polyacrylamide gels, 389–390
 polyacrylamide gel preparation, 386–387
 power, 384
 sample preparation, 380
 staining with ethidium bromide,
  384–385
 standards/markers, 380–381
 documentation, 379
 drying, 378
 fixing, 378
 formats, 375
 gel properties, 375–377
 molecular weight determination, 379
 power supplies, 377–378
 principle, 373
 protein gels
  buffers, 396
  formats, 394–395
  gels, 395–396
  power, 396
  sample preparation, 392–394
  staining, 397
  standards/markers, 394
 RNA gels
  buffers, 391
  formats, 391
  gels, 392
  power, 392
  sample preparation, 390–391
  staining with ethidium bromide, 392
  standards/markers, 391
 sample preparation, 374
 staining, 378–379
 standards/markers, 374–375, 380
Electroporator, overview, 36
Equipment
 alarm
  importance, 38
  response, 38–39
 basic rules, 37–38

 purchasing guidelines, 39–40
 room organization, 27–29
Ethanol precipitation
 DNA, 286–288
 oligonucleotides, 294
 RNA, 297
Eukaryotic cell culture
 antibiotics, 215–217
 area organization, 25, 27
 aseptic technique. *See* Aseptic technique
 carbon dioxide incubator
  alarms, 236–237
  Fyrite gas analyzer, 237–239
  gas cylinders, 239–242
  maintenance, 236–237
 classification of cultures
  by manner of growth, 207–208
  by origin, 206–207
 commonly used cell lines, 207
 contamination
  cross contamination, 235–236
  macroscopic features, 231–232
  microscopic features, 232–233
  mycoplasma, 234–235
 continuous cell sources, 212–213
 counting with hemocytometer, 225–228
 freezing and storage, 228–231
 frozen cells, thawing and culture, 213–214
 hybridomas, 207
 medium
  additives, 219
  phenol red as pH indicator, 219
  warming, 219–220
 microscopic observation, 209–210, 215,
  232–233
 passaging (splitting), 206, 215
  importance, 221
  adherent cells, 221–224
  suspension cells, 224
 primary cell sources, 211–212
 serum
  heat inactivation, 220
  sources, 221
  variables, 220
 suspension versus adherent cells, 208–209
 transformed cells, characteristics, 207
 vessels, 216, 218
Experiment

background research, 73
controls. *See* Controls
initial, 11, 69
mistakes in setup, 72
philosophical considerations, 69–71
planning, 71–73, 130–131
protocol
    examples, 80–82
    kits, 78
    modification, 78–79
    sources, 77–78
result interpretation, 83
small versus large, 71
solution preparation, 130–131
troubleshooting, 84
Eye protection, 133

F

Filter sterilization
    disposable cup filtering, 194–196
    filter types, 157–158
    syringe filtering, 194
First week, attitude and activities, 11–14
Fixation, light microscopy specimens, 419
Fluorescence microscopy
    applications, 420–421
    microscope features, 421
    overview, 407
    tips, 422
Freezer
    defrosting, 173–175
    guidelines, 172–173
Fume hood, operation, 133–134
Fyrite gas analyzer
    measuring carbon dioxide levels, 237–238
    precautions for using Fyrite, 239

G

Gas cylinder
    changing in carbon dioxide incubator, 242
    precautions in use, 241
    regulator, 240–241
Geiger counter, operation, 34, 325–326
Glassware
    buffer storage, 136
    mixing of solutions, 135

Gloves, 132, 179
Gossip, control in laboratory, 103–104
Graduate student, function in lab, 6
Grant
    politics in submission, 123, 125
    process to funding, 124

H

Harassment, response, 104
Hemocytometer, cell counting, 225–228
High performance liquid chromatography
    (HPLC), overview, 34
Hood. *See* Fume hood; Laminar flow hood
Hours, expectations for laboratory work, 7–8,
    105
HPLC. *See* High performance liquid chro-
    matography

I

Immersion oils
    condenser lens, 413–414
    objective lens, 413
    types, 412
Incubator
    function, 32, 35
    shaking motion, 33
Internet access, 62

J

Journal club. *See also* Seminar
    format, 9–10, 116–117
    presentation guidelines, 116
    topic selection, 117

K

Kitchen, organization, 28–29
Koehler illumination, 414–417

L

Laboratory aide, function in lab, 6–7
Laboratory meeting. *See also* Seminar
    format, 9–10
Laboratory notebook
    bound notebook features, 90–91
    content for each experiment, 92–93
    ethics, 96–98

Laboratory notebook (*continued*)
  importance, 89
  integrity of data, 97–98
  maintenance, 93, 96
  sample pages, 94–95
  security, 89–90, 97
  types, advantages and drawbacks, 89–90
Laboratory supervisor, function in lab, 7
Laminar flow hood
  aseptic technique, 198, 200–202
  contamination sources, 200
  maintenance, 202
Light microscopy. *See* Microscopy
Light-sensitive reagents, storage, 168–169
Liquid nitrogen, handling and freezing of cells,
        230–231
Liquid scintillation counting
  channels, 337
  cocktails, 337
  disposal of vials, 338, 341
  efficiency of counting, 337
  principle, 336
Literature update software, 62
Lowry assay, 306

M
Magnesium chloride, stock solution prepara-
        tion, 143
Manuscript
  abused phrases in, 122–123
  planning, 121
  process to publication, 124
  review, 121–122
Mask, 133
Materials Safety Data Sheet (MSDS), 131–132,
        165
Medium
  bacteria culture
    liquids, 251–252
    plates, 252–254
    slants, 254–255
  eukaryotic cell culture
    additives, 219
    phenol red as pH indicator, 219
    serum addition, 220–221
    warming, 219–220
Meetings. *See* Journal club; Laboratory meeting;
        Seminar

2-Mercaptoethanol, stock solution preparation,
        143
Microscopy
  bright-field microscopy, 406
  cleaning of microscope, 414
  components of light microscope, 410–411
  confocal microscopy, 407–408
  dark-field microscopy, 406
  differential interference contrast microscopy,
        407
  electron microscopy
    scanning electron microscopy, 408–409
    transmission electron microscopy, 408
  eukaryotic cell culture, 209–210, 215,
        232–233
  fixation of specimens, 419
  fluorescence microscopy
    applications, 420–421
    microscope features, 421
    overview, 407
    tips, 422
  immersion oils
    condenser lens, 413–414
    objective lens, 413
    types, 412
  inverted microscopy, 407
  Koehler illumination, 414–417
  light sources, 410–411
  measurement of samples, 412
  numerical aperture, 404
  objective lens types, 411–412
  phase-contrast microscopy, 406
  photography
    exposure protocol, 423–424
    film formats, 424–425
    film storage, 426
    filters, 425
    processing, 426
  refractive index, 404
  resolution, 403–404
  selection of light microscopy method,
        405–408
  shared facilities, 426
  smear preparation, 418–419
  staining of specimens, 420
  working rules, 409
Microwave, lab functions, 35, 385–386
Middle eastern blot, 397

Mixing
    glassware for, 135
    protocol, 149–150
Molarity, calculation and preparation of solutions, 136–138
Molecular biology. *See specific techniques*
MSDS. *See* Materials Safety Data Sheet

N

Needles, disposal, 179
Normality, calculation and preparation of solutions, 138
Northern blot, 397
Notebook. *See* Laboratory notebook
Numerical aperture, 404
Nutator
    function, 32
    motion, 33

O

Objective lens, types, 411–412
Oligonucleotides
    design, 293–294
    ethanol precipitation, 294
Oral presentation. *See also* Seminar
    execution, 110
    preparation, 110
Ordering
    equipment, 39–40
    radioisotopes, 319–320
    supplies and reagents, 45–47
Oxygen-sensitive reagents, storage, 169–170

P

Paper management, 58–60
Passaging, cell cultures, 206, 215
    adherent cells, 221–224
    importance, 221
    suspension cells, 224
PCR. *See* Polymerase chain reaction
Pellets
    handling, 357
    washing, 365–366
Percent solution, calculation and preparation, 139
Petroff Hausser counting chamber, protocol for use, 265–267

pH
    common stock solutions, 142
    measurement area, organization, 26–27
    phenol red as indicator in medium, 219
    temperature dependence, 151, 154
pH meter
    calibration, 151–152
    electrodes, 150–151
    operation, 152–154
    troubleshooting, 154–155
Phase-contrast microscopy, 406
Phenol
    disposal, 179
    DNA extraction, 284–286
    equilibration, 145–146
    safety in handling, 145
Phenol:chloroform:isoamyl alcohol, preparation, 146
Phenylmethylsulfonyl fluoride, stock solution preparation, 143
Phosphate-buffered saline, stock solution preparation, 143
Photocopying, excess in first week, 13
Photography. *See* Microscopy
Pipet
    aids, 52–53, 56
    aseptic technique pipeting
        disposable pipets, 192
        reusable glass pipets, 190–192
    disposal, 179–180
    types, 52
Pipettor
    maintenance, 57
    types and operation, 51–52, 141
Plasmid. *See* DNA
Plasticware
    buffer storage, 136
    mixing of solutions, 135
Plate reader
    overview, 34
    supernatant removal, 363–365
Polyacrylamide gel electrophoresis. *See* Electrophoresis
Polymerase chain reaction (PCR)
    basic rules, 293
    contamination sources, 293
    principle, 290–292
Postdoc, function in lab, 5

Poster session, presentation, 107
Potassium acetate, stock solution preparation, 143–144
Principal investigator
    communication with, 102
    difficulty with, 103
    favorite subordinates, 103
    function in lab, 5
Probability test, 76
Project
    assignment, 10
    switching indications, 84–86
Protease inhibitors, 304
Protein purification
    basic rules, 299
    cell lysis
        detergent lysis, 303–304
        physical lysis methods, 303
        protease inhibitors, 304
    chromatography types, 299–300
    concentration assays
        absorption at 280 nm, 306
        bicinchonic assay, 305
        Biuret assay, 306
        Bradford assay, 305–306
        detergent removal, 306–308
        Lowry assay, 306
    dialysis
        principle, 300
        setup and buffer changes, 302
        tubing preparation, 301
    gel electrophoresis. *See* Electrophoresis
Protocol. *See* Experiment
Publication. *See* Manuscript
Purchasing. *See* Ordering

R
Radioactive waste, disposal, 180, 182, 327–328, 338–342
Radioactivity. *See also* Radioisotope
    alternatives
        chemiluminescent assay, 342–343
        colorimetry, 342
    basic rules in handling, 320–321, 326–329
    Cerenkov counting of phosphorous-32, 338
    detection. *See* Autoradiography; Geiger counter; Liquid scintillation counting

    emission types, 313–314
    metabolic labeling, 316–317
    nucleic acid probe selection for in situ hybridization, 317
    purchasing, 319–320
    safety issues
        distance from source, 325
        duration of exposure, 325
        monitoring, 325–326, 329
        overview, 321–322
        pregnancy, 322
        protective clothing, 324
        shielding, 323
    specific activity, 314, 318–319
    storage, 338–339
    units of measure, 314
Radioisotope
    certification, 315
    half-lives and emission energies, 318–319
    selection of isotope for molecular biology experiments, 317–319
Reasoning, approaches, 70
Recommendation letter, 105
Refractive index, 404
Refrigerator, guidelines, 172–173
Research, types in lab definition, 4
Resident, function in lab, 6
Resolution, light microscopy, 403–404
Restriction enzymes, buffers and handling, 290–291
RNA isolation
    basic rules in handling, 296
    concentration determination by ultraviolet spectroscopy, 298
    ethanol precipitation, 297
    gel electrophoresis. *See* Electrophoresis
    kits, 297
    messenger RNA, 298
    selective RNA precipitation, 297–298
Rotation student, function in lab, 6
Rotor. *See* Centrifugation

S
Safety
    radiation safety, 321–326, 329
    reagent handling, 131–134
    universal laboratory rules, 17–18

Safety officer
    function in lab, 7
    initial orientation, 10–11
Secretary, function in lab, 6
Seminar. *See also* Oral presentation
    attendance, 108
    controlling tactics, 115
    formal seminar
        answering questions, 114
        characteristics, 111
        data presentation, 114
        introduction, 113
        objectives, 113
    informal seminar
        answering questions, 113
        characteristics, 111–112
        data presentation, 112–113
        introduction, 112
        objectives, 112
    presentation tools
        overhead projector, 118–119
        photocopies, 119
        slides, 119–120
    question asking, 109
    ten-minute talk, 115
Serum, cell culture
    heat inactivation, 220
    sources, 221
    variables, 220
Shaker
    function, 32
    motion, 33
Sharps, disposal, 180
Sink, organization and equipment placement,
        24, 26
Slides, seminar guidelines, 119–120
Smear preparation, 418–419
Sodium acetate, stock solution preparation,
        144
Sodium chloride, stock solution preparation,
        144
Sodium dodecyl sulfate, stock solution prepara-
        tion, 144
Solvents, disposal, 180
Sonicator
    cell lysis, 303
    overview, 36
Southern blot, 397

Southwestern blot, 397
Spectrophotometer
    DNA concentration determination by ultra-
            violet spectroscopy, 288–289
    overview, 34, 38
    protein assays, 305–306
    RNA concentration determination by ultra-
            violet spectroscopy, 298
    turbidity measurement of bacteria growth,
            270–271
Speed vac
    operation, 287–288
    overview, 35
Splitting. *See* Aliquoting; Passaging
SSC, stock solution preparation, 144
SSPE, stock solution preparation, 144
Standard deviation, 76
Standard error, 76
Statistics
    applicability to different research types,
            75–76
    tests, 76–77
Sterilization. *See* Aseptic technique; Autoclave;
            Filter sterilization
Stock buffer dilution
    calculations, 139–140
    serial dilution, 140–141
Stock solution, preparation, 143–144
Storage
    aliquoting, 170–172
    desiccated materials, 166–168
    emergency storage of various reactions,
            163–165
    light-sensitive reagents, 168–169
    oxygen-sensitive reagents, 169–170
    radioactivity, 338–339
    refrigerators and freezers, 172–175
    sources for reagent sources, 165–166
Streaking
    multiple strains, 261–262
    single strains, 259–260
Student's *t*-test, 77
Summer student, function in lab, 6
Supernatants
    aspirating, 364–365
    decanting, 363
    disposal, 180
Syringes, disposal, 181

T

Task assignment, 9

Technician, function in lab, 5–6

Temperature cycler, overview, 35, 291

Thermometers, disposal, 181

Tissue culture. *See also* Eukaryotic cell culture

Transfection, overview of techniques, 295–296

Transformation, overview of techniques, 294–295

Trichloroacetic acid, stock solution preparation, 144

Tris-buffered saline, stock solution preparation, 144

Tris

pH adjustment, 154

stock solution preparation, 144

V

Vacation policy, 105

Vacuum concentrator. *See* Speed vac

Viable plate counting, 263–264, 267–270

Vials, opening, 255

Visiting faculty, definition, 6

W

Warm room, organization, 31

Waste disposal, 175–182, 339–342

Water

classification, 134–135

distillation, 135

Water bath, maintenance, 57

Weighing

accessories, 146–147

area, organization, 26–27

protocol, 147–149

Western blot, 397

Word processing software, 61

Work space. *See also* Bench; Desk

assignment, 10–11

organization, 11

X

Xylene cyanol, migration in gels, 380

Also from the author of *At the Bench:*

At the Helm: A Laboratory Navigator

by Kathy Barker, *The Institute for Systems Biology, Seattle*

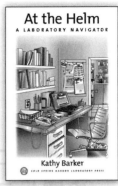

Newly appointed principal research investigators have to recruit, motivate, and lead a research team, manage personnel and institutional responsibilities, and compete for funding, while maintaining the outstanding scientific record that got them their position in the first place. Small wonder, then, that many principal investigators feel ill-prepared. In this book, a successor to her best-selling manual for new recruits to experimental science, *At the Bench,* Kathy Barker provides a guide for newly appointed leaders of research teams, and those who aspire to that role. With extensive use of interviews and a text enlivened with quotes and real-life examples, Dr. Barker discusses a wide range of management challenges and the skills that promote success. Her book is a unique and much-needed contribution to the literature of science.

What the reviewers have to say:

"The numerous practical ideas make *At the Helm* a valuable read for many scientists embarking on their careers. But Barker also offers, implicitly, a compelling argument that young researchers have the right—and, indeed, the responsibility—to chart their own course, deciding for themselves how to do good work while seeking rich and meaningful professional and personal lives."   —*Science*

"In her new book, *At the Helm: A Laboratory Navigator,* Kathy Barker provides a handbook to guide new PI past some of the pitfalls and problems of starting and managing a research laboratory. She skillfully weaves material from interviews, scientific memoirs and management theory into a valuable and unique discourse on the many challenges facing the laboratory head, with practical guidance and suggestions for meeting these challenges. . . . The major strength of the book lies in its near comprehensive treatment of the issues pertaining to laboratory personnel, and it is in these sections that the book should prove invaluable to inexperienced lab managers."   —*Trends in Genetics*

2002, 352 pp., illus., index
Hardcover $45

ISBN 0-87969-583-8

CONTENTS

Chapter 1: Know What You Want

Chapter 2: You as a Leader

Chapter 3: Choose Your People

Chapter 4: Starting and Keeping New
Lab Members

Chapter 5: Make Research the Foundation

Chapter 6: Organizing the Lab to Support
the Research

Chapter 7: Communication as the Glue

Chapter 8: Dealing with a Group

Chapter 9: For the Long Run

To order or request additional information:

Call: 1-800-843-4388 (Continental US and Canada)   516-422-4100 (All other locations)

FAX: 516-422-4097

Online ordering at http://www.cshlpress.com   E-mail: cshpress@cshl.edu

Write: Cold Spring Harbor Laboratory Press, 500 Sunnyside Blvd, Woodbury, NY 11797-2924

CSHL PRESS